Injury & Trauma Sourcebook

Learning Disabilities Sourcebook,
  2nd Edition

Leukemia Sourcebook

Liver Disorders Sourcebook

Lung Disorders Sourcebook

Medical Tests Sourcebook, 2nd Edition

Men's Health Concerns Sourcebook,
  2nd Edition

Mental Health Disorders Sourcebook,
  3rd Edition

Mental Retardation Sourcebook

Movement Disorders Sourcebook

Muscular Dystrophy Sourcebook

Obesity Sourcebook

Osteoporosis Sourcebook

Pain Sourcebook, 2nd Edition

Pediatric Cancer Sourcebook

Physical & Mental Issues in Aging
  Sourcebook

Podiatry Sourcebook, 2nd Edition

Pregnancy & Birth Sourcebook,
  2nd Edition

Prostate Cancer Sourcebook

Prostate & Urological Disorders
  Sourcebook

Rehabilitation Sourcebook

Respiratory Diseases & Disorders
  Sourcebook

Sexually Transmitted Diseases
  Sourcebook, 3rd Edition

Sleep Disorders Sourcebook,
  2nd Edition

Smoking Concerns Sourcebook

Sports Injuries Sourcebook, 3rd Edition

Stress-Related Disorders Sourcebook

Stroke Sourcebook

Substance Abuse Sourcebook

Surgery Sourcebook

Thyroid Disorders Sourcebook

Transplantation Sourcebook

Traveler's Health Sourcebook

Urinary Tract & Kidney Diseases &
  Disorders Sourcebook, 2nd Edition

Teen Health Series

Abuse & Violence Information
  for Teens

Alcohol Information for Teens

Allergy Information for Teens

Asthma Information for Teens

Body Information for Teens

Cancer Information for Teens

Complementary & Alternative
  Medicine Information for
  Teens

Diabetes Information for Teens

Diet Information for Teens,
  2nd Edition

Drug Information for Teens,
  2nd Edition

Eating Disorders Information
  for Teens

Fitness Information for Teens

Learning Disabilities Information
  for Teens

Mental Health Information for
  Teens, 2nd Edition

Pegnancy Information for Teens

Sexual Health Information for
  Teens

Skin Health Information for
  Teens

Sports Injuries Information
  for Teens

Suicide Information for Teens

Tobacco Information for Teens

AIDS
SOURCEBOOK
Fourth Edition

Health Reference Series

Fourth Edition

AIDS
SOURCEBOOK

Basic Consumer Health Information about Human
Immunodeficiency Virus (HIV) and Acquired
Immunodeficiency Syndrome (AIDS), Featuring Updated
Statistics and Facts about Risks, Prevention, Screening,
Diagnosis, Treatments, Side Effects, and Complications, and
Including a Section about the Impact of HIV/AIDS on the
Health of Women, Children, and Adolescents

Along with Tips on Managing Life with AIDS, Reports on
Current Research Initiatives and Clinical Trials, a Glossary
of Related Terms, and Resource Directories for Further Help
and Information

Edited by
Ivy L. Alexander

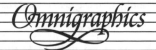

Omnigraphics

P.O. Box 31-1640, Detroit, MI 48231

Bibliographic Note

Because this page cannot legibly accommodate all the copyright notices, the Bibliographic Note portion of the Preface constitutes an extension of the copyright notice.

Edited by Ivy L. Alexander

Health Reference Series
Karen Bellenir, *Managing Editor*
David A. Cooke, M.D., *Medical Consultant*
Elizabeth Collins, *Research and Permissions Coordinator*
Cherry Stockdale, *Permissions Assistant*
EdIndex, Services for Publishers, *Indexers*

* * *

Omnigraphics, Inc.
Matthew P. Barbour, *Senior Vice President*
Kay Gill, *Vice President—Directories*
Kevin M. Hayes, *Operations Manager*

* * *

Peter E. Ruffner, *Publisher*

Copyright © 2008 Omnigraphics, Inc.

ISBN 978-0-7808-0997-0

Library of Congress Cataloging-in-Publication Data

AIDS sourcebook : basic consumer health information about human immunodeficiency virus (HIV) and acquired immunodeficiency syndrome (AIDS), featuring updated statistics and facts about risks, prevention, screening, diagnosis, treatments, side effects, and complications, and including a section about the impact of HIV/AIDS on the health of women, children, and adolescents, along with tips on managing life with AIDS, reports on current research initiatives and clinical trials, a glossary of related terms, and resource directories for further help and information / edited by Ivy L. Alexander. -- 4th ed.
  p. cm. -- (Health reference series)
  Summary: "Provides basic consumer health information about transmission, testing, and treatment of HIV and related complications, along with tips on living with HIV/AIDS. Includes index, glossary of related terms and directory of resources"--Provided by publisher.
  Includes bibliographical references and index.
  ISBN 978-0-7808-0997-0 (hardcover : alk. paper) 1. AIDS (Disease)--Popular works. I. Alexander, Ivy L.
  RC606.64.A337 2007
  362.196'9792--dc22
                                                          2007034967

Table of Contents

Visit www.healthreferenceseries.com to view *A Contents Guide to the Health Reference Series*, a listing of more than 13,000 topics and the volumes in which they are covered.

Part III: Strategies for Preventing HIV Transmission

Part IV: Screening, Diagnosis, and Treatment of HIV/AIDS

Part VI: Issues for Women, Children, and Adolescents with HIV/AIDS

Part VII: Living with HIV/AIDS

Part VIII: Research Initiatives and Clinical Trials

Preface

About This Book

The first acquired immunodeficiency syndrome (AIDS) cases were reported in the United States a quarter of a century ago. Since that time, AIDS has become the world's leading cause of death among both men and women between the ages of 15 and 59. In recent years, new drug treatments have decreased mortality rates by 70 percent and enabled those infected with human immunodeficiency virus (HIV) to stay relatively healthy and symptom free for years. Despite such advances, however, 40,000 new HIV infections are reported in the United States annually. These disproportionately affect minorities and women. In addition, approximately 25 percent of HIV-infected people in the United States do not know they are infected and, despite educational efforts, a large percentage of Americans still are not aware of how it is transmitted.

AIDS Sourcebook, Fourth Edition, provides updated information about HIV and AIDS and how it is transmitted, diagnosed, and treated. Information about prevention, risks, screening, treatments, complications, and tips on living with AIDS are included, along with a special section on the needs of HIV-infected women and children. Reports on current research initiatives and clinical trials, a glossary of related terms, and directories for further help and information are also provided.

How to Use This Book

This book is divided into parts and chapters. Parts focus on broad areas of interest. Chapters are devoted to single topics within a part.

Part I: Understanding the Human Immunodeficiency Virus (HIV) and Acquired Immunodeficiency Syndrome (AIDS) provides an overview of HIV/AIDS with specific information about how HIV causes AIDS, the various types of HIV, and myths and misunderstandings about AIDS.

Part II: HIV/AIDS Transmission: Statistics, Trends, and Risk Factors reports on the latest statistical information regarding HIV/AIDS cases in the United States and around the world. Various risk factors for contracting the disease are described, including genetics, alcohol and drug abuse, and sexual orientation. In addition, emerging trends, especially among minority populations, are discussed.

Part III: Strategies for Preventing HIV Transmission discusses ways to reduce the risk of contracting the virus, including modifying risky behaviors. It also presents information about current research into the development of a vaccine and other medical advances, and it offers prevention guidelines for health care workers. Blood supply safeguards and barriers to prevention are also discussed.

Part IV: Screening, Diagnosis, and Treatment of HIV/AIDS covers testing, including home and rapid tests, treatment options, and drug regimens. The latest advances in treatments, as well as alternative therapies, are discussed.

Part V: Complications Associated with HIV/AIDS looks at the various infections and conditions which occur in connection with the disease and its treatment. Tips on managing the side effects of anti-HIV medications are also included.

Part VI: Issues for Women, Children, and Adolescents with HIV/AIDS provides information on how HIV/AIDS specifically affects women's health and the health of babies born to HIV-positive mothers. Methods for preventing mother-to-child transmission of HIV are discussed, and information about pediatric AIDS is presented.

Part VII: Living with HIV/AIDS offers patients and caregivers updated information on coping with the day-to-day concerns of living with HIV/AIDS. Ways to stay healthy while living with the disease, including nutrition, exercise, food safety, emotional health, and adherence to therapy regimens, are discussed. A chapter on caring for someone with AIDS at home contains information and suggestions for caregivers, and legal issues for both patient and caregiver are discussed.

Part VIII: Research Initiatives and Clinical Trials focuses on current developments and future possibilities in the areas of prevention and potential cures, including the hoped-for development of a vaccine. Information is also provided for people who may be interested in participating in ongoing medical research.

Part IX: Additional Help and Information offers a glossary of related terms and acronyms associated with HIV/AIDS and facts about government support services, including Social Security benefits, drug assistance programs, and housing assistance. A directory of other resources and suggestions for further reading are also included.

Bibliographic Note

This volume contains documents and excerpts from publications issued by the following U.S. government agencies: Agency for Healthcare Research and Quality (AHRQ), Centers for Disease Control and Prevention (CDC); National Heart, Lung, and Blood Institute (NHLBI); National Institute of Dental and Craniofacial Research (NIDCR); National Institute on Aging (NIA); National Institute on Alcohol Abuse and Alcoholism (NIAAA); National Institute of Allergy and Infectious Diseases (NIAID); National Institute on Drug Abuse (NIDA); National Institutes of Health (NIH); National Institute of Mental Health (NIMH); National Institute of Neurological Disorders and Stroke (NINDS); National Prevention Information Network (NPIN); National Women's Health Information Center (NWHIC); Oak Ridge Institute for Science and Education (ORISE); Office of Minority Health; Office of the Press Secretary—The White House; Social Security Administration (SSA); U.S. Agency for International Development; U.S. Department of Health and Human Services (AIDSinfo); U.S. Department of Housing and Urban Development (HUD); U.S. Department of Veterans Affairs (VA); U.S. Food and Drug Administration (FDA).

In addition, this volume contains copyrighted documents from the following organizations: A.D.A.M. Inc.; AIDS Alliance for Children, Youth, and Families; AIDS Education and Training Centers National Resource Center; American Academy of Family Physicians; American Association for Clinical Chemistry; American Lung Association; American Psychiatric Association; AMFAR, The Foundation for AIDS Research; AVERT; Body Health Resources Foundation; Directors of Health Promotion and Education; Elizabeth Glaser Pediatric AIDS Foundation; Global Alliance for Tuberculosis Drug Development; Henry J. Kaiser Family Foundation; Illinois Department of Public

Health; International AIDS Vaccine Initiative; Monogram Biosciences, Inc.; NAM Publications; National Coalition for the Homeless; National Health Policy Forum; New Mexico AIDS InfoNet; New York State Department of Health; New Zealand Dermatological Society; Project Inform; Rural Center for AIDS/STD Prevention; UNAIDS (Joint United Nations Programme on HIV/AIDS); University of Pennsylvania Health System; Voice of America; ScoutNews, LLC; Washington State University Department of Food Science and Human Nutrition.

Full citation information is provided on the first page of each chapter or section. Every effort has been made to secure all necessary rights to reprint the copyrighted material. If any omissions have been made, please contact Omnigraphics to make corrections for future editions.

Acknowledgements

Thanks go to the many organizations, agencies, and individuals who have contributed materials for this *Sourcebook* and to medical consultant Dr. David Cooke and document engineer Bruce Bellenir. Special thanks go to managing editor Karen Bellenir and permissions specialist Liz Collins for their help and support.

About the Health Reference Series

The *Health Reference Series* is designed to provide basic medical information for patients, families, caregivers, and the general public. Each volume takes a particular topic and provides comprehensive coverage. This is especially important for people who may be dealing with a newly diagnosed disease or a chronic disorder in themselves or in a family member. People looking for preventive guidance, information about disease warning signs, medical statistics, and risk factors for health problems will also find answers to their questions in the *Health Reference Series*. The *Series*, however, is not intended to serve as a tool for diagnosing illness, in prescribing treatments, or as a substitute for the physician/patient relationship. All people concerned about medical symptoms or the possibility of disease are encouraged to seek professional care from an appropriate health care provider.

A Note about Spelling and Style

Health Reference Series editors use *Stedman's Medical Dictionary* as an authority for questions related to the spelling of medical terms and the *Chicago Manual of Style* for questions related to grammatical structures, punctuation, and other editorial concerns. Consistent adherence is not always possible, however, because the individual volumes within the *Series* include many documents from a wide variety of different producers and copyright holders, and the editor's primary goal is to present material from each source as accurately as is possible following the terms specified by each document's producer. This sometimes means that information in different chapters or sections may follow other guidelines and alternate spelling authorities. For example, occasionally a copyright holder may require that eponymous terms be shown in possessive forms (Crohn's disease *vs.* Crohn disease) or that British spelling norms be retained (leukaemia *vs.* leukemia).

Locating Information within the Health Reference Series

The *Health Reference Series* contains a wealth of information about a wide variety of medical topics. Ensuring easy access to all the fact sheets, research reports, in-depth discussions, and other material contained within the individual books of the *Series* remains one of our highest priorities. As the *Series* continues to grow in size and scope, however, locating the precise information needed by a reader may become more challenging.

A *Contents Guide to the Health Reference Series* was developed to direct readers to the specific volumes that address their concerns. It presents an extensive list of diseases, treatments, and other topics of general interest compiled from the Tables of Contents and major index headings. To access *A Contents Guide to the Health Reference Series*, visit www.healthreferenceseries.com.

Medical Consultant

Medical consultation services are provided to the *Health Reference Series* editors by David A. Cooke, M.D. Dr. Cooke is a graduate of Brandeis University, and he received his M.D. degree from the University of Michigan. He completed residency training at the University of Wisconsin Hospital and Clinics. He is board-certified in Internal Medicine. Dr. Cooke currently works as part of the University of Michigan Health System and practices in Ann Arbor, MI. In his free time, he enjoys writing, science fiction, and spending time with his family.

Our Advisory Board

We would like to thank the following board members for providing guidance to the development of this *Series*:

- Dr. Lynda Baker, Associate Professor of Library and Information Science, Wayne State University, Detroit, MI

- Nancy Bulgarelli, William Beaumont Hospital Library, Royal Oak, MI

- Karen Imarisio, Bloomfield Township Public Library, Bloomfield Township, MI

- Karen Morgan, Mardigian Library, University of Michigan-Dearborn, Dearborn, MI

- Rosemary Orlando, St. Clair Shores Public Library, St. Clair Shores, MI

Health Reference Series *Update Policy*

The inaugural book in the *Health Reference Series* was the first edition of *Cancer Sourcebook* published in 1989. Since then, the *Series* has been enthusiastically received by librarians and in the medical community. In order to maintain the standard of providing high-quality health information for the layperson the editorial staff at Omnigraphics felt it was necessary to implement a policy of updating volumes when warranted.

Medical researchers have been making tremendous strides, and it is the purpose of the *Health Reference Series* to stay current with the most recent advances. Each decision to update a volume is made on an individual basis. Some of the considerations include how much new information is available and the feedback we receive from people who use the books. If there is a topic you would like to see added to the update list, or an area of medical concern you feel has not been adequately addressed, please write to:

Editor
Health Reference Series
Omnigraphics, Inc.
P.O. Box 31-1640
Detroit, MI 48231
E-mail: editorial@omnigraphics.com

Part One

Understanding the Human Immunodeficiency Virus (HIV) and Acquired Immunodeficiency Syndrome (AIDS)

Chapter 1

HIV Infection and AIDS: An Overview

Introduction

AIDS (acquired immunodeficiency syndrome) was first reported in the United States in 1981 and has since become a major worldwide epidemic. AIDS is caused by HIV (human immunodeficiency virus). By killing or damaging cells of the body's immune system, HIV progressively destroys the body's ability to fight infections and certain cancers. People diagnosed with AIDS may get life-threatening diseases called opportunistic infections, which are caused by microbes such as viruses or bacteria that usually do not make healthy people sick.

More than 900,000 cases of AIDS have been reported in the United States since 1981. As many as 950,000 Americans may be infected with HIV, one-quarter of whom are unaware of their infection. The epidemic is growing most rapidly among minority populations and is a leading killer of African American males ages 25 to 44. According to the Centers for Disease Control and Prevention (CDC), AIDS affects nearly seven times more African Americans and three times more Hispanics than whites. In recent years, an increasing number of African American women and children are being affected by HIV/AIDS. In 2003, two-thirds of U.S. AIDS cases in both women and children were among African Americans.

Produced by the National Institute of Allergy and Infectious Diseases (www.niaid.nih.gov), a component of the National Institutes of Health (NIH), March 2005.

Transmission

HIV is spread most commonly by having unprotected sex with an infected partner. The virus can enter the body through the lining of the vagina, vulva, penis, rectum, or mouth during sex.

Risky Behavior

HIV can infect anyone who practices the following risky behaviors:

- sharing drug needles or syringes
- having sexual contact, including oral, with an infected person without using a condom
- having sexual contact with someone whose HIV status is unknown

Infected Blood

HIV also is spread through contact with infected blood. Before donated blood was screened for evidence of HIV infection and before heat-treating techniques to destroy HIV in blood products were introduced, HIV was transmitted through transfusions of contaminated blood or blood components. Today, because of blood screening and heat treatment, the risk of getting HIV from such transfusions is extremely small.

Contaminated Needles

HIV is frequently spread among injection drug users by the sharing of needles or syringes contaminated with very small quantities of blood from someone infected with the virus.

It is rare, however, for a patient to give HIV to a health care worker or vice-versa by accidental sticks with contaminated needles or other medical instruments.

Mother to Child

Women can transmit HIV to their babies during pregnancy or birth. Approximately one-quarter to one-third of all untreated pregnant women infected with HIV will pass the infection to their babies. HIV also can be spread to babies through the breast milk of mothers infected with the virus. If the mother takes certain drugs during pregnancy, she can significantly reduce the chances that her baby will get infected with HIV. If health care providers treat HIV-infected pregnant women and deliver their babies by cesarean section, the chances of the baby being infected can be reduced to a rate of 1 percent. HIV infection of newborns has been almost eradicated in the United States due to appropriate treatment.

A study sponsored by the National Institute of Allergy and Infectious Diseases (NIAID) in Uganda found a highly effective and safe drug for preventing transmission of HIV from an infected mother to her newborn. Independent studies have also confirmed this finding. This regimen is more affordable and practical than any other examined to date. Results from the study show that a single oral dose of the antiretroviral drug nevirapine (NVP) given to an HIV-infected woman in labor and another to her baby within three days of birth reduces the transmission rate of HIV by half compared with a similar short course of AZT (azidothymidine). For more information on preventing transmission from mother to child, go to http://aidsinfo.nih.gov/guidelines.

Saliva

Although researchers have found HIV in the saliva of infected people, there is no evidence that the virus is spread by contact with saliva. Laboratory studies reveal that saliva has natural properties that limit the power of HIV to infect, and the amount of virus in saliva appears to be very low. Research studies of people infected with HIV have found no evidence that the virus is spread to others through saliva by kissing. The lining of the mouth, however, can be infected by HIV, and instances of HIV transmission through oral intercourse have been reported.

Scientists have found no evidence that HIV is spread through sweat, tears, urine, or feces.

Casual Contact

Studies of families of HIV-infected people have shown clearly that HIV is not spread through casual contact such as the sharing of food utensils, towels and bedding, swimming pools, telephones, or toilet seats.

HIV is not spread by biting insects such as mosquitoes or bedbugs.

Sexually Transmitted Infections

If you have a sexually transmitted disease (STD) such as syphilis, genital herpes, chlamydial infection, gonorrhea, or bacterial vaginosis appears, you may be more susceptible to getting HIV infection during sex with infected partners.

Early Symptoms of HIV Infection

If you are like many people, you will not have any symptoms when you first become infected with HIV. You may, however, have a flu-like illness within a month or two after exposure to the virus. This illness may include the following:

- fever

- headache

- tiredness

- enlarged lymph nodes (glands of the immune system easily felt in the neck and groin)

These symptoms usually disappear within a week to a month and are often mistaken for those of another viral infection. During this period, people are very infectious, and HIV is present in large quantities in genital fluids.

More persistent or severe symptoms may not appear for ten years or more after HIV first enters the body in adults, or within two years in children born with HIV infection. This period of "asymptomatic" infection varies greatly in each individual. Some people may begin to have symptoms within a few months, while others may be symptom-free for more than ten years.

Even during the asymptomatic period, the virus is actively multiplying, infecting, and killing cells of the immune system. The virus can also hide within infected cells and lay dormant. The most obvious effect of HIV infection is a decline in the number of CD4 positive T cells (CD4+) found in the blood—the immune system's key infection fighters. The virus slowly disables or destroys these cells without causing symptoms.

As the immune system worsens, a variety of complications start to take over. For many people, the first signs of infection are large lymph nodes or "swollen glands" that may be enlarged for more than three months. Other symptoms often experienced months to years before the onset of AIDS include the following:

- lack of energy

- weight loss

- frequent fevers and sweats

- persistent or frequent yeast infections (oral or vaginal)

- persistent skin rashes or flaky skin
- pelvic inflammatory disease in women that does not respond to treatment
- short-term memory loss

Some people develop frequent and severe herpes infections that cause mouth, genital, or anal sores, or a painful nerve disease called shingles. Children may grow slowly or be sick a lot.

What Is AIDS?

The term *AIDS* applies to the most advanced stages of HIV infection. CDC developed official criteria for the definition of AIDS and is responsible for tracking the spread of AIDS in the United States.

CDC's definition of AIDS includes all HIV-infected people who have fewer than 200 CD4+ T cells per cubic millimeter of blood. (Healthy adults usually have CD4+ T-cell counts of 1,000 or more.) In addition, the definition includes 26 clinical conditions that affect people with advanced HIV disease. Most of these conditions are opportunistic infections that generally do not affect healthy people. In people with AIDS, these infections are often severe and sometimes fatal because the immune system is so ravaged by HIV that the body cannot fight off certain bacteria, viruses, fungi, parasites, and other microbes.

Symptoms of opportunistic infections common in people with AIDS include the following:

- coughing and shortness of breath
- seizures and lack of coordination
- difficult or painful swallowing
- mental symptoms such as confusion and forgetfulness
- severe and persistent diarrhea
- fever
- vision loss
- nausea, abdominal cramps, and vomiting
- weight loss and extreme fatigue
- severe headaches
- coma

Children with AIDS may get the same opportunistic infections as do adults with the disease. In addition, they also have severe forms of the typically common childhood bacterial infections, such as conjunctivitis (pink eye), ear infections, and tonsillitis.

People with AIDS are also particularly prone to developing various cancers, especially those caused by viruses such as Kaposi sarcoma and cervical cancer, or cancers of the immune system known as lymphomas. These cancers are usually more aggressive and difficult to treat in people with AIDS. Signs of Kaposi sarcoma in light-skinned people are round brown, reddish, or purple spots that develop in the skin or in the mouth. In dark-skinned people, the spots are more pigmented.

During the course of HIV infection, most people experience a gradual decline in the number of CD4+ T cells, although some may have abrupt and dramatic drops in their CD4+ T-cell counts. A person with CD4+ T cells above 200 may experience some of the early symptoms of HIV disease. Others may have no symptoms even though their CD4+ T-cell count is below 200.

Many people are so debilitated by the symptoms of AIDS that they cannot hold a steady job or do household chores. Other people with AIDS may experience phases of intense life-threatening illness followed by phases in which they function normally.

A small number of people first infected with HIV ten or more years ago have not developed symptoms of AIDS. Scientists are trying to determine what factors may account for their lack of progression to AIDS, such as the following:

- whether their immune systems have particular characteristics
- whether they were infected with a less aggressive strain of the virus
- if their genes may protect them from the effects of HIV

Scientists hope that understanding the body's natural method of controlling infection may lead to ideas for protective HIV vaccines and use of vaccines to prevent the disease from progressing.

Diagnosis

Because early HIV infection often causes no symptoms, your health care provider usually can diagnose it by testing your blood for the presence of antibodies (disease-fighting proteins) to HIV. HIV antibodies generally do not reach noticeable levels in the blood for one to three months following infection. It may take the antibodies as long as six months to be produced in quantities large enough to show up in standard blood tests. Hence, to determine whether you have been recently infected (acute infection), your health care provider can screen you for the presence of HIV genetic material. Direct screening of HIV is extremely critical in order to prevent transmission of HIV from recently infected individuals.

If you have been exposed to the virus, you should get an HIV test as soon as you are likely to develop antibodies to the virus—within six weeks to twelve months after possible exposure to the virus. By getting tested early, if infected, you can discuss with your health care provider when you should start treatment to help your immune system combat HIV and help prevent the emergence of certain opportunistic infections (see section on treatment). Early testing also alerts you to avoid high-risk behaviors that could spread the virus to others.

Most health care providers can do HIV testing and will usually offer you counseling at the same time. Of course, you can be tested anonymously at many sites if you are concerned about confidentiality.

Health care providers diagnose HIV infection by using two different types of antibody tests: ELISA and Western blot. If you are highly likely to be infected with HIV but have been tested negative for both tests, your health care provider may request additional tests. You also may be told to repeat antibody testing at a later date, when antibodies to HIV are more likely to have developed.

Babies born to mothers infected with HIV may or may not be infected with the virus, but all carry their mothers' antibodies to HIV for several months. If these babies lack symptoms, a doctor cannot make a definitive diagnosis of HIV infection using standard antibody. Health care providers are using new technologies to detect HIV to more accurately determine HIV infection in infants between ages three months and fifteen months. They are evaluating a number of blood tests to determine which ones are best for diagnosing HIV infection in babies younger than three months.

Treatment

When AIDS first surfaced in the United States, there were no medicines to combat the underlying immunodeficiency and few treatments existed for the opportunistic diseases that resulted. Researchers, however, have developed drugs to fight both HIV infection and its associated infections and cancers.

HIV Infection

The Food and Drug Administration (FDA) has approved a number of drugs for treating HIV infection. The first group of drugs used to treat HIV infection, called nucleoside reverse transcriptase (RT) inhibitors, interrupts an early stage of the virus making copies of itself. These drugs may slow the spread of HIV in the body and delay the start of opportunistic infections. This class of drugs, called nucleoside analogs, includes the following:

- AZT (azidothymidine)
- ddC (zalcitabine)
- ddI (dideoxyinosine)
- d4T (stavudine)

- 3TC (lamivudine)
- abacavir (Ziagen)
- tenofovir (Viread)
- Emtriva (emtricitabine)

Health care providers can prescribe non-nucleoside reverse transcriptase inhibitors (NNRTIs), such as these:

- delavirdine (Rescriptor)
- nevirapine (Viramune)

- efavirenz (Sustiva) (in combination with other antiretroviral drugs)

FDA also has approved a second class of drugs for treating HIV infection. These drugs, called protease inhibitors, interrupt the virus from making copies of itself at a later step in its life cycle. They include the following:

- ritonavir (Norvir)
- saquinavir (Invirase)
- indinavir (Crixivan)
- amprenavir (Agenerase)

- nelfinavir (Viracept)
- lopinavir (Kaletra)
- atazanavir (Reyataz)
- fosamprenavir (Lexiva)

FDA also has introduced a third new class of drugs, known as fusion inhibitors, to treat HIV infection. Fuzeon (enfuvirtide or T-20), the first approved fusion inhibitor, works by interfering with HIV-1's ability to enter into cells by blocking the merging of the virus with the cell membranes. This inhibition blocks HIV's ability to enter and infect the human immune cells. Fuzeon is designed for use in combination with other anti-HIV treatment. It reduces the level of HIV infection in the blood and may be active against HIV that has become resistant to current antiviral treatment schedules.

Because HIV can become resistant to any of these drugs, health care providers must use a combination treatment to effectively suppress the virus. When multiple drugs (three or more) are used in combination, it is referred to as highly active antiretroviral therapy, or HAART, and can be used by people who are newly infected with HIV as well as people with AIDS.

Researchers have credited HAART as being a major factor in significantly reducing the number of deaths from AIDS in this country. While HAART is not a cure for AIDS, it has greatly improved the health of many people with AIDS and it reduces the amount of virus circulating in the blood to nearly undetectable levels. Researchers, however, have shown that HIV remains present in hiding places, such as the lymph nodes, brain, testes, and retina of the eye, even in people who have been treated.

Side effects: Despite the beneficial effects of HAART, there are side effects associated with the use of antiviral drugs that can be severe. Some of the nucleoside RT inhibitors may cause a decrease of red or white blood cells, especially when taken in the later stages of the disease. Some may also cause inflammation of the pancreas and painful nerve damage. There have been reports of complications and other severe reactions, including death, to some of the antiretroviral nucleoside analogs when used alone or in combination. Therefore, health care experts recommend that you be routinely seen and followed by your health care provider if you are on antiretroviral therapy.

The most common side effects associated with protease inhibitors include nausea, diarrhea, and other gastrointestinal symptoms. In addition, protease inhibitors can interact with other drugs resulting in serious side effects. Fuzeon may also cause severe allergic reactions such as pneumonia, trouble breathing, chills and fever, skin rash, blood in urine, vomiting, and low blood pressure. Local skin reactions are also possible since it is given as an injection underneath the skin.

If you are taking HIV drugs, you should contact your health care provider immediately if you have any of these symptoms.

Opportunistic Infections

A number of available drugs help treat opportunistic infections. These drugs include the following:

- foscarnet and ganciclovir to treat CMV (cytomegalovirus) eye infections
- fluconazole to treat yeast and other fungal infections

- trimethoprim/sulfamethoxazole (TMP/SMX) or pentamidine to treat PCP (*Pneumocystis carinii/jiroveci* pneumonia)

Cancers

Health care providers use radiation, chemotherapy, or injections of alpha interferon—a genetically engineered protein that occurs naturally in the human body—to treat Kaposi sarcoma or other cancers associated with HIV infection.

Prevention

Because no vaccine for HIV is available, the only way to prevent infection by the virus is to avoid behaviors that put you at risk of infection, such as sharing needles and having unprotected sex.

Many people infected with HIV have no symptoms. Therefore, there is no way of knowing with certainty whether your sexual partner is infected unless he or she has repeatedly tested negative for the virus and has not engaged in any risky behavior. You should either abstain from having sex or use male latex condoms or female polyurethane condoms, which may offer partial protection, during oral, anal, or vaginal sex. Only water-based lubricants should be used with male latex condoms.

Although some laboratory evidence shows that spermicides can kill HIV, researchers have not found that these products can prevent you from getting HIV.

Research

NIAID-supported investigators are conducting an abundance of research on all areas of HIV infection, including developing and testing preventive HIV vaccines and new treatments for HIV infection and AIDS-associated opportunistic infections. Researchers also are investigating exactly how HIV damages the immune system. This research is identifying new and more effective targets for drugs and vaccines. NIAID-supported investigators also continue to trace how the disease progresses in different people.

Scientists are investigating and testing chemical barriers, such as topical microbicides, that people can use in the vagina or in the rectum during sex to prevent HIV transmission. They also are looking at other ways to prevent transmission, such as controlling STDs and modifying personal behavior, as well as ways to prevent transmission from mother to child.

Chapter 2

Understanding HIV Infection

Chapter Contents

Section 2.1

What Is HIV Infection?

"HIV Infection," © 2007 A.D.A.M., Inc. Reprinted with permission.

Alternative names: Human immunodeficiency virus infection

Definition: HIV infection is a viral infection caused by the human immunodeficiency virus (HIV) that gradually destroys the immune system, resulting in infections that are hard for the body to fight.

Causes, Incidence, and Risk Factors

Acute HIV infection may be associated with symptoms resembling mononucleosis or the flu within two to four weeks of exposure. HIV seroconversion (converting from HIV negative to HIV positive) usually occurs within three months of exposure.

People who become infected with HIV may have no symptoms for up to ten years, but they can still transmit the infection to others. Meanwhile, their immune system gradually weakens until they are diagnosed with AIDS. Acute HIV infection progresses over time to asymptomatic HIV infection and then to early symptomatic HIV infection and later, to AIDS (advanced HIV infection).

Most individuals infected with HIV will progress to AIDS if not treated. However, there is a tiny subset of patients who develop AIDS very slowly, or never at all. These patients are called long-term non-progressors.

HIV has spread throughout the United States. Higher concentrations of the disease are found in inner cities.

Symptoms

Any symptoms of illness may occur, since infections can occur throughout the body. Special symptoms relating to HIV infection include:

- sore throat;
- mouth sores, including candidal infection;

- muscular stiffness or aching;
- headache;
- diarrhea;
- swollen lymph glands;
- fever;
- fatigue;
- rash of various types, including seborrheic dermatitis;
- frequent vaginal yeast infections.

Note: At the time of diagnosis with HIV infection, many people have not experienced any symptoms.

Signs and Tests

- HIV ELISA/Western blot may show positive HIV antibody. If it is negative and the patient has definite risk factor for HIV infection, the test should be repeated in three months.
- Lower-than-normal CD4 cell count may show suppression of the immune system by the virus.
- HIV RNA viral load indicates the amount of virus in the bloodstream.
- Blood differential may show abnormalities.

Treatment

Drug therapy is often recommended for patients who are committed to taking all their medications and have a CD4 count between 200 and 350 (indicating immune system suppression).

It is extremely important that patients take all doses of their medications, otherwise the virus will rapidly become resistant to the medications. Therapy is always given with a combination of antiviral drugs.

People with HIV infection need to receive education about the disease and treatment so that they can be active partners in decision making with their health care provider.

Support Groups

The stress of illness can often be helped by joining a support group where members share common experiences and problems.

Expectations (Prognosis)

HIV is a chronic medical condition that can be treated, but not yet cured. There are effective means of preventing complications and delaying, but not preventing, progression to AIDS. At the present time, not all persons infected with HIV have progressed to AIDS, but time has shown that the vast majority do.

Complications

- Opportunistic infections
  - *Pneumocystis carinii* [also called *jiroveci*] pneumonia
  - candidiasis
  - Cytomegalovirus infection
  - toxoplasmosis
  - *Cryptococcus*
  - *Cryptosporidium enterocolitis* (or other protozoal)
  - *Mycobacterium avium* complex (MAC)
  - tuberculosis
  - bacillary angiomatosis
  - *Salmonella* infection in the bloodstream
  - progressive multifocal leukoencephalopathy (viral infection of the brain)
- HIV dementia
- malignancies (cancers)
- HIV lipodystrophy
- chronic wasting from HIV infection

Calling Your Health Care Provider

Call for an appointment with your health care provider if you have had a possible or actual exposure to AIDS or HIV infection.

Prevention

- Use protection when having sexual contact with persons known or suspected of being infected with HIV.

- If you have sex with numerous people or with people who have multiple partners, always use protection.

- Avoid intravenous (IV) drugs. If IV drugs are used, avoid sharing needles or syringes. Always use new needles. (Boiling or cleaning them with alcohol does not guarantee sterility.)

- If you have sex with people who use IV drugs, always use protection.

- People with AIDS or who have had positive HIV antibody tests may pass the disease on to others. They should not donate blood, plasma, body organs, or sperm. They should not exchange genital fluids during sexual activity.

- Avoid oral, vaginal, or anal contact with semen from HIV-infected individuals.

- Avoid unprotected anal intercourse, since it causes small abrasions in the rectal tissues, through which HIV in an infected partner's semen may be injected directly into the recipient's blood.

- Safer sex behaviors may reduce the risk of acquiring the infection. There is a slight risk of acquiring the infection even if "safe sex" is practiced with the use of condoms, due to the possibility of the condom breaking. Abstinence is the only sure way to prevent sexual transmission of the virus.

Section 2.2

How HIV Causes AIDS

National Institute of Allergy and Infectious Diseases (www.niaid.nih.gov), a component of the National Institutes of Health (NIH), November 2004.

Untreated HIV disease is characterized by a gradual deterioration of immune function. Most notably, crucial immune cells called CD4 positive (CD4+) T cells are disabled and killed during the typical course of infection. These cells, sometimes called "T-helper cells," play a central role in the immune response, signaling other cells in the immune system to perform their special functions.

A healthy, uninfected person usually has 800 to 1,200 CD4+ T cells per cubic millimeter (mm^3) of blood. During untreated HIV infection, the number of these cells in a person's blood progressively declines. When the CD4+ T-cell count falls below 200/mm^3, a person becomes particularly vulnerable to the opportunistic infections and cancers that typify AIDS, the end stage of HIV disease. People with AIDS often suffer infections of the lungs, intestinal tract, brain, eyes, and other organs, as well as debilitating weight loss, diarrhea, neurologic conditions, and cancers such as Kaposi sarcoma and certain types of lymphomas.

Most scientists think that HIV causes AIDS by directly inducing the death of CD4+ T cells or interfering with their normal function, and by triggering other events that weaken a person's immune function. For example, the network of signaling molecules that normally regulates a person's immune response is disrupted during HIV disease, impairing a person's ability to fight other infections. The HIV-mediated destruction of the lymph nodes and related immunologic organs also plays a major role in causing the immunosuppression seen in people with AIDS. Immunosuppression by HIV is confirmed by the fact that medicines, which interfere with the HIV life-cycle, preserve CD4+ T cells and immune function as well as delay clinical illness.

Scope of the HIV Epidemic

Although HIV was first identified in 1983, studies of previously stored blood samples indicate that the virus entered the U.S. population sometime in the late 1970s. In the United States, 886,575 cases of AIDS, and 501,669 deaths among people with AIDS had been reported to the Centers for Disease Control and Prevention (CDC) by the end of 2002. Approximately 40,000 new HIV infections occur each year in the United States, 70 percent of them among men and 30 percent among women. Of the new infections, approximately 40 percent are from male-to-male contact, 30 percent from heterosexual contact, and 25 percent from injection drug use. Minority groups in the United States have also been disproportionately affected by the epidemic.

Worldwide, an estimated 38 million people were living with HIV/AIDS as of December 2003, according to the Joint United Nations Programme on HIV/AIDS (UNAIDS). Through 2003, cumulative AIDS-associated deaths worldwide numbered more than 20 million. Globally, approximately 5 million new HIV infections and approximately 3 million AIDS-related deaths, including an estimated 490,000 children under 15 years old, occurred in the year 2003 alone.

HIV Is a Retrovirus

HIV belongs to a class of viruses called retroviruses. Retroviruses are RNA (ribonucleic acid) viruses, and in order to replicate (duplicate) they must make a DNA (deoxyribonucleic acid) copy of their RNA. It is the DNA genes that allow the virus to replicate.

Like all viruses, HIV can replicate only inside cells, commandeering the cell's machinery to reproduce. Only HIV and other retroviruses, however, once inside a cell, use an enzyme called reverse transcriptase to convert their RNA into DNA, which can be incorporated into the host cell's genes.

Slow Viruses

HIV belongs to a subgroup of retroviruses known as lentiviruses, or "slow" viruses. The course of infection with these viruses is characterized by a long interval between initial infection and the onset of serious symptoms.

Other lentiviruses infect nonhuman species. For example, the feline immunodeficiency virus (FIV) infects cats and the simian immunodeficiency virus (SIV) infects monkeys and other nonhuman primates. Like IIIV in humans, these animal viruscs primarily infect immune system cells, often causing immunodeficiency and AIDS-like symptoms. These viruses and their hosts have provided researchers with useful, albeit imperfect, models of the HIV disease process in people.

Structure of HIV

The Viral Envelope

HIV has a diameter of 1/10,000 of a millimeter and is spherical in shape. The outer coat of the virus, known as the viral envelope, is composed of two layers of fatty molecules called lipids, taken from the membrane of a human cell when a newly formed virus particle buds from the cell. Evidence from the National Institute of Allergy and Infectious Diseases (NIAID)-supported research indicates that HIV may enter and exit cells through special areas of the cell membrane known as "lipid rafts." These rafts are high in cholesterol and glycolipids and may provide a new target for blocking HIV.

Embedded in the viral envelope are proteins from the host cell, as well as 72 copies (on average) of a complex HIV protein (frequently called "spikes") that protrudes through the surface of the virus particle (virion). This protein, known as Env, consists of a cap made of three molecules called glycoprotein (gp) 120, and a stem consisting of three gp41 molecules that anchor the structure in the viral envelope. Much of the research to develop a vaccine against HIV has focused on these envelope proteins.

The Viral Core

Within the envelope of a mature HIV particle is a bullet-shaped core or capsid [virion], made of 2,000 copies of another viral protein, p24. The capsid [virion] surrounds two single strands of HIV RNA, each of which has a copy of the virus's nine genes. Three of these genes, *gag, pol,* and *env,* contain information needed to make structural proteins for new virus particles. The *env* gene, for example, codes for a protein called gp160 that is broken down by a viral enzyme to form gp120 and gp41, the components of Env.

Six regulatory genes, *tat, rev, nef, vif, vpr,* and *vpu,* contain information necessary to produce proteins that control the ability of HIV to infect a cell, produce new copies of virus, or cause disease. The protein encoded by *nef,* for instance, appears necessary for the virus to replicate efficiently, and the *vpu*-encoded protein influences the release of new virus particles from infected cells. Recently, researchers discovered that Vif (the protein encoded by the *vif* gene) interacts with an antiviral defense protein in host cells (APOBEC3G), causing inactivation of the antiviral effect and enhancing HIV replication. This interaction may serve as a new target for antiviral drugs.

The ends of each strand of HIV RNA contain an RNA sequence called the long terminal repeat (LTR). Regions in the LTR act as switches to control production of new viruses and can be triggered by proteins from either HIV or the host cell.

The core of HIV also includes a protein called p7, the HIV nucleocapsid protein. Three enzymes carry out later steps in the virus's life cycle: reverse transcriptase, integrase, and protease. Another HIV protein called p17, or the HIV matrix protein, lies between the viral core and the viral envelope.

Replication Cycle of HIV

Entry of HIV into Cells

Infection typically begins when an HIV particle, which contains two copies of the HIV RNA, encounters a cell with a surface molecule called cluster designation 4 (CD4). Cells carrying this molecule are known as CD4+ cells.

One or more of the virus's gp120 molecules binds tightly to CD4 molecule(s) on the cell's surface. The binding of gp120 to CD4 results in a conformational change in the gp120 molecule allowing it to bind to a second molecule on the cell surface known as a co-receptor. The envelope of the virus and the cell membrane then fuse, leading to entry of the virus into the cell. The gp41 of the envelope is critical to the fusion process. Drugs that block either the binding or the fusion process are being developed and tested in clinical trials. The Food and Drug Administration (FDA) has approved one of the so-called fusion inhibitors, T20, for use in HIV-infected people.

Studies have identified multiple co-receptors for different types of HIV strains. These co-receptors are promising targets for new anti-HIV drugs, some of which are now being tested in preclinical and clinical studies. Agents that block the co-receptors are showing particular promise as potential microbicides that could be used in gels or creams to prevent HIV transmission. In the early stage of HIV disease, most people harbor viruses that use, in addition to CD4, a receptor called CCR5 to enter their target cells. With disease progression, the spectrum of co-receptor usage expands in approximately 50 percent of patients to include other receptors, notably a molecule called CXCR4. Virus that uses CCR5 is called R5 HIV and virus that uses CXCR4 is called X4 HIV.

Although CD4+ T cells appear to be the main targets of HIV, other immune system cells with and without CD4 molecules on their surfaces are infected as well. Among these are long-lived cells called monocytes and macrophages, which apparently can harbor large quantities of the virus without being killed, thus acting as reservoirs of HIV. CD4+ T cells also serve as important reservoirs of HIV; a small proportion of these cells harbor HIV in a stable, inactive form. Normal immune processes may activate these cells, resulting in the production of new HIV virions.

Cell-to-cell spread of HIV also can occur through the CD4-mediated fusion of an infected cell with an uninfected cell.

Reverse Transcription

In the cytoplasm of the cell, HIV reverse transcriptase converts viral RNA into DNA, the nucleic acid form in which the cell carries its genes. Fifteen of the 26 antiviral drugs approved in the United States for treating people with HIV infection work by interfering with this stage of the viral life cycle.

Integration

The newly made HIV DNA moves to the cell's nucleus, where it is spliced into the host's DNA with the help of HIV integrase. HIV DNA that enters the DNA of the cell is called a provirus. Several drugs that target the integrase enzyme are in the early stages of development and are being investigated for their potential as antiretroviral agents.

Transcription

For a provirus to produce new viruses, RNA copies must be made that can be read by the host cell's protein-making machinery. These copies are called messenger RNA (mRNA), and production of mRNA is called transcription, a process that involves the host cell's own enzymes. Viral genes in concert with the cellular machinery control this process; the *tat* gene, for example, encodes a protein that accelerates transcription. Genomic RNA is also transcribed for later incorporation in the budding virion (see assembly and budding).

Cytokines, proteins involved in the normal regulation of the immune response, also may regulate transcription. Molecules such as tumor necrosis factor (TNF)-alpha and interleukin (IL)-6, secreted in elevated levels by the cells of HIV-infected people, may help to activate HIV proviruses. Other infections, by organisms such as *Mycobacterium tuberculosis*, also may enhance transcription by inducing the secretion of cytokines.

Translation

After HIV mRNA is processed in the cell's nucleus, it is transported to the cytoplasm. HIV proteins are critical to this process; for example, a protein encoded by the *rev* gene allows mRNA encoding HIV structural proteins to be transferred from the nucleus to the cytoplasm. Without the rev protein, structural proteins are not made. In the cytoplasm, the virus co-opts the cell's protein-making machinery—including structures called ribosomes—to make long chains of viral proteins and enzymes, using HIV mRNA as a template. This process is called translation.

Assembly and Budding

Newly made HIV core proteins, enzymes, and genomic RNA gather inside the cell and an immature viral particle forms and buds off from the cell, acquiring an envelope that includes both cellular and HIV proteins from the cell membrane. During this part of the viral life cycle, the core of the virus is immature and the virus is not yet infectious. The long chains of proteins and enzymes that make up the immature viral core are now cut into smaller pieces by a viral enzyme called protease.

This step results in infectious viral particles. Drugs called protease inhibitors interfere with this step of the viral life cycle. FDA has approved eight such drugs—saquinavir, ritonavir, indinavir, amprenavir, nelfinavir, fosamprenavir, atazanavir, and lopinavir—for marketing in the United States. Recently, an HIV inhibitor that targets a unique step in the viral life cycle, very late in the process of viral maturation, has been identified and is currently undergoing further development.

Recently, researchers have discovered that virus budding from the host cell is much more complex than previously thought. Binding between the HIV Gag protein and molecules in the cell directs the accumulation of HIV components in special intracellular sacs, called multivesicular bodies (MVB), that normally function to carry proteins out of the cell. In this way, HIV actively hitchhikes out of the cell in the MVB by hijacking normal cell machinery and mechanisms. Discovery of this budding pathway has revealed several potential points for intervening in the viral replication cycle.

Transmission of HIV

Among adults, HIV is spread most commonly during sexual intercourse with an infected partner. During intercourse, the virus can enter the body through the mucosal linings of the vagina, vulva, penis, or rectum or, rarely, via the mouth and possibly the upper gastrointestinal tract after oral sex. The likelihood of transmission is increased by factors that may damage these linings, especially other sexually transmitted infections that cause ulcers or inflammation.

Research suggests that immune system cells of the dendritic cell type, which live in the mucosa, may begin the infection process after sexual exposure by binding to and carrying the virus from the site of infection to the lymph nodes where other immune system cells become infected. A molecule on the surface of dendritic cells, DC-SIGN, may be critical for this transmission process.

HIV also can be transmitted by contact with infected blood, most often by the sharing of needles or syringes contaminated with minute quantities of blood containing the virus. The risk of acquiring HIV from blood transfusions is extremely small in the United States, as all blood products in this country are screened routinely for evidence of the virus.

Almost all HIV-infected children in the United States get the virus from their mothers before or during birth. In the United States, approximately 25 percent of pregnant HIV-infected women not receiving antiretroviral therapy have passed on the virus to their babies. In 1994, researchers showed that a specific regimen of the drug AZT (zidovudine) can reduce the risk of transmission of HIV from mother to baby by two-thirds. The use of combinations of antiretroviral drugs and simpler drug regimens has further reduced the rate of mother-to-child HIV transmission in the United States.

In developing countries, cheap and simple antiviral drug regimens have been proven to significantly reduce mother-to-child transmission at birth in resource-poor settings. Unfortunately, the virus also may be transmitted from an HIV-infected mother to her infant via breastfeeding. Moreover, due to the use of medicines to prevent transmission at delivery, breastfeeding may become the most common mode of HIV infection in infants. Thus, development of affordable alternatives to breastfeeding is greatly needed.

Early Events in HIV Infection

Once it enters the body, HIV infects a large number of CD4+ cells and replicates rapidly. During this acute or primary phase of infection, the blood contains many viral particles that spread throughout the body, seeding various organs, particularly the lymphoid organs.

Two to four weeks after exposure to the virus, up to 70 percent of HIV-infected people suffer flu-like symptoms related to the acute infection. Their immune system fights back with killer T cells (CD8+ T cells) and B-cell-produced antibodies, which dramatically reduce HIV levels. A person's CD4+ T-cell count may rebound somewhat and even approach its original level. A person may then remain free of HIV-related symptoms for years despite continuous replication of HIV in the lymphoid organs that had been seeded during the acute phase of infection.

One reason that HIV is unique is the fact that despite the body's aggressive immune responses, which are sufficient to clear most viral infections, some HIV invariably escapes. This is due in large part to the high rate of mutations that occur during the process of HIV replication. Even when the virus does not avoid the immune system by mutating, the body's best soldiers in the fight against HIV—certain subsets of killer T cells that recognize HIV—may be depleted or become dysfunctional.

In addition, early in the course of HIV infection, people may lose HIV-specific CD4+ T-cell responses that normally slow the replication of viruses. Such responses include the secretion of interferons and other antiviral factors, and the orchestration of CD8+ T cells.

Finally, the virus may hide within the chromosomes of an infected cell and be shielded from surveillance by the immune system. Such cells can be considered as a latent reservoir of the virus. Because the antiviral agents currently in our therapeutic arsenal attack actively replicating virus, they are not effective against hidden, inactive viral DNA (so-called provirus). New strategies to purge this latent reservoir of HIV have become one of the major goals for current research efforts.

Course of HIV Infection

Among people enrolled in large epidemiologic studies in Western countries, the median time from infection with HIV to the development of AIDS-related symptoms has been approximately ten to twelve years in the absence of antiretroviral therapy. Researchers, however, have observed a wide variation in disease progression. Approximately 10 percent of HIV-infected people in these studies have progressed to AIDS within the first two to three years following infection, while up to 5 percent of individuals in the studies have stable CD4+ T-cell counts and no symptoms even after 12 or more years.

Factors such as age or genetic differences among individuals, the level of virulence of an individual strain of virus, and co-infection with other microbes may influence the rate and severity of disease progression. Drugs that fight the infections associated with AIDS have improved and prolonged the lives of HIV-infected people by preventing or treating conditions such as *Pneumocystis carinii/jiroveci* pneumonia, cytomegalovirus disease, and diseases caused by a number of fungi.

HIV Co-Receptors and Disease Progression

Recent research has shown that most infecting strains of HIV use a co-receptor molecule called CCR5, in addition to the CD4 molecule, to enter certain of its target cells. HIV-infected people with a specific mutation in one of their two copies of the gene for this receptor may have a slower disease course than people with two normal copies of the gene. Rare individuals with two mutant copies of the CCR5 gene appear, in most cases, to be completely protected from HIV infection. Mutations in the gene for other HIV co-receptors also may influence the rate of disease progression.

Viral Burden and Disease Progression

Numerous studies show that people with high levels of HIV in their bloodstream are more likely to develop new AIDS-related symptoms or die than those with lower levels of virus. For instance, in the Multicenter AIDS Cohort Study (MACS), investigators showed that the level of HIV in an untreated person's plasma six months to a year after infection—the so-called viral "set point"—is highly predictive of the rate of disease progression; that is, patients with high levels of virus are much more likely to get sicker faster than those with low levels of virus. The MACS and other studies have provided the rationale for providing aggressive antiretroviral therapy to HIV-infected people, as well as for routinely using newly available blood tests to measure viral load when initiating, monitoring, and modifying anti-HIV therapy.

Potent combinations of three or more anti-HIV drugs known as highly active antiretroviral therapy, or HAART, can reduce a person's "viral burden" (amount of virus in the circulating blood) to very low levels and in many cases delay the progression of HIV disease for prolonged periods. Before the introduction of HAART therapy, 85 percent of patients survived an average of three years following AIDS diagnosis. Today, 95 percent of patients who start therapy before they get AIDS survive on average three years following their first AIDS diagnosis. For those who start HAART after their first AIDS event, survival is still very high at 85 percent, averaging three years after AIDS diagnosis.

Antiretroviral regimens, however, have yet to completely and permanently suppress the virus in HIV-infected people. Recent studies have shown that, in addition to the latent HIV reservoir discussed above, HIV persists in a replication-competent form in resting CD4+

T cells even in people receiving aggressive antiretroviral therapy who have no readily detectable HIV in their blood. Investigators around the world are working to develop the next generation of anti-HIV drugs that can stop HIV, even in these biological scenarios.

A treatment goal, along with reduction of viral burden, is the reconstitution of the person's immune system, which may have become sufficiently damaged that it cannot replenish itself. Various strategies for assisting the immune system in this regard are being tested in clinical trials in tandem with HAART, such as the Evaluation of Subcutaneous Proleukin in a Randomized International Trial (ESPRIT) trial exploring the effects of the T-cell growth factor, IL-2 [interleukin-2].

HIV Is Active in the Lymph Nodes

Although HIV-infected people often show an extended period of clinical latency with little evidence of disease, the virus is never truly completely latent although individual cells may be latently infected. Researchers have shown that even early in disease, HIV actively replicates within the lymph nodes and related organs, where large amounts of virus become trapped in networks of specialized cells with long, tentacle-like extensions. These cells are called follicular dendritic cells (FDCs). FDCs are located in hot spots of immune activity in lymphoid tissue called germinal centers. They act like flypaper, trapping invading pathogens (including HIV) and holding them until B cells come along to start an immune response.

Over a period of years, even when little virus is readily detectable in the blood, significant amounts of virus accumulate in the lymphoid tissue, both within infected cells and bound to FDCs. In and around the germinal centers, numerous CD4+ T cells are probably activated by the increased production of cytokines such as TNF-alpha and IL-6 by immune system cells within the lymphoid tissue. Activation allows uninfected cells to be more easily infected and increases replication of HIV in already infected cells.

While greater quantities of certain cytokines such as TNF-alpha and IL-6 are secreted during HIV infection, other cytokines with key roles in the regulation of normal immune function may be secreted in decreased amounts. For example, CD4+ T cells may lose their capacity to produce IL-2, a cytokine that enhances the growth of other T cells and helps to stimulate other cells' response to invaders. Infected cells also have low levels of receptors for IL-2, which may reduce their ability to respond to signals from other cells.

Breakdown of Lymph Node Architecture

Ultimately, with chronic cell activation and secretion of inflammatory cytokines, the fine and complex inner structure of the lymph node breaks down and is replaced by scar tissue. Without this structure, cells in the lymph node cannot communicate and the immune system cannot function properly. Investigators also have reported recently that this scarring reduces the ability of the immune system to replenish itself following antiretroviral therapy that reduces the viral burden.

Role of CD8+ T Cells

CD8+ T cells are critically important in the immune response to HIV. These cells attack and kill infected cells that are producing virus. Thus, vaccine efforts are directed toward eliciting or enhancing these killer T cells, as well as eliciting antibodies that will neutralize the infectivity of HIV.

CD8+ T cells also appear to secrete soluble factors that suppress HIV replication. Several molecules, including RANTES, MIP-1alpha, MIP-1beta, and MDC appear to block HIV replication by occupying the co-receptors necessary for many strains of HIV to enter their target cells. There may be other immune system molecules—including the so-called CD8 antiviral factor (CAF), the defensins (type of antimicrobials), and others yet undiscovered—that can suppress HIV replication to some degree.

Rapid Replication and Mutation of HIV

HIV replicates rapidly; several billion new virus particles may be produced every day. In addition, the HIV reverse transcriptase enzyme makes many mistakes while making DNA copies from HIV RNA. As a consequence, many variants or strains of HIV develop in a person, some of which may escape destruction by antibodies or killer T cells. Additionally, different strains of HIV can recombine to produce a wide range of variants.

During the course of HIV disease, viral strains emerge in an infected person that differ widely in their ability to infect and kill different cell types, as well as in their rate of replication. Scientists are investigating why strains of HIV from people with advanced disease appear to be more virulent and infect more cell types than strains obtained earlier from the same person. Part of the explanation may be the expanded ability of the virus to use other co-receptors, such as CXCR4.

Theories of Immune System Cell Loss in HIV Infection

Researchers around the world are studying how HIV destroys or disables CD4+ T cells, and many think that a number of mechanisms may occur simultaneously in an HIV-infected person. Data suggest that billions of CD4+ T cells may be destroyed every day, eventually overwhelming the immune system's capacity to regenerate.

Direct Cell Killing

Infected CD4+ T cells may be killed directly when large amounts of virus are produced and bud out from the cell surface, disrupting the cell membrane, or when viral proteins and nucleic acids collect inside the cell, interfering with cellular machinery.

Apoptosis

Infected CD4+ T cells may be killed when the regulation of cell function is distorted by HIV proteins, probably leading to cell suicide by a process known as programmed cell death or apoptosis. Recent reports indicate that apoptosis occurs to a greater extent in HIV-infected people, both in their bloodstream and lymph nodes. Apoptosis is closely associated with the aberrant cellular activation seen in HIV disease.

Uninfected cells also may undergo apoptosis. Investigators have shown in cell cultures that the HIV envelope alone or bound to antibodies sends an inappropriate signal to CD4+ T cells causing them to undergo apoptosis, even if not infected by HIV.

Innocent Bystanders

Uninfected cells may die in an innocent bystander scenario: HIV particles may bind to the cell surface, giving them the appearance of an infected cell and marking them for destruction by killer T cells after antibody attaches to the viral particle on the cell. This process is called antibody-dependent cellular cytotoxicity.

Killer T cells also may mistakenly destroy uninfected cells that have consumed HIV particles and that display HIV fragments on their surfaces. Alternatively, because HIV envelope proteins bear some resemblance to certain molecules that may appear on CD4+ T cells, the body's immune responses may mistakenly damage such cells as well.

Anergy

Researchers have shown in cell cultures that CD4+ T cells can be turned off by activation signals from HIV that leaves them unable to respond to further immune stimulation. This inactivated state is known as anergy.

Damage to Precursor Cells

Studies suggest that HIV also destroys precursor cells that mature to have special immune functions, as well as the microenvironment of the bone marrow and the thymus needed for developing such cells. These organs probably lose the ability to regenerate, further compounding the suppression of the immune system.

Central Nervous System Damage

Although monocytes and macrophages can be infected by HIV, they appear to be relatively resistant to being killed by the virus. These cells, however, travel throughout the body and carry HIV to various organs, including the brain, which may serve as a hiding place or "reservoir" for the virus that may be relatively resistant to most anti-HIV drugs.

Neurologic manifestations of HIV disease are seen in up to 50 percent of HIV-infected people, to varying degrees of severity. People infected with HIV often experience the following:

- cognitive symptoms, including impaired short-term memory, reduced concentration, and mental slowing

- motor symptoms such as fine motor clumsiness or slowness, tremor, and leg weakness

- behavioral symptoms including apathy, social withdrawal, irritability, depression, and personality change

More serious neurologic manifestations in HIV disease typically occur in patients with high viral loads, generally when a person has advanced HIV disease or AIDS.

Neurologic manifestations of HIV disease are the subject of many research projects. Current evidence suggests that although nerve cells do not become infected with HIV, supportive cells within the brain, such as astrocytes and microglia (as well as monocyte/macrophages that have migrated to the brain) can be infected with the virus. Researchers postulate that infection of these cells can cause a disruption of normal neurologic functions by altering cytokine levels, by delivering aberrant signals, and by causing the release of toxic products in the brain. The use of anti-HIV drugs frequently reduces the severity of neurologic symptoms, but in many cases does not, for reasons that are unclear. The impact of long-term therapy and long-term HIV disease on neurologic function is also unknown and under intensive study.

Role of Immune Activation in HIV Disease

During a normal immune response, many parts of the immune system are mobilized to fight an invader. CD4+ T cells, for instance, may quickly multiply and increase their cytokine secretion, thereby signaling other cells to perform their special functions. Scavenger cells called macrophages may double in size and develop numerous organelles, including lysosomes that contain digestive enzymes used to process ingested pathogens. Once the immune system clears the foreign antigen, it returns to a relative state of quiescence.

Paradoxically, although it ultimately causes immunodeficiency, HIV disease for most of its course is characterized by immune system hyperactivation, which has negative consequences. As noted above, HIV replication and spread are much more efficient in activated CD4+ cells. Chronic immune system activation during HIV disease also may result in a massive stimulation of B cells, impairing the ability of these cells to make antibodies against other pathogens.

Chronic immune activation also can result in apoptosis, and an increased production of cytokines that not only may increase HIV replication but also have other deleterious effects. Increased levels of TNF-alpha, for example, may be at least partly responsible for the severe weight loss or wasting syndrome seen in many HIV-infected people.

The persistence of HIV and HIV replication plays an important role in the chronic state of immune activation seen in HIV-infected people. In addition, researchers have shown that infections with other organisms activate immune system cells and increase production of the virus in HIV-infected people. Chronic immune activation due to persistent infections, or the cumulative effects of multiple episodes of immune activation and bursts of virus production, likely contribute to the progression of HIV disease.

31

New Clinical Signs of HIV in the Era of HAART Therapy

The clinical spectrum of disease among people with HIV has changed dramatically in the era of HAART. NIAID and its grantees are actively studying the new clinical syndrome of disease among persons on long-term therapy. Research is concentrating on the impact of HIV over the long term, the toxicity of the medicines used to control HIV, and the effects of aging on HIV disease progression. People with HIV have a variety of conditions including diabetes, heart disease, neurocognitive decline, and cancers that may, or may not, be directly due to HIV or its treatment. Long-term studies of people with HIV in the United States and abroad are underway.

NIAID Research on the Pathogenesis of AIDS

NIAID-supported scientists conduct research on HIV pathogenesis in laboratories on the campus of the National Institutes of Health (NIH) in Bethesda, Maryland; at the Institute's Rocky Mountain Laboratories in Hamilton, Montana; and at universities and medical centers in the United States and abroad.

An NIAID-supported resource, the NIH AIDS Research and Reference Reagent Program, in collaboration with the World Health Organization, provides critically needed AIDS-related research materials free to qualified researchers around the world.

The NIH Centers for AIDS Research, supported by NIAID in collaboration with six other NIH Institutes, fosters and facilitates development of infrastructure and interdisciplinary collaboration of HIV researchers at major medical and research centers across the United States.

In addition, the Institute convenes groups of investigators and advisory committees to exchange scientific information, clarify research priorities, and bring research needs and opportunities to the attention of the scientific community.

Chapter 3

HIV Types, Groups, and Subtypes

Introduction to HIV Types, Groups, and Subtypes

HIV is a highly variable virus which mutates very readily. This means there are many different strains of HIV, even within the body of a single infected person.

Based on genetic similarities, the numerous virus strains may be classified into types, groups, and subtypes.

What is the difference between HIV-1 and HIV-2?

There are two types of HIV: HIV-1 and HIV-2. Both types are transmitted by sexual contact, through blood, and from mother to child, and they appear to cause clinically indistinguishable AIDS. However, it seems that HIV-2 is less easily transmitted, and the period between initial infection and illness is longer in the case of HIV-2.

Worldwide, the predominant virus is HIV-1, and generally when people refer to HIV without specifying the type of virus they will be referring to HIV-1. The relatively uncommon HIV-2 type is concentrated in West Africa and is rarely found elsewhere.

How many subtypes of HIV-1 are there?

The strains of HIV-1 can be classified into three groups: the "major" group M, the "outlier" group O, and the "new" group N. These three groups may represent three separate introductions of simian immunodeficiency virus into humans.

Group O appears to be restricted to west-central Africa and group N—discovered in 1998 in Cameroon—is extremely rare. More than 90 percent of HIV-1 infections belong to HIV-1 group M and, unless specified, the rest of this section will relate to HIV-1 group M only.

Within group M there are known to be at least nine genetically distinct subtypes (or clades) of HIV-1. These are subtypes A, B, C, D, F, G, H, J, and K.

Occasionally, two viruses of different subtypes can meet in the cell of an infected person and mix together their genetic material to create a new hybrid virus (a process similar to sexual reproduction, and sometimes called "viral sex").[1] Many of these new strains do not survive for long, but those that infect more than one person are known as "circulating recombinant forms" or CRFs. For example, the CRF A/B is a mixture of subtypes A and B.

The classification of HIV strains into subtypes and CRFs is a complex issue and the definitions are subject to change as new discoveries are made. Some scientists talk about subtypes A1, A2, A3, F1, and F2 instead of A and F, though others regard the former as sub-subtypes.

What about subtypes E and I?

One of the CRFs is called A/E because it is thought to have resulted from hybridization between subtype A and some other "parent" subtype E. However, no one has ever found a pure form of subtype E. Confusingly, many people still refer to the CRF A/E as "subtype E" (in fact it is most correctly called CRF01_AE).[2]

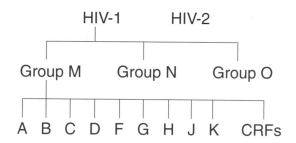

Figure 3.1. *This diagram illustrates the different levels of HIV classification. Each type is divided into groups, and each group is divided into subtypes and CRFs.*

A virus isolated in Cyprus was originally placed in a new subtype I, before being reclassified as a recombinant form A/G/I. It is now thought that this virus represents an even more complex CRF comprised of subtypes A, G, H, K, and unclassified regions. The designation "I" is no longer used.[3]

Where are the different subtypes and CRFs found?

The HIV-1 subtypes and CRFs are very unevenly distributed throughout the world, with the most widespread being subtypes B and C.

Subtype C is largely predominant in southern and eastern Africa, India, and Nepal. It has caused the world's worst HIV epidemics and is responsible for around half of all infections.

Historically, subtype B has been the most common subtype/CRF in Europe, the Americas, Japan, and Australia. Although this remains the case, other subtypes are becoming more frequent and now account for at least 25 percent of new infections in Europe.

Subtype A and CRF A/G predominate in west and central Africa, with subtype A possibly also causing much of the Russian epidemic.[4] Subtype D is generally limited to east and central Africa; A/E is prevalent in Southeast Asia, but originated in central Africa; F has been found in central Africa, South America, and eastern Europe; G and A/G have been observed in western and eastern Africa and central Europe.

Subtype H has only been found in central Africa; J only in central America; and K only in the Democratic Republic of Congo and Cameroon.

Are more subtypes likely to "appear"?

It is almost certain that new HIV genetic subtypes and CRFs will be discovered in the future, and indeed that new ones will develop as virus recombination and mutation continue to occur. The current subtypes and CRFs will also continue to spread to new areas as the global epidemic continues.

The Implications of Variability

Does subtype affect disease progression?

A study presented in 2006 found that Ugandans infected with subtype D or recombinant strains incorporating subtype D developed AIDS sooner than those infected with subtype A, and also died sooner. The study's authors suggested that subtype D is more virulent because it is more effective at binding to immune cells.[5] This result was supported by another study presented in 2007, which found that Kenyan women infected with subtype D had more than twice the risk of death over six years compared with those infected with subtype A.[6] An earlier study of sex workers in Senegal, published in 1999, found that women infected with subtype C, D, or G were more likely to develop AIDS within five years of infection than those infected with subtype A.[7]

Are there differences in transmission?

It has been observed that certain subtypes/CRFs are predominantly associated with specific modes of transmission. In particular, subtype B is spread mostly by homosexual contact and intravenous drug use (essentially via blood), while subtype C and CRF A/E tend to fuel heterosexual epidemics (via a mucosal route).

Whether there are biological causes for the observed differences in transmission routes remains the subject of debate. Some scientists, such as Dr. Max Essex of Harvard, believe such causes do exist. Among their claims are that subtype C and CRF A/E are transmitted much more efficiently during heterosexual sex than subtype B.[8,9] However, this theory has not been conclusively proven.[10,11]

More recent studies have looked for variation between subtypes in rates of mother-to-child transmission. One of these found that such transmission is more common with subtype D than subtype A.[12] Another reached the opposite conclusion (A worse than D), and also found that subtype C was more often transmitted than subtype D.[13] A third study concluded that subtype C is more transmissible than either D or A.[14] Other researchers have found no association between subtype and rates of mother-to-child transmission.[15,16,17,18]

Is it possible to be infected more than once?

Until about 1994, it was generally thought that individuals do not become infected with multiple distinct HIV-1 strains. Since then, many cases of people co-infected with two or more strains have been documented.

All cases of co-infection were once assumed to be the result of people being exposed to the different strains more or less simultaneously, before their immune systems had had a chance to react. However, it is now thought that "superinfection" is also occurring. In these cases, the second infection occurred several months after the first. It would appear that the body's immune response to the first virus is sometimes not enough to prevent infection with a second strain, especially with a virus belonging to a different subtype. It is not yet known how commonly superinfection occurs, or whether it can take place only in special circumstances.[19,20]

Do HIV antibody tests detect all types, groups, and subtypes?

Initial tests for HIV are usually conducted using the EIA [enzyme immunoassay] (or ELISA [enzyme-linked immunosorbent assay]) antibody test or a rapid antibody test.

EIA tests which can detect either one or both types of HIV have been available for a number of years. According to the U.S. Centers for Disease Control and Prevention, current HIV-1 EIAs "can accurately identify infections with nearly all non-B subtypes and many infections with group O HIV subtypes."[21] However, because HIV-2 and group O infections are extremely rare in most countries, routine screening programs might not be designed to test for them. Anyone who believes they may have contracted HIV-2, HIV-1 group O, or one of the rarer subtypes of group M should seek expert advice.

Rapid tests—which can produce a result in less than an hour—are becoming increasingly popular. Most modern rapid HIV-1 tests are capable of detecting all the major subtypes of group M.[22] Rapid tests which can detect HIV-2 are also now available.[23]

What are the treatment implications?

Most current HIV-1 antiretroviral drug regimens were designed for use against subtype B, and so hypothetically might not be equally effective in Africa or Asia where other strains are more common. At present, there is no compelling evidence that subtypes differ in their sensitivity to antiretroviral drugs. However, some subtypes may occasionally be more likely to develop resistance to certain drugs. In some situations, the types of mutations associated with resistance may vary. This is an important subject for future research.

The effectiveness of HIV-1 treatment is monitored using viral load tests. It has been demonstrated that some such tests are sensitive only to subtype B and can produce a significant underestimate of viral load if used to process other strains. The latest tests do claim to produce accurate results for most group M subtypes, though not necessarily for group O. It is important that health workers and patients are aware of the subtype/CRF they are testing for and of the limitations of the test they are applying.

Not all of the drugs used to treat HIV-1 infection are as effective against HIV-2. In particular, HIV-2 has a natural resistance to NNRTI antiretroviral drugs and they are therefore not recommended. As yet there is no FDA-licensed viral load test for HIV-2 and those designed for HIV-1 are not reliable for monitoring the other type. Instead, response to treatment may be monitored by following CD4+ T-cell counts and indicators of immune system deterioration. More research and clinical experience is needed to determine the most effective treatment for HIV-2.[24]

What are the implications for an AIDS vaccine?

The development of an AIDS vaccine is affected by the range of virus subtypes as well as by the wide variety of human populations who need protection and who differ, for example, in their genetic make-up and their routes of exposure to HIV. In particular, the occurrence of superinfection indicates that an immune response triggered by a vaccine to prevent infection by one strain of HIV may not protect against all other strains. The effectiveness of a vaccine is likely to vary in different populations unless some innovative method is developed which guards against many virus strains.

Inevitably, different types of candidate vaccines will have to be tested against various viral strains in multiple vaccine trials, conducted in both high-income and developing countries.

Sources

UNAIDS Questions and Answers II, Section I, July 2004.

"HIV-1 Subtype Distribution and the Problem of Drug Resistance" by Mark A. Wainberg, *AIDS 2004,* Volume 18, Supplement 3, 3 June 2004.

References

1. "Recombination of HIV: An Important Viral Evolutionary Strategy" by Burke DS, *Emerging Infectious Diseases* Volume 3 Number 3, July–September 1997.

2. "The Circulating Recombinant Forms (CRFs)," Los Alamos National Laboratory website, http://www.hiv.lanl.gov/content/hiv-db/CRFs/CRFs.html, accessed 15 November 2004.

3. "An Isolate of Human Immunodeficiency Virus Type 1 Originally Classified as Subtype I Represents a Complex Mosaic Comprising Three Different Group M Subtypes (A, G, and I)"

by Feng G, Robertson DL, Carruthers CD et al, *Journal of Virology* Volume 72 Number 12, December 1998.

4. "Temporal trends in the HIV-1 epidemic in Russia: predominance of subtype A" by Bobkov AF, Kazennova EV, Selimova LM et al, *J Med Virol*, October 2004.

5. "The Effect of HIV Subtype on Rapid Disease Progression in Rakai, Uganda" by Laeyendecker O, Li X, Arroyo M et al, 13th Conference on Retroviruses and Opportunistic Infections (abstract no. 44LB), February 2006.

6. "HIV-1 subtype D infection is associated with faster disease progression than subtype A, in spite of similar HIV-1 plasma viral loads" by Baeten D et al, 14th Conference on Retroviruses and Opportunistic Infections (abstract no. 68), February 2007.

7. "Human Immunodeficiency Virus Type 1 Subtypes Differ in Disease Progression" by Kanki PJ, Hamel DJ, Sankale J-L et al, *Journal of Infectious Diseases* Volume 179 Number 1, January 1999.

8. "In vivo identification of Langerhans and related dendritic cells infected with HIV-1 subtype E in vaginal mucosa of asymptomatic patients" by Bhoopat L, Eiangleng L, Rugpao S et al, *Mod Pathol*, December 2001.

9. "Retroviral vaccines: challenges for the developing world" by Essex M, *AIDS Res Hum Retroviruses,* 20 March 1996.

10. "Human immunodeficiency virus type 1 strains of subtypes B and E replicate in cutaneous dendritic cell-T-cell mixtures without displaying subtype-specific tropism" by Pope M, Frankel SS, Mascola JR et al, *J Virol,* October 1997.

11. "Langerhans cell tropism of human immunodeficiency virus type 1 subtype A through F isolates derived from different transmission groups" by Dittmar MT, Simmons G, Hibbitts S et al, *J Virol,* October 1997.

12. "Genetic diversity of HIV-1 in western Kenya: subtype-specific differences in mother-to-child transmission" by Yang, Li, Newman et al, *AIDS 2003* Volume 17 Number 11, 25 July 2003.

13. "HIV-1 LTR subtype and perinatal transmission" by Blackard, Renjifo et al, *Virology 2001* Volume 287 Number 2, 1 September 2001.

14. "Preferential in-utero transmission of HIV-1 type C as compared to HIV-1 subtype A or D" by Renjifo B, Gilbert P, Chaplin B et al, *AIDS 2004* Volume 18 Number 12, 20 August 2004.

15. "Effect of human immunodeficiency virus (HIV) type 1 viral genotype on mother-to-child transmission of HIV-1" by Murray, Embree et al, *Journal Infectious Diseases* Volume 181 Number 2, February 2000.

16. "Maternal humoral factors associated with perinatal human immunodeficiency virus type-1 transmission in a cohort from Kigali, Rwanda, 1988–1994" by Tranchat, Van de Perre et al, *J Infect* Volume 39 Number 3, November 1999.

17. "Influence of human immunodeficiency virus type 1 subtype on mother-to-child transmission" by Tapia, Franco et al, *Journal of General Virology* Volume 84, 2003.

18. "Determinants of HIV-1 Mother-to-Child transmission in Southern Brazil" by Martinez, Da Hora et al, *Anais da Academia Brasileira de Ciencias* Volume 78 Number 1, 2006.

19. "HIV-1 superinfection and viral diversity" by Gross KL, Porco TC and Grant RM, *AIDS 2004* Volume 18 Number 11, 23 July 2004.

20. "HIV-1 superinfections: omens for vaccine efficacy?" by Fultz PN, *AIDS 2004* Volume 18 Number 1, 2 January 2004.

21. "Revised Guidelines for HIV Counseling, Testing, and Referral," *Morbidity and Mortality Weekly Report 50*(RR19);1–58, 9 November 2001.

22. "Diagnosis of Human Immunodeficiency Virus Type 1 Infection with Different Subtypes Using Rapid Tests" by Phillips S, Granade TC, Pau C-P et al, *Clinical and Diagnostic Laboratory Immunology,* July 2000.

23. "OraQuick Rapid HIV Test for Oral Fluid—Frequently Asked Questions," Centers for Disease Control and Prevention, 2 November 2004.

24. "Human Immunodeficiency Virus Type 2", CDC website, accessed 23 November 2004.

Chapter 4

Testing HIV Positive: What Does It Mean?

I tested HIV positive. What does this mean? Does it mean I have AIDS?

A positive HIV test result means that you are infected with HIV (human immunodeficiency virus), the virus that causes AIDS (acquired immunodeficiency syndrome). Being infected with HIV does not mean that you have AIDS right now. However, if left untreated, HIV infection damages a person's immune system and can progress to AIDS.

What is AIDS?

AIDS is the most serious stage of HIV infection. It results from the destruction of the infected person's immune system.

Your immune system is your body's defense system. Cells of your immune system fight off infection and other diseases. If your immune system does not work well, you are at risk for serious and life-threatening infections and cancers. HIV attacks and destroys the disease-fighting cells of the immune system, leaving the body with a weakened defense against infections and cancer.

"Testing HIV Positive—Do I Have AIDS?" AIDSinfo, a service of the U.S. Department of Health and Human Services (http://www.aidsinfo.nih.gov), reviewed August 2006.

Which disease-fighting cells does HIV attack?

CD4 cells are a type of white blood cell that fights infections. They are also called CD4 + T cells or CD4 T lymphocytes. A CD4 count is the number of CD4 cells in a sample of blood.

When HIV enters a person's CD4 cells, it uses the cells to make copies of itself. This process destroys the CD4 cells, and the CD4 count goes down. As you lose CD4 cells, your immune system becomes weak. A weakened immune system makes it harder for your body to fight infections and cancer.

How will I know if I have AIDS?

AIDS is not a diagnosis you can make yourself; it is diagnosed when the immune system is severely weakened. If you are infected with HIV and your CD4 count drops below 200 cells/mm³, or if you develop an AIDS-defining condition (an illness that is very unusual in someone who is not infected with HIV), you have AIDS.

What are the AIDS-defining conditions?

In December 1992, the Centers for Disease Control and Prevention (CDC) published the most current list of AIDS-defining conditions. The AIDS-defining conditions are listed below:

- candidiasis

- cervical cancer (invasive)

- coccidioidomycosis, cryptococcosis, cryptosporidiosis

- Cytomegalovirus disease

- encephalopathy (HIV-related)

- herpes simplex (severe infection)

- histoplasmosis

- isosporiasis

- Kaposi sarcoma

- lymphoma (certain types)

- *Mycobacterium avium* complex

- *Pneumocystis carinii/jiroveci* pneumonia

- pneumonia (recurrent)

- progressive multifocal leukoencephalopathy
- Salmonella septicemia (recurrent)
- toxoplasmosis of the brain
- tuberculosis
- wasting syndrome

People who are not infected with HIV may also develop these diseases; this does not mean they have AIDS. To be diagnosed with AIDS, a person must be infected with HIV.

What is HIV treatment?

HIV treatment is the use of medications to keep an HIV infected person healthy. Treatment can help people at all stages of HIV disease. Although anti-HIV medications can treat HIV infection, they cannot cure HIV infection. HIV treatment is complicated and must be tailored to you and your needs.

For More Information

Contact your doctor or an AIDSinfo health information specialist at 800-448-0440 or http://aidsinfo.nih.gov.

Chapter 5

Basic Information about AIDS

Alternative names: Acquired immune deficiency syndrome

Definition: AIDS (acquired immunodeficiency syndrome) is the final and most serious stage of HIV disease, which causes severe damage to the immune system.

According to the Centers for Disease Control and Prevention, AIDS begins when a person with HIV infection has a CD4 cell count below 200. CD4 cells are also called "T cells" or "helper cells"; they are a type of immune cell. AIDS is also defined by numerous opportunistic infections and cancers that occur in the presence of HIV infection.

Causes, Incidence, and Risk Factors

AIDS is the fifth leading cause of death among persons between ages 25 and 44 in the United States, down from number one in 1995. About 25 million people worldwide have died from this infection since the start of the epidemic, and 40.3 million people are currently living with HIV/AIDS globally.

Human immunodeficiency virus (HIV) causes AIDS. The virus attacks the immune system and leaves the body vulnerable to a variety of life-threatening infections and cancers.

Common bacteria, yeast, parasites, and viruses that ordinarily do not cause serious disease in people with healthy immune systems can cause fatal illnesses in people with AIDS.

HIV has been found in saliva, tears, nervous system tissue and spinal fluid, blood, semen (including pre-seminal fluid), vaginal fluid, and breast milk. However, only blood, semen, vaginal secretions, and breast milk generally transmit infection to others.

Transmission of the virus occurs:

- through sexual contact, including oral, vaginal, and anal sex;

- through blood, via blood transfusions (now extremely rare in the U.S.) or needle sharing;

- from mother to child, a pregnant woman can transmit the virus to her fetus through their shared blood circulation, or a nursing mother can transmit it to her baby in her milk.

Other transmission methods are rare and include accidental needle injury, artificial insemination with donated semen, and organ transplants.

HIV infection is not spread by casual contact such as hugging, by touching items previously touched by a person infected with the virus, during participation in sports, or by mosquitoes.

It is not transmitted to a person who donates blood or organs. Those who donate organs are not in direct contact with those who receive them. Likewise, a person who donates blood is not in contact with the person receiving it. In all these procedures, sterile needles and instruments are used.

However, HIV can be transmitted to a person receiving blood or organs from an infected donor. This is why blood banks and organ donor programs screen donors, blood, and tissues thoroughly.

Those at highest risk include:

- persons engaging in unprotected sex;

- sexual partners of those who participate in high-risk activities (such as anal sex);

- intravenous drug users who share needles;

- infants born to mothers with HIV who don't receive HIV therapy during pregnancy;

- people who received blood transfusions or clotting products between 1977 and 1985 (prior to the beginning standard screening for the virus in the blood).

AIDS begins with HIV infection. People infected with HIV may have no symptoms for ten years or longer, but they can still transmit the infection to others during this symptom-free period. Meanwhile, if the infection is not detected and treated, the immune system gradually weakens, and AIDS develops.

Acute HIV infection progresses over time to asymptomatic HIV infection and then to early symptomatic HIV infection. Later, it progresses to AIDS (defined as very advanced HIV infection with T-cell count below 200).

Most individuals infected with HIV, if not treated, will develop AIDS. There is a small group of patients who develop AIDS very slowly, or never at all. These patients are called non-progressors, and many seem to have a genetic difference that prevents the virus from attaching to certain immune receptors.

Symptoms

The symptoms of AIDS are primarily the result of infections that do not normally develop in individuals with healthy immune systems. These are called opportunistic infections.

Patients with AIDS have had their immune system depleted by HIV and are very susceptible to such opportunistic infections. Common symptoms are fevers, sweats (particularly at night), swollen glands, chills, weakness, and weight loss.

See the signs and tests section for a list of common opportunistic infections and major symptoms associated with them.

Note: Initial infection with HIV can produce no symptoms. Most people, however, do experience flu-like symptoms with fever, rash, sore throat, and swollen lymph nodes, usually two weeks after contracting the virus. Some people with HIV infection remain without symptoms for years between the time of exposure and development of AIDS.

Signs and Tests

The following is a list of AIDS-related infections and cancers that people with AIDS acquire as their CD4 count decreases. Previously, having AIDS was defined as having HIV infection and getting one of these additional diseases. Now it is additionally defined as a CD4 count below 200, even without an opportunistic infection. Many other illnesses and corresponding symptoms may develop in addition to those listed here.

Common with CD4 Count below 350 Cells/ml

- **Herpes simplex virus:** Causes ulcers/vesicles in the mouth or genitals, occurring more frequently and more severely in an HIV-infected patient than before HIV infection

- **Tuberculosis:** Infection by the tuberculosis bacteria that predominately affects the lungs, but can affect other organs such as the bowel, lining of the heart or lungs, brain, or lining of the central nervous system

- **Oral or vaginal thrush:** Yeast infection of the mouth or genitals

- **Herpes zoster (shingles):** Ulcers/vesicles over a discrete patch of skin caused by the varicella-zoster virus

- **Non-Hodgkin lymphoma:** Cancer of the lymph glands

- **Kaposi sarcoma:** Cancer of the skin, lungs, and bowel, associated with a herpes virus (HHV-8). Can occur at any CD4 count, but more likely at lower CD4 counts, and more common in men than women

CD4 Count below 200 Cells/ml

- ***Pneumocystis carinii* pneumonia (PCP),** now called *Pneumocystis jiroveci* pneumonia

- **Candida esophagitis:** Painful yeast infection of the esophagus

- **Bacillary angiomatosis:** Skin lesions caused by a bacteria called *Bartonella*, which is usually acquired from cat scratches

CD4 Count below 100 Cells/ml

- **Cryptococcal meningitis:** Infection of the lining of the brain by a yeast

- **AIDS dementia:** Worsening and slowing of mental function, caused by HIV itself

- **Toxoplasmosis encephalitis:** Infection of the brain by a parasite, which is frequently found in cat feces; causes discrete lesions in the brain

- **Progressive multifocal leukoencephalopathy:** A viral disease of the brain caused by a virus (called the JC virus) that results in a severe decline in cognitive and motor functions

- **Wasting syndrome:** Extreme weight loss and loss of appetite, caused by HIV

- ***Cryptosporidium* diarrhea:** Extreme diarrhea caused by one of several related parasites

CD4 Count below 50/ml

- *Mycobacterium avium:* A blood infection by a bacterium related to tuberculosis

- **Cytomegalovirus infection:** A viral infection that can affect almost any organ system, especially the large bowel and the eyes

In addition to the CD4 count, HIV RNA load, and basic screening lab tests, regular vaginal Pap smears are important to monitor in HIV infection, due to the increased risk of cervical cancer in immunocompromised patients. Anal Pap smears to detect potential cancers may also be important in both HIV infected men and women.

Treatment

There is no cure for AIDS at this time. However, a variety of treatments are available that can delay the progression of disease for many years, and improve the quality of life of those who have developed symptoms.

Antiretroviral therapy suppresses the replication of the HIV virus in the body. A combination of several antiretroviral agents, termed highly active antiretroviral therapy (HAART), has been highly effective in reducing the number of HIV particles in the blood stream, as measured by a blood test called the viral load. This can help the immune system recover from the HIV infection and improve T-cell counts.

Although not a cure for HIV, and people on HAART with suppressed levels of HIV can still transmit the virus to others through sex or sharing of needles, these treatments have been enormously effective for the past ten years. There is good evidence that if the levels of HIV remain suppressed and the CD4 count remains high (above 200), life can be significantly prolonged and improved. However, HIV may become resistant to HAART in patients who do not take their medications on schedule every day. Genetic tests are now available to determine whether a particular strain is resistant to a particular drug—these may be useful in determining the best drug combination, and adjusting the regimen if it starts to fail. These tests should be performed for any failing treatment course, and prior to starting therapy.

When HIV becomes resistant to HAART, salvage therapy is required to try to suppress the resistant strain of HIV. Different combinations of medications are used to try to reduce viral load, and there are a variety of new drugs coming out on the market for the treatment of drug-resistant HIV.

Treatment with HAART is not without complications. HAART is a collection of different medications, each with its own side effects. Some common side effects are nausea, headache, weakness, malaise, and fat accumulation on the back and abdomen ("buffalo hump"). When used long-term, these medications increase the risk of heart attack by affecting fat breakdown, specifically through increasing lipids and glucose levels.

Any doctor prescribing HAART should carefully follow the patient for possible side effects associated with the combination of medications the patient takes. In addition, routine blood tests measuring CD4 counts and HIV viral load (a blood test that measures how much virus is in the blood) should be taken every three to four months. The goal is to get the CD4 count as close to normal as possible, and to suppress the HIV viral load to an undetectable level.

Other antiviral agents are in investigational stages and many new drugs are in development. In addition, growth factors that stimulate cell growth, such as Epogen (erythropoietin) and G-CSF are sometimes used to treat anemia and low white blood cell counts associated with AIDS.

Medications are also used to prevent opportunistic infections (such as *Pneumocystis carinii* pneumonia) if the CD4 count is low enough. This keeps AIDS patients healthier for longer periods of time. Opportunistic infections are treated as they occur.

Support Groups

Joining support groups where members share common experiences and problems can often help the emotional stress of devastating illnesses.

Expectations (Prognosis)

At the present time, there is no cure for AIDS. It is always fatal if no treatment is provided. In the U.S., most patients survive many years following diagnosis because of the availability of HAART. HAART has dramatically increased the time from diagnosis to death, and research continues in the areas of drug treatments and vaccine development. Unfortunately, HIV medications are not always available in the developing world, where the bulk of the epidemic is raging, due to socio-economic reasons.

Complications

When a person is infected with HIV, the virus slowly begins to destroy that person's immune system. How fast this occurs differs in each individual. Treatment with HAART can help slow and even halt the destruction of the immune system.

Once the immune system is severely damaged, that person has AIDS, and is now susceptible to infections and cancers that most healthy adults would not get. However, antiretroviral treatment can still be very effective, even at that stage of illness.

Calling Your Health Care Provider

Call for an appointment with your health care provider if you have any of the risk factors for HIV infection, or if symptoms of AIDS are present. By law, AIDS testing must be kept confidential. Your health care provider will review results of your testing with you.

Prevention

1. See the article on safe sex [in chapter 24] to learn how to reduce the chance of acquiring or spreading HIV, and other sexually transmitted diseases.

2. Try not to use intravenous drugs. If IV drugs are used, do not share needles or syringes. Many communities now have needle exchange programs, where used syringes can be disposed of and new, sterile needles obtained for free. These programs can also provide referrals to addiction treatment.

3. Avoid contact with another person's blood when the HIV status of the bleeding individual is unknown. Protective clothing, masks, and goggles may be appropriate when caring for people who are injured.

4. Anyone who tests positive for HIV can pass the disease to others and should not donate blood, plasma, body organs, or sperm. An infected person should warn any prospective sexual partner of their HIV-positive status, should not exchange body fluids during sexual activity, and should use whatever preventive measures (such as condoms) will afford the partner the most protection.

5. HIV-positive women who wish to become pregnant should seek counseling about the risk to unborn children, and medical

advances which may help prevent the fetus from becoming infected. Use of certain medications can dramatically reduce the chances that the baby will become infected during pregnancy.

6. Mothers who are HIV positive should not breastfeed their babies.

7. Safe-sex practices, such as latex condoms, are highly effective in preventing HIV transmission. However, there remains a risk of acquiring the infection even with the use of condoms, if the condom breaks. Abstinence is the only sure way to prevent sexual transmission of HIV.

The riskiest sexual behavior is unprotected receptive anal intercourse—the least risky sexual behavior is receiving oral sex. Performing oral sex on a man is associated with some risk of HIV transmission, but this is less risky than unprotected vaginal intercourse. Female-to-male transmission of the virus is much less likely than male-to-female transmission. Performing oral sex on a woman who does not have her period carries low risk of transmission.

HIV-positive patients who are taking antiretroviral medications are less likely to transmit the virus. For example, pregnant women who are on effective treatment at the time of delivery with undetectable viral loads transmit HIV to the infant less than 1 percent of the time, compared to approximately 20 percent if medications are not used.

The U.S. blood supply is among the safest in the world. Nearly all people infected with HIV through blood transfusions received those transfusions before 1985, the year HIV testing began for all donated blood. Currently, the risk of infection with HIV through a blood transfusion or blood products is vanishingly low in the United States, even in geographic areas with high HIV prevalence.

If you believe you have been exposed to HIV, seek medical attention immediately. There is some evidence that an immediate course of antiviral drugs can reduce the chances that you will be infected. This is called post-exposure prophylaxis (PEP), and has been used to treat health care workers injured by needlesticks, to prevent ultimate transmission.

There is less information on the effectiveness of PEP for people exposed via sexual activity or intravenous drug use. However, if you believe you have been exposed, you should discuss the possibility with a knowledgeable specialist (check local AIDS organizations for the latest information) as soon as possible. Anyone who has been raped should be offered PEP and should consider its potential risks and benefits in their particular case.

Chapter 6

AIDS Myths and Misunderstandings

Why Are There So Many AIDS Myths?

When AIDS first became known, it was a very mysterious disease. It caused the death of many people. There are still many unanswered questions about the disease. Many people reacted with fear and came up with stories to back up their fear. Most of these had to do with how easy it was to become infected with HIV. Most of these are not true.

Transmission Myths

Many people believed that HIV and AIDS could be transmitted by a mosquito bite, by sharing a drinking glass with someone with AIDS, by being around someone with AIDS who was coughing, by hugging or kissing someone with AIDS, and so on. Transmission can only occur if someone is exposed to blood, semen, vaginal fluid, or mother's milk from an infected person. There is no documentation of transmission from the tears or saliva of an infected person.

Myth: A woman with HIV infection can't have children without infecting them.

Reality: Without any treatment, HIV-infected mothers pass HIV to their newborns about 25 percent of the time. However, with modern treatments, this rate has dropped to only about 2 percent.

"AIDS Myths and Misunderstandings," Fact Sheet 158, © 2007 AIDS InfoNet. Reprinted with permission. Fact sheets are regularly updated. Check http://www.aidsinfonet.org for the most recent information.

53

Myth: HIV is being spread by needles left in theater seats or vending machine coin returns.

Reality: There is no documented case of this type of transmission.

Myths about a Cure

It can be very scary to have HIV infection or AIDS. The course of the disease is not very predictable. Some people get very sick in just a few months. Others live healthy lives for 20 years or more. The treatments can be difficult to take, with serious side effects. Not everyone can afford the medications. It's not surprising that scam artists have come up with several "cures" for AIDS that involve a variety of substances. Unfortunately, none of these "cures" work.

A very unfortunate myth in some parts of the world is that having sex with a virgin will cure AIDS. As a result, many young girls have been exposed to HIV and have developed AIDS. There is no evidence to support this belief.

Myth: Current medications can cure AIDS. It's no big deal if you get infected.

Reality: Today's medications have cut the death rate from AIDS by about 80 percent. They are also easier to take than they used to be. However, they still have side effects, are very expensive, and have to be taken every day for the rest of your life. If you miss too many doses, HIV can develop resistance to the drugs you are taking and they'll stop working.

AIDS Is a Death Sentence

In the 1980s, there was a very high death rate from AIDS. However, medications have improved dramatically and so has the life span of people with HIV infection. If you have access to ARVs [anti-retrovirals] and to medical monitoring, there's no reason you can't live a long life even with HIV infection or AIDS.

The Government Developed AIDS to Reduce Minority Populations

The world's best researchers in government and in private pharmaceutical companies are working hard to try to stop AIDS. The government doesn't have the capability to create a virus.

Many minorities do not trust the government, especially regarding health care. A recent study in Texas found that as many as 30 percent of Latinos and African Americans believed that HIV is a government conspiracy to kill minorities. However, it seems that minorities receive a lower level of health care due to the same factors as anyone else: low income, inconvenient health care offices, and so on. Attitudes about health care and health care providers were much less important.

Myths about Medications

It has been very challenging for doctors to choose the best anti-HIV medications (ARVs) for their patients. When the first drugs were developed, they had to be taken as many as three times a day. Some drugs had complicated requirements about storage, or what kind of food they had to be taken with (or how long you had to wait after eating before taking a dose.) The reality of ARVs has changed dramatically. However, there are still some myths:

Myth: You have to take your doses exactly 12 (or 8, or 24) hours apart.

Reality: Medications today are fairly forgiving. Although you will have the most consistent blood levels of your drugs if they are taken at even intervals through the day, they won't stop working if you're off by an hour or two. However, people taking Crixivan® (indinavir) without ritonavir need to be very careful about timing.

Myth: You have to take 100 percent of your doses on time or else they'll stop working.

Reality: It's very important to take AIDS medications correctly. In fact, if you miss more than about 5 percent of your doses, HIV has an easier time developing resistance and possibly being able to multiply even when you're taking ARVs. However, 100 percent adherence is not realistic for just about anyone. Do the best you can and be sure to let your health care provider know what's going on.

Myth: Current drugs are so strong that you can stop taking them (take a drug holiday) with no problem.

Reality: Ever since the first AIDS drugs were developed, patients have wanted to stop taking them due to side effects or just being reminded that they had AIDS. There have been many studies of "treatment interruptions" and all of them have shown that stopping your ARVs is very likely to cause problems. You could give the virus a chance to multiply or your count of CD4 cells could drop, a sign of immune damage.

Myth: AIDS drugs are poison and are more dangerous than the HIV virus.

Reality: When the first AIDS drugs became available, they weren't as good as current medications. People still died of AIDS-related conditions. It's true that some people get serious side effects from AIDS medications, but the death rate in the U.S. has dropped by about 80 percent. Researchers are working hard to make HIV treatments easier and safer to use.

Chapter 7

AIDS: A Historical Perspective

Twenty-Five Years Ago

On June 5,1981, the first cases of a new and fatal disease now known as acquired immunodeficiency syndrome (AIDS) were reported in the Centers for Disease Control and Prevention (CDC) publication *Morbidity and Mortality Weekly Report.*

AIDS was first recognized in homosexual men, but it was soon determined that the virus that causes AIDS can spread through sexual contact, blood and blood products, and from mother to infant during pregnancy, delivery, and breastfeeding.

AIDS is caused by the human immunodeficiency virus (HIV). By killing or damaging cells of the body's immune system, HIV progressively destroys the body's ability to fight infections and certain cancers. People diagnosed with AIDS may get life-threatening diseases called opportunistic infections, which are caused by microbes such as viruses or bacteria that usually do not make healthy people sick.

At the beginning of the AIDS pandemic, treatment was confined to palliative care and management of opportunistic infections.

Today

Today, HIV/AIDS is a global catastrophe. According to the Joint United Nations Programme on HIV/AIDS (UNAIDS), approximately

"HIV/AIDS Fact Sheet," National Institutes of Health (http://www.nih.gov), updated October 2006.

38.6 million people worldwide are living with HIV/AIDS, and more than 4 million people were newly infected in 2005—about 11,000 each day. In the United States, more than 1 million people are living with HIV/AIDS, with one-quarter of the people unaware of their status, and approximately 40,000 new infections occurring each year. Worldwide, more than 25 million people with HIV died since the pandemic began, including more than 520,000 in the United States. In 2005, there were an estimated 2.8 million deaths worldwide due to HIV/AIDS.

As shocking as these numbers are, they do not begin to adequately reflect the physical and emotional devastation to individuals, families, and communities coping with HIV/AIDS, and of the terrible impact of HIV/AIDS on regional and global security and the global economy.

Today, the National Institutes of Health (NIH) effort represents the largest public investment in HIV/AIDS research anywhere in the world. In FY 2006, the budget for NIH HIV/AIDS and HIV/AIDS-related research was $2.9 billion.

The NIH supports a comprehensive biomedical research program of basic, clinical, and behavioral research on HIV infection, its associated co-infections, opportunistic infections, malignancies, and other complications. This represents a unique trans-NIH and global research program that strives to better understand the basic biology of HIV, develop effective therapies to treat and control HIV disease, and design interventions to prevent new infections.

The risk factors associated with HIV transmission are now well defined, providing the foundation for prevention efforts. In virtually all developed nations and in a growing number of developing countries, prevention programs are slowing the spread of HIV infection, although rates of new infections, even in countries considered to be "success stories," continue at an unacceptably high level.

Scientists around the world illuminated the structure and genetic make up of HIV and made rapid advances in understanding its disease-causing mechanisms. These advances in turn facilitated the rapid development and testing of potent anti-HIV drugs and guidelines for the use of these medications.

Many HIV-infected people are living with the benefits resulting from NIH-supported therapeutics research. Combination antiretroviral therapy, also known as highly active antiretroviral therapy or HAART, plays a major role in the dramatic decreases in HIV-related morbidity and mortality where these medications are available and used. A recent study indicates that AIDS drugs saved 3 million years of life in the United States. In addition, certain antiretroviral drug regimens dramatically reduce the risk of HIV transmission from mother to child.

However, the use of antiretroviral therapy is now associated with a series of serious side effects and long-term complications that may have a negative impact on mortality rates. More deaths occurring from liver failure, kidney disease, and cardiovascular complications are being observed in this patient population. About one-quarter of the HIV-infected population in the United States is also co-infected with hepatitis C virus (HCV). The appearance of multi-drug resistant strains of HIV presents an additional serious public health concern.

The AIDS research investment provides benefits for people with other infectious, malignant, neurologic, autoimmune, and metabolic diseases, and led to an entirely new paradigm to treat other viral infections. For example, the drug 3TC, developed to treat AIDS, is now a widely used and effective therapy for chronic hepatitis B infection. Drugs developed to prevent and treat AIDS-associated opportunistic infections also provide benefit to patients undergoing cancer chemotherapy or receiving anti-transplant rejection therapy. In addition, AIDS research is providing a new understanding of the relationship between viruses and cancer.

Despite advances in HIV/AIDS research, the pandemic continues to undermine lives, communities, and societies. There is no cure for AIDS or a vaccine to prevent infection. Scientific, medical, logistical, and operational challenges remain to make HIV therapies, prevention services, and other interventions available to poor countries.

If left unchecked, HIV/AIDS will continue to have devastating consequences around the world for decades to come in every sector of society.

Tomorrow

Personalized Approaches

The increasing incidence of HIV drug resistance and drug-related complications in patients underscores the critical need for new and better treatment regimens.

Improved regimens also are needed to reduce drug interactions between HIV treatments and treatments for opportunistic co-infections, including hepatitis B and C, and problems with adherence to complicated treatment regimens.

A high priority of NIH-sponsored AIDS therapeutics research continues to be the development of drugs and therapeutic regimens that limit the development of drug resistance, can enter viral reservoirs to inhibit viral replication, are less toxic with fewer side effects, facilitate easier adherence, and are less expensive and more readily accessible.

Preventing Infections: Pre-Empting HIV

NIH is committed to the development of preventive interventions to protect individuals against HIV infection.

The ultimate defeat of HIV/AIDS will require a multi-pronged effort—difficult, if not impossible, without a safe and effective HIV vaccine. Over the past five years, NIH devoted approximately $2 billion to HIV/AIDS vaccine research. The development of an HIV vaccine is a complex research challenge because HIV is unusually well equipped to elude immune defenses, due to its ability to vary extensively, to persist in viral reservoirs, and to eventually overcome the immune system.

NIH has now conducted or initiated approximately 80 Phase I, two Phase II, and one Phase III clinical trials of nearly 50 vaccine candidates, individually or in combination, in collaboration with partners in academia and industry. Among these is a vaccine targeted to multiple HIV subtypes found worldwide that is in the second phase of clinical testing.

NIH is supporting the development of topical microbicides, which include creams, gels, or other substances that could be applied topically to prevent the transmission of HIV and other sexually transmitted infections. It is believed that topical microbicides might be more effective than condoms in preventing HIV infection because they would be easier to use and women would not have to negotiate their use, as they often must do with condoms.

Prevention priorities also include improved prevention of mother-to-child transmission, behavioral research strategies, interventions related to drug and alcohol use, and newer areas of promising investigation, such as circumcision, early treatment of co-infections, use of antiretroviral therapy as prevention, cervical barrier methods, and combination prevention strategies.

NIH places high priority on the need for affordable and sustainable prevention and treatment approaches that can be implemented in resource-limited nations.

Part Two

HIV/AIDS Transmission: Statistics, Trends, and Risk Factors

Chapter 8

Statistics on HIV/AIDS Cases in the United States

Basic Statistics

AIDS Cases

In 2005, the estimated number of diagnoses of AIDS in the United States and dependent areas was 45,669. Of these, 44,198 were in the 50 states and District of Columbia and 1,096 were in the dependent areas. In the 50 states and District of Columbia, adult and adolescent AIDS cases totaled 44,140 with 32,430 cases in males and 11,710 cases in females, and 58 cases estimated in children under age 13.

The cumulative estimated number of diagnoses of AIDS through 2005 in the United States and dependent areas was 988,376. Of these, 956,666 were in the 50 states and District of Columbia and 30,523 were in the dependent areas. In the 50 states and District of Columbia, adult and adolescent AIDS cases totaled 947,585 with 764,763 cases in males and 182,822 cases in females, and 9,078 cases estimated in children under age 13.[1]

AIDS Cases by Age

Of the estimated number of AIDS cases in the 50 states and District of Columbia, person's age at time of diagnosis were distributed as shown in Table 8.1.

This chapter includes text from "Basic Statistics," Centers for Disease Control and Prevention (CDC; http://www.cdc.gov), March 19, 2007; and "A Glance at the HIV/AIDS Epidemic," CDC, May 3, 2007.

Table 8.1. Distribution of AIDS cases by age at time of diagnosis.

Age	Estimated Number of AIDS Cases in 2005	Cumulative Estimated Number of AIDS Cases from Beginning of Epidemic through 2005
Under 13:	58	9,089
Ages 13–14:	66	1,015
Ages 15–19:	476	5,309
Ages 20–24:	2,004	34,987
Ages 25–29:	3,739	114,519
Ages 30–34:	5,635	194,529
Ages 35–39:	7,867	209,210
Ages 40–44:	8,925	165,497
Ages 45–49:	6,953	103,326
Ages 50–54:	4,277	57,336
Ages 55–59:	2,237	30,631
Ages 60–64:	1,068	16,611
Ages 65 or older:	894	14,606

AIDS Cases by Race/Ethnicity

Centers for Disease Control and Prevention (CDC) tracks HIV/AIDS information on five racial and ethnic groups: white, black (African American), Hispanic, Asian/Pacific Islander, and American Indian/Alaska Native.

Table 8.2. Estimated numbers of diagnoses of AIDS in the 50 states and District of Columbia by race or ethnicity.

Race or Ethnicity	Estimated Number of AIDS Cases in 2005	Cumulative Estimated Number of AIDS Cases from Beginning of Epidemic through 2005
White, not Hispanic	12,689	386,552
Black, not Hispanic	22,030	399,637
Hispanic	8,432	156,026
Asian/Pacific Islander	549	7,739
American Indian/ Alaska Native	196	3,251

AIDS Cases by Transmission Category

Six common transmission categories are male-to-male sexual contact, injection drug use, male-to-male sexual contact and injection drug use, heterosexual (male-female) contact, mother-to-child (perinatal) transmission, and other (includes blood transfusions and unknown cause).

In the following two tables is the distribution of the estimated number of diagnoses of AIDS among adults and adolescents by transmission category in the 50 states and District of Columbia. A breakdown by sex is provided where appropriate.

Table 8.3. Estimated number of AIDS cases among adults and adolescents by transmission category in 2005.

Transmission Category	Adult and Adolescent Male	Adult and Adolescent Female	Total
Male-to-male sexual contact	18,939	–	18,939
Injection drug use	5,806	3,179	8,985
Male-to-male sexual contact and injection drug use	2,190	–	2,190
High-risk heterosexual contact*	5,208	8,278	13,486
Other**	287	253	540

*Heterosexual contact with a person known to have, or to be at high risk for, HIV infection.

**Includes hemophilia, blood transfusion, perinatal, and risk not reported or not identified.

Table 8.4. Estimated number of AIDS cases by transmission category among adults and adolescents, from beginning of the epidemic through 2005.

Transmission Category	Adult and Adolescent Male	Adult and Adolescent Female	Total
Male-to-male sexual contact	454,106	–	454,106
Injection Drug Use	168,695	73,311	242,006
Male-to-male sexual contact and injection drug use	66,081	–	66,081
High-risk heterosexual contact*	61,914	102,936	164,850
Other**	13,967	6,575	20,542

*Heterosexual contact with a person known to have, or to be at high risk for, HIV infection.

**Includes hemophilia, blood transfusion, perinatal, and risk not reported or not identified.

The distribution of the estimated number of diagnoses of AIDS, among children (the term "children" refers to persons under age 13 at the time of diagnosis) in the 50 states and District of Columbia, by transmission categories is shown in Table 8.5.

Top Ten AIDS Cases by State/Dependent Area

Following are the ten states or dependent areas reporting the highest number of AIDS cases in 2005. The number of cumulative AIDS cases is shown in Table 8.6.

New York: 6,299

Florida: 4,960

California: 4,088

Texas: 3,113

Georgia: 2,333

Illinois: 1,922

Maryland: 1,595

Pennsylvania: 1,510

New Jersey: 1,278

Puerto Rico: 1,033

Table 8.5. Distribution of the estimated number of diagnoses of AIDS among children.

Transmission Category	Estimated Number of AIDS Cases in 2005	Cumulative Estimated Number of AIDS Cases from Beginning of Epidemic through 2005
Perinatal	57	8,438
Other*	1	640

*Includes hemophilia, blood transfusion, and risk not reported or not identified.

Table 8.6. Number of cumulative AIDS cases from beginning of epidemic through 2005 by state/dependent area.

State/Dependent Area	Adults or Adolescents	Children (under age 13)	Total
New York	170,035	2,342	172,377
California	138,361	658	139,019
Florida	99,290	1,519	100,809
Texas	66,836	391	67,227
New Jersey	47,659	772	48,431
Illinois	32,314	281	32,595
Pennsylvania	31,619	358	31,977
Georgia	30,179	226	30,405
Maryland	28,804	312	29,116
Puerto Rico	28,693	399	29,092

Persons Living with AIDS

In 2005, the estimated number of persons living with AIDS in the United States and dependent areas was 437,982. In the 50 states and District of Columbia, this included 422,143 adults and adolescents, and 3,764 children under age 13.[1,2]

Deaths of Persons with AIDS

In 2005, the estimated number of deaths of persons with AIDS in the United States and dependent areas was 17,011. In the 50 states and District of Columbia, this included 16,316 adults and adolescents, and seven children under age 13.

The cumulative estimated number of deaths of persons with AIDS in the United States and dependent areas, through 2005, was 550,394. In the 50 states and District of Columbia, this included 525,442 adults and adolescents, and 4,865 children under age 13.[1]

HIV/AIDS Cases

In 2005, the estimated number of cases of HIV/AIDS in the 33 states and four dependent areas with confidential name-based HIV infection reporting was 38,133. Of these, 38,096 were in the 33 states and 37 were in the four dependent areas. In the 33 states, adult and adolescent HIV/ AIDS cases totaled 37,930 with 28,037 cases in males and 9,893 cases in females, and 166 cases estimated in children under age 13.[1,2]

HIV/AIDS Cases by Age

Of the estimated number of HIV/AIDS cases in the 33 states with confidential name-based HIV infection reporting, person's age at time of diagnosis were distributed as follows.[2]

Under Age 13: 166
Ages 13–14: 43
Ages 15–19: 1,225
Ages 20–24: 3,904
Ages 25–29: 4,641

Ages 30–34: 5,207
Ages 35–39: 6,247
Ages 40–44: 6,201
Ages 45–49: 4,524

Ages 50–54: 2,879
Ages 55–59: 1,581
Ages 60–64: 799
Ages 65 or older: 679

HIV/AIDS Cases by Race/Ethnicity

CDC tracks HIV/AIDS information on five racial and ethnic groups: white, black (African American), Hispanic, Asian/Pacific Islander, and

American Indian/Alaska Native. The estimated numbers of diagnoses of HIV/AIDS in the 33 states with confidential name-based HIV infection reporting, by race or ethnicity are shown in Table 8.7.

Table 8.7. Distribution of HIV/AIDS cases by race/ethnicity.

Race or Ethnicity	Estimated Number of HIV/AIDS Cases in 2005
White, not Hispanic	11,758
Black, not Hispanic	18,510
Hispanic	6,944
Asian/Pacific Islander	429
American Indian/Alaska Native	198

Table 8.8. Estimated number of diagnoses of HIV/AIDS among adults and adolescents in 2005 by transmission category.

Transmission Category	Adult and Adolescent Male	Adult and Adolescent Female	Total
Male-to-male sexual contact	18,722	–	18,722
Injection Drug Use	3,506	1,879	5,385
Male-to-male sexual contact and injection drug use	1,336	–	1,336
High-risk heterosexual contact*	4,333	7,886	12,219
Other**	141	128	269

*Heterosexual contact with a person known to have, or to be at high risk for, HIV infection.

**Includes hemophilia, blood transfusion, perinatal, and risk not reported or not identified.

Table 8.9. Estimated number of HIV/AIDS cases among children in 2005 by transmission category.

Transmission Category	Estimated Number of HIV/AIDS Cases in 2005
Perinatal	141
Other (includes hemophilia, blood transfusion, and risk not reported or not identified.)	26

HIV/AIDS Cases by Transmission Category

Six common transmission categories are male-to-male sexual contact, injection drug use, male-to-male sexual contact and injection drug use, heterosexual (male-female) contact, mother-to-child (perinatal) transmission, and other (includes blood transfusions and unknown cause).

Following is the distribution of the estimated number of diagnoses of HIV/AIDS among adults and adolescents in the 33 states with confidential name-based HIV infection reporting, by transmission category. A breakdown by sex is provided where appropriate.

The distribution of the estimated number of diagnoses of HIV/AIDS, among children in the 33 states with confidential name-based HIV infection reporting, by transmission categories is shown in Table 8.9.

Persons Living with HIV/AIDS

In 2005, the estimated number of persons living with HIV/AIDS in the 33 states and dependent areas with confidential name-based HIV/AIDS infection reporting was 476,749. In the 33 states only, this included 469,298 adults and adolescents, and 6,792 children under age 13.[1,2]

State-by-State HIV/AIDS Data

Statehealthfacts.org provides state-by-state information about new and cumulative AIDS cases, AIDS case rates, persons living with AIDS, AIDS deaths, HIV infections, HIV testing statistics and policies, additional AIDS-related state policies, Ryan White funding and funding for HIV prevention, and AIDS Drug Assistance Programs, including budget, client, and expenditure data from the Kaiser Family Foundation.

International Statistics

For the most up-to-date information in international HIV and AIDS statistics, visit the Joint United Nations Programme on HIV/AIDS online at http://www.unaids.org.

For current statistics on the number of reported AIDS cases in North, Central, and South America, please contact the Pan American Health Organization (PAHO) which is the regional office for the Americas of the World Health Organization, online at http://www.paho.org.

A Glance at the HIV/AIDS Epidemic

HIV/AIDS Diagnoses

At the end of 2003, an estimated 1,039,000 to 1,185,000 persons in the United States were living with HIV/AIDS.[3] (The term *HIV/AIDS* refers to three categories of diagnoses collectively: (1) a diagnosis of HIV infection (not AIDS), (2) a diagnosis of HIV infection with a later diagnosis of AIDS, and (3) concurrent diagnoses of HIV infection and AIDS.) In 2005, 38,096 cases of HIV/AIDS in adults, adolescents, and children were diagnosed in the 33 states with long-term, confidential name-based HIV reporting.[4] CDC has estimated that approximately 40,000 persons in the United States become infected with HIV each year.[5]

By Transmission Category

In 2005, the largest estimated proportion of HIV/AIDS diagnoses were for men who have sex with men (MSM), followed by adults and adolescents infected through heterosexual contact.

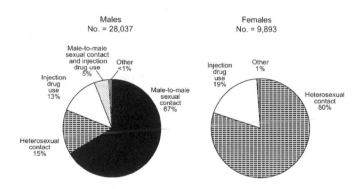

Figure 8.1. *Transmission categories of adults and adolescents with HIV/AIDS diagnosed during 2005 (based on data from 33 states with long-term, confidential name-based HIV reporting).*

By Sex

In 2005, almost three-quarters of HIV/AIDS diagnoses were for male adolescents and adults.

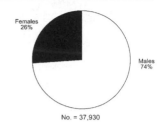

Figure 8.2. *Sex of adults and adolescents with HIV/AIDS diagnosed during 2005 (based on data from 33 states with long-term, confidential name-based HIV reporting).*

By Race/Ethnicity

In 2005, African Americans, who make up approximately 12 percent of the U.S. population, accounted for almost half of the estimated number of HIV/AIDS cases diagnosed.

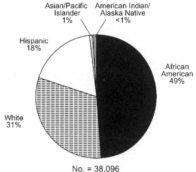

Figure 8.3. *Race/ethnicity of persons (including children) with HIV/AIDS diagnosed during 2005 (based on data from 33 states with long-term, confidential name-based HIV reporting).*

Trends in AIDS Diagnoses and Deaths

During the mid- to late-1990s, advances in treatment slowed the progression of HIV infection to AIDS and led to dramatic decreases in deaths among persons with AIDS. The decrease in the estimated number of deaths of persons with AIDS continued, but the number of AIDS cases diagnosed during that same period increased.[2] The reasons for the increase in the number of AIDS diagnoses are unclear but may be due to increased emphasis on testing; the fact that more people are living with HIV and thus are experiencing the development of AIDS; and technical issues in the statistical process used in estimating the number of AIDS diagnoses.

Better treatments have also led to an increase in the number of persons in the United States who are living with AIDS. From 2001 through 2005, the estimated number of persons in the United States living with AIDS increased from 331,512 to 425,910—an increase of 28 percent.[2]

Table 8.10. Estimated numbers of AIDS diagnoses, deaths, and persons living with AIDS, 2001–2005.

	2001	2002	2003	2004	2005	Cumulative (1981-2005)
AIDS diagnoses	38,016	38,513	39,728	39,775	44,198	956,666
Deaths of persons with AIDS	16,980	16,641	17,404	17,453	16,316	530,756
Persons living with AIDS	331,512	353,384	375,707	398,029	425,910	NA*

*not applicable, the values given for each year are cumulative

Notes

1. Totals include persons of unknown race or multiple races, persons of unknown sex, and persons of unknown state of residence. Because totals were calculated independently of the values for the subpopulations, subpopulation values may not equal the totals.

2. These numbers do not represent reported case counts. Rather, these numbers are point estimates, which result from adjustments of reported case counts. The reported case counts have been adjusted for reporting delays and for redistribution of cases in persons initially reported without an identified risk factor, but not for incomplete reporting.

3. Glynn M, Rhodes P. Estimated HIV prevalence in the United States at the end of 2003. National HIV Prevention Conference; June 2005; Atlanta. Abstract T1-B1101. Available at http://www.aegis.com/conferences/NHIVPC/2005/T1-B1101.html. Accessed January 11, 2007.

4. CDC. *HIV/AIDS Surveillance Report, 2005. Vol. 17.* Atlanta: U.S. Department of Health and Human Services, CDC; 2006: 1–46. Accessed January 11, 2007.

5. CDC. Guidelines for National Human Immunodeficiency Virus Case Surveillance, Including Monitoring for Human Immunodeficiency Virus Infection and Acquired Immunodeficiency Syndrome. *MMWR 1999*; 48 (RR-13): 1–28.

Chapter 9

HIV and AIDS:
Global Facts and Figures

- To date around 65 million people have been infected with HIV and AIDS has killed more than 25 million people since it was first recognized in 1981. The vast majority of the 38.6 million people living with HIV in 2005 are unaware of their status. AIDS is among the greatest development and security issues facing the world today.

- In 2005 AIDS claimed the lives of 2.8 million people and over 4 million people were newly infected with the virus.

- At around 17.3 million, women make up almost half of the total number of people living with the virus, 13.2 million of which live in sub-Saharan Africa (76 percent of all women living with HIV).

- Sub-Saharan Africa remains the most affected region in the world. Two-thirds of all people living with HIV are in sub-Saharan Africa where 24.5 million people were living with HIV in 2005.

- Growing epidemics are underway in eastern Europe and central Asia where 220,000 people were newly infected with HIV in 2005.

- Declines in HIV prevalence have been noted in Kenya, Zimbabwe, urban parts of Haiti and Burkina Faso, and four Indian states, including Tamil Nadu.

"Global Facts and Figures," reproduced with kind permission from UNAIDS, 2006. UNAIDS (Joint United Nations Programme on HIV/AIDS) can be found online at http://www.unaids.org.

Prevention

- There are more new HIV infections every year than AIDS-related deaths and as more people become infected with HIV, more people will die of AIDS-related illnesses.

- Worldwide, less than one in five people at risk of becoming infected with HIV has access to basic prevention services. Across the world, only one in eight people who want to be tested are currently able to do so.

- Each day, 1,500 children worldwide become infected with HIV, the vast majority of them newborns. In 2005, 9 percent of pregnant women in low- and middle-income countries were offered services to prevent transmission to their newborns.

- To get ahead of the epidemic, HIV prevention efforts must be scaled up and intensified, as part of a comprehensive response that simultaneously expands access to treatment and care.

- Scaling up available prevention strategies in 125 low- and middle-income countries would avert an estimated 28 million new infections between 2005 and 2015, more than half of those that are projected to occur during this period and would save $24 billion in associated treatment costs.

- Simultaneous scaling up of both prevention and treatment would avert 29 million new infections by the end of 2020.

Treatment

- According to the latest Joint United Nations Programme on HIV/AIDS (UNAIDS)/World Health Organization (WHO) '3 by 5' progress report, around 1.3 million people living with HIV are receiving anti-retroviral (ARV) therapy in low- and middle-income countries—this means that 20 percent of those in need of treatment are now receiving it.

- The number of people receiving antiretroviral treatment in low- and middle-income countries has tripled since the end of 2001.

Resource Needs

- In 2005, a total of $8.3 billion was estimated to be available for AIDS funding; this figure is estimated to rise to $8.9 billion in

Table 9.1. Regional statistics.

	People living with HIV	New infections 2005	AIDS deaths 2005	Adult prevalence percentage
Sub-Saharan Africa	24.5 million	2.7 million	2 million	6.1 percent
Asia	8.3 million	930,000	600,000	0.4 percent
Latin America	1.6 million	140,000	59,000	0.5 percent
North America and Western and Central Europe	2 million	65,000	30,000	0.5 percent
Eastern Europe and Central Asia	1.5 million	220,000	53,000	0.8 percent
Middle East and North Africa	440,000	64,000	37,000	0.2 percent
Caribbean	330,000	37,000	27,000	1.6 percent
Oceania	78,000	7,200	3,400	0.3 percent
Total	**38.6 million**	**4.1 million**	**2.8 million**	**1 percent**

Table 9.2. Treatment.

Geographical region	Estimated number of people receiving ARV therapy, December 2005	Estimated number of people needing ARV therapy, December 2005	ARV therapy coverage, December 2005
Sub-Saharan Africa	810,000	4,700,000	17 percent
Latin America and Caribbean	315,000	465,000	68 percent
East, South, and Southeast Asia	180,000	1,100,000	16 percent
Europe and Central Asia	21,000	160,000	13 percent
Middle East and North Africa	4,000	75,000	5 percent
Total	**1,330,000**	**6.5 million**	**20 percent**

Note: Some numbers do not add up due to rounding.

2006 and $10 billion in 2007. But it falls short of what is needed—$14.9 billion in 2006, $18.1 billion in 2007, and $22.1 billion in 2008.

- For treatment and care, about 55 percent of these resources will be needed in Africa, 20 percent in Asia and the Pacific, 17 percent in Latin America and the Caribbean, 7 percent in Eastern Europe, and 1 percent in North Africa and the Near East.

Table 9.3. AIDS resource needs (US$ billion).

	2006	2007	2008	Totals for 2006–2008
Prevention	8.4	10.0	11.4	29.8
Treatment and care	3.0	4.0	5.3	12.3
Orphans and vulnerable children	1.6	2.1	2.7	6.4
Program costs	1.5	1.4	1.8	4.6
Human resources	0.4	0.6	0.9	1.9
Total	**14.9**	**18.1**	**22.1**	**55.1**

Chapter 10

Genetic Factors
Influence HIV Infection Risk

People with more copies of a gene that helps to fight HIV are less likely to become infected with the virus or to develop AIDS than those of the same geographical ancestry, such as European Americans, who have fewer copies of the gene, according to a study funded by the National Institute of Allergy and Infectious Diseases (NIAID), part of the National Institutes of Health (NIH). The findings help to explain why some people are more prone to HIV/AIDS than others.

Scientists believe that this discovery could lead to a screening test that identifies people who have a higher or lower susceptibility to HIV/AIDS, potentially enabling clinicians to adapt treatment regimens, vaccine trials, and other studies accordingly. The research appears January 6, [2005], in *Science Express*, an online publication of the journal *Science*.

"Individual risk of acquiring HIV and experiencing rapid disease progression is not uniform within populations," says Anthony S. Fauci, MD, director of NIAID. "This important study identifies genetic factors of particular groups that either mitigate or enhance one's susceptibility to infection and disease onset. In a broader sense, it also suggests how the immune systems of individuals with different geographical ancestries might have evolved in response to microbial stresses and how

"Scientists Discover Key Genetic Factor in Determining HIV/AIDS Risk," National Institute of Allergy and Infectious Disease (http://www.niaid.nih.gov), a component of the National Institutes of Health (http://www.nih.gov), January 6, 2005.

these differences in the immune system might result in medical approaches to thwart HIV/AIDS or other infections that vary among groups."

The study focused on the gene that encodes *CCL3L1,* a potent HIV-blocking protein that interacts with *CCR5*—a major receptor protein that HIV uses as a doorway to enter and infect cells. The senior authors are Sunil K. Ahuja, MD, of the University of Texas Health Science Center and the Veterans Administration Center for AIDS and HIV-1 Infection in San Antonio, and Matthew J. Dolan, MD, of the U.S. Air Force's Wilford Hall Medical Center and Brooks City-Base in San Antonio.

The researchers analyzed blood samples from more than 4,300 HIV-positive and HIV-negative people of different ancestral origins to determine the average number of *CCL3L1* gene copies in each group. They found that, for example, HIV-negative African American adults had an average of four *CCL3L1* copies, while HIV-negative European and Hispanic American adults averaged two and three copies, respectively.

This does not mean that European Americans are more prone to HIV/AIDS than other populations. Rather, using the average *CCL3L1* gene copy number as a reference point for each group, the authors found that individuals with fewer *CCL3L1* copies than their population's average were more susceptible to HIV infection and rapid progression to AIDS. People with greater-than-average *CCL3L1* gene copies, in contrast, were less prone to infection by HIV or to rapid progression to AIDS.

Depending on the study population, each additional *CCL3L1* copy lowered the risk of acquiring HIV by between 4.5 and 10.5 percent. Additionally, below-average *CCL3L1* copy numbers were associated with a 39 to 260 percent higher risk of rapid progression to AIDS.

To further test the impact of *CCL3L1* copies on HIV/AIDS risk, the researchers then studied variations in the *CCR5* gene that they had previously linked to varying rates of AIDS progression. They found that individuals who possessed a low *CCL3L1* copy number along with disease-accelerating *CCR5* variants had an even higher risk of HIV acquisition and rate of progression to AIDS.

"This work adds significantly to our understanding of the central role that molecules that interact with the *CCR5* co-receptor play in influencing susceptibility to HIV/AIDS," says Carl W. Dieffenbach, PhD, who oversees basic research at NIAID's Division of AIDS. "In addition, by examining the duplication of a specific gene, this study further emphasizes the significance of defining all existing types of genetic variation and the impact that these variations may have on human susceptibility to infectious diseases."

The study is the result of collaboration between NIAID-supported researchers and investigators from the U.S. Military's Tri-Service AIDS Clinical Consortium. "This partnership highlights the importance of inter- and multi-disciplinary research teams in clinical genomic research, a theme heavily emphasized in the NIH Roadmap," says NIAID's Dr. Dieffenbach.

The research also received support from the National Institute of Mental Health, another NIH component; the Veterans Administration Center for AIDS and HIV-1 Infection; the Elizabeth Glaser Pediatric AIDS Foundation; and the Burroughs Wellcome Fund.

NIAID is a component of the National Institutes of Health, an agency of the U.S. Department of Health and Human Services. NIAID supports basic and applied research to prevent, diagnose and treat infectious diseases such as HIV/AIDS and other sexually transmitted infections, influenza, tuberculosis, malaria and illness from potential agents of bioterrorism. NIAID also supports research on transplantation and immune-related illnesses, including autoimmune disorders, asthma and allergies. News releases, fact sheets and other NIAID-related materials are available on the NIAID website at http://www3.niaid.nih.gov.

Reference

Gonzalez, E, et al. The influence of *CCL3L1* gene-containing segmental duplications on HIV-1/AIDS susceptibility. *Science* DOI: 10.1126/science.1101160.

Chapter 11

HIV/AIDS among Youth

Young people in the United States are at persistent risk for HIV infection. This risk is especially notable for youth of minority races and ethnicities. Continual HIV prevention, outreach, and education efforts, including programs on abstinence and on delaying the initiation of sex, are required as new generations replace the generations that benefited from earlier prevention strategies. Unless otherwise noted, this chapter defines youth, or young people, as persons who are 13–24 years of age.

Statistics

HIV/AIDS in 2004

The following are based on data from the 35 areas with long-term, confidential name-based HIV reporting.

- An estimated 4,883 young people received a diagnosis of HIV infection or AIDS, representing about 13 percent of the persons given a diagnosis during that year.

- HIV infection progressed to AIDS more slowly among young people than among all persons with a diagnosis of HIV infection. The following are the proportions of persons in whom HIV

From "HIV/AIDS among Youth," Centers for Disease Control and Prevention (CDC), June 2006. The complete text of this document, including references, is available online at http://www.cdc.gov/hiv/resources/factsheets/youth.htm.

infection did not progress to AIDS within 12 months after diagnosis of HIV infection:

- 81 percent of persons aged 15–24
- 70 percent of persons aged 13–14
- 61 percent of all persons

- African Americans were disproportionately affected by HIV infection, accounting for 55 percent of all HIV infections reported among persons aged 13–24.

- Young men who have sex with men (MSM), especially those of minority races or ethnicities, were at high risk for HIV infection. In the seven cities that participated in CDC's Young Men's Survey during 1994–1998, 14 percent of African American MSM and 7 percent of Hispanic MSM aged 15–22 were infected with HIV.

- During 2001–2004, in the 33 states with long-term, confidential name-based HIV reporting, 62 percent of the 17,824 persons 13–24 years of age given a diagnosis of HIV/AIDS were males, and 38 percent were females.

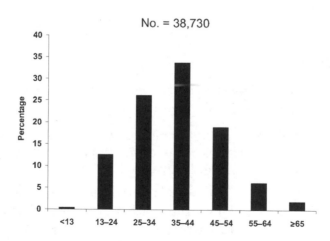

Figure 11.1. *Age of persons with HIV infection or AIDS diagnosed during 2004 (based on data from 35 areas with long-term, confidential name-based HIV reporting).*

- An estimated 2,174 young people received a diagnosis of AIDS (5.1 percent of the estimated total of 42,514 AIDS diagnoses), and 232 young people with AIDS died.

- An estimated 7,761 young people were living with AIDS, a 42 percent increase since 2000, when 5,457 young people were living with AIDS.

- Young people for whom AIDS was diagnosed during 1996–2004 lived longer than persons with AIDS in any other age group except those younger than 13 years. Nine years after receiving a diagnosis of AIDS, 76 percent of those aged 13–24 were alive, compared with the following age groups:

  - 81 percent of those younger than age 13
  - 74 percent of those aged 25–34
  - 70 percent of those aged 35–44
  - 63 percent of those aged 45–54
  - 53 percent of those aged 55 and older

- Since the beginning of the epidemic, an estimated 40,059 young people in the United States had received a diagnosis of AIDS, and an estimated 10,129 young people with AIDS had died. They accounted for about 4 percent of the estimated total of 944,306 AIDS diagnoses and 2 percent of the 529,113 deaths of people with AIDS.

Risk Factors and Barriers to Prevention

Sexual Risk Factors

Early age at sexual initiation: According to the Centers for Disease Control (CDC)'s Youth Risk Behavioral Survey (YRBS), many young people begin having sexual intercourse at early ages: 47 percent of high school students have had sexual intercourse, and 7.4 percent of them reported first sexual intercourse before age 13. HIV/AIDS education needs to take place at correspondingly young ages, before young people engage in sexual behaviors that put them at risk for HIV infection.

Heterosexual transmission: Young women, especially those of minority races or ethnicities, are increasingly at risk for HIV infection

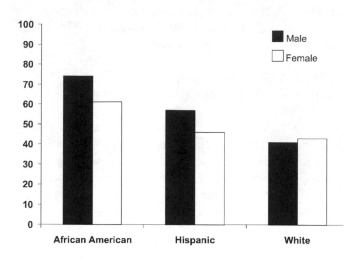

Figure 11.2. High school students reporting ever having had sexual intercourse, 2003 (Source: CDC's Youth Risk Behavioral Survey, 2003).

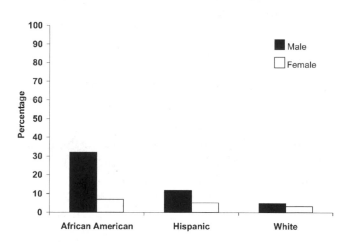

Figure 11.3. High school students reporting sexual intercourse for the first time before age 13, 2003 (Source: CDC's Youth Risk Behavioral Survey, 2003).

through heterosexual contact. According to data from a CDC study of HIV prevalence among disadvantaged youth during the early to mid-1990s, the rate of HIV prevalence among young women aged 16–21 was 50 percent higher than the rate among young men in that age group. African American women in this study were seven times as likely as white women and eight times as likely as Hispanic women to be HIV positive. Young women are at risk for sexually transmitted HIV for several reasons, including biologic vulnerability, lack of recognition of their partners' risk factors, inequality in relationships, and having sex with older men who are more likely to be infected with HIV.

MSM: Young MSM are at high risk for HIV infection, but their risk factors and the prevention barriers they face differ from those of persons who become infected through heterosexual contact. According to a CDC study of 5,589 MSM, 55 percent of young men (aged 15–22) did not let other people know they were sexually attracted to men. MSM who do not disclose their sexual orientation are less likely to seek HIV testing, so if they become infected, they are less likely to know it. Further, because MSM who do not disclose their sexual orientation are likely to have one or more female sex partners, MSM who become infected may transmit the virus to women as well as to men. In a small study of African American MSM college students and nonstudents in North Carolina, the participants had sexual risk factors for HIV infection, and 20 percent had a female sex partner during the preceding 12 months.

Sexually transmitted diseases (STDs): The presence of an STD greatly increases a person's likelihood of acquiring or transmitting HIV. Some of the highest STD rates in the country are those among young people, especially young people of minority races and ethnicities.

Substance Abuse

Young people in the United States use alcohol, tobacco, and other drugs at high rates. Both casual and chronic substance users are more likely to engage in high-risk behaviors, such as unprotected sex, when they are under the influence of drugs or alcohol. Runaways and other homeless young people are at high risk for HIV infection if they are exchanging sex for drugs or money.

Lack of Awareness

Research has shown that a large proportion of young people are not concerned about becoming infected with HIV. Adolescents need accurate, age-appropriate information about HIV infection and AIDS, including how to talk with their parents or other trusted adults about HIV and AIDS, how to reduce or eliminate risk factors, how to talk with a potential partner about risk factors, where to get tested for HIV, how to use a condom correctly. Information should also include the concept that abstinence is the only 100 percent effective way to avoid infection.

Poverty and Out-of-School Youth

Nearly one in four African Americans and one in five Hispanics live in poverty. The socioeconomic problems associated with poverty, including lack of access to high-quality health care, can directly or indirectly increase the risk for HIV infection. Young people who have dropped out of school are more likely to become sexually active at younger ages and to fail to use contraception.

The Coming of Age of HIV-Positive Children

Many young people who contracted HIV through perinatal transmission are facing decisions about becoming sexually active. They will require ongoing counseling and prevention education to ensure that they do not transmit HIV.

Prevention

In the United States, the annual number of new HIV infections has declined from a peak of more than 150,000 in the mid-1980s and has stabilized since the late 1990s at approximately 40,000. Populations of minority races or ethnicities are disproportionately affected by the HIV epidemic. To reduce further the incidence of HIV, CDC announced a new initiative, Advancing HIV Prevention, in 2003. This initiative comprises four strategies: making HIV testing a routine part of medical care, implementing new models for diagnosing HIV infections outside medical settings, preventing new infections by working with HIV-infected persons and their partners, and further decreasing perinatal HIV transmission.

Through the Minority AIDS Initiative, CDC explores ways to reduce health disparities in communities made up of persons of minority races or ethnicities who are at high risk for HIV. These funds are used to address the high-priority HIV prevention needs in such communities.

CDC provides nine awards to community-based organizations (CBOs) that focus primarily on youth and provides indirect funding through state, territorial, and local health departments to organizations serving youth. Of these nine awards, five are focused on African Americans, three on Hispanics, one on Asians and Pacific Islanders, and one on whites. The following are some CDC-tested prevention programs that state and local health departments and CBOs can provide for youth.

- Teens Linked to Care is focused on young people aged 13–29 who are living with HIV.

- Street Smart is an HIV/AIDS and STD prevention program for runaway and homeless youth.

- PROMISE (Peers Reaching Out and Modeling Intervention Strategies for HIV/AIDS Risk Reduction in their Community) is a community-level HIV prevention intervention that relies on role-model stories and peers from the community.

- Adult Identity Mentoring project, which encourages students to articulate personal goals and then teaches them the skills required to achieve those goals, can be effective in helping at-risk youth delay the initiation of sex.

CDC research has shown that early, clear parent-child communication regarding values and expectations about sex is an important step in helping adolescents delay sexual initiation and make responsible decisions about sexual behaviors later in life. Parents are in a unique position to engage their children in conversations about HIV, STD, and teen pregnancy prevention because the conversations can be ongoing and timely.

Schools also can be important partners for reaching youth before high-risk behaviors are established, as evidenced by the YRBS finding that 88 percent of high school students in the United States reported having been taught about AIDS or HIV infection in school.

Overall, a multifaceted approach to HIV/AIDS prevention, which includes individual, peer, familial, school, church, and community programs, is necessary to reduce the incidence of HIV/AIDS in young people. For *Guidelines for Effective School Health Education to Prevent the Spread of AIDS,* visit http://www.cdc.gov/HealthyYouth/ sexualbehaviors/guidelines/guidelines.htm.

Chapter 12

HIV/AIDS among Women

Early in the epidemic, HIV infection and AIDS were diagnosed for relatively few women and female adolescents (although we know now that many women were infected with HIV through injection drug use but that their infections were not diagnosed). Today, women account for more than one-quarter of all new HIV/AIDS diagnoses. Women of color are especially affected by HIV infection and AIDS. In 2004 (the most recent year for which data are available), HIV infection was:

- the leading cause of death for black women aged 25–34 years.
- the third leading cause of death for black women aged 35–44 years.
- the fourth leading cause of death for black women aged 45–54 years.
- the fourth leading cause of death for Hispanic women aged 35–44 years.

In the same year, HIV infection was the fifth leading cause of death among all women aged 35–44 years and the sixth leading cause of death among all women aged 25–34 years. The only diseases causing more deaths of women were cancer and heart disease.

Centers for Disease Control and Prevention (CDC), reviewed/modified March 20, 2007. References and examples of prevention programs are available online at http://www.cdc.gov/hiv/topics/women/resources/factsheets/women.htm.

Statistics

HIV/AIDS in 2005

The following bullets, except for the last one, are based on data from 33 states with long-term, confidential name-based HIV reporting.

- HIV/AIDS was diagnosed for an estimated 9,893 women.

- High-risk heterosexual contact was the source of 80 percent of these newly diagnosed infections.

- Women accounted for 26 percent of the estimated 37,930 diagnoses for adults and adolescents.

- Of the 127,150 women living with HIV/AIDS, 64 percent were black, 19 percent were white, 15 percent were Hispanic, 1 percent were Asian or Pacific Islander, and less than 1 percent were American Indian or Alaska Native.

- The number of reported cases of HIV/AIDS in female adults or adolescents decreased from 11,934 in 2001 to 9,893 in 2005.

- According to a recent Centers for Disease Control and Prevention (CDC) study of more than 19,500 patients with HIV in ten U.S. cities, women were slightly less likely than men to receive prescriptions for the most effective treatments for HIV infection.

AIDS in 2005

- Of 44,198 AIDS diagnoses in the 50 states and the District of Columbia, 11,710 (26 percent) were for women.

- The rate of AIDS diagnosis for black women (49.9/100,000 women) was approximately 24 times the rate for white women (2.1/100,000) and 4 times the rate for Hispanic women (12.2/100,000).

- An estimated 96,978 women were living with AIDS, representing 23 percent of the estimated 425,910 people living with AIDS in the 50 states and the District of Columbia.

- An estimated 4,128 women with AIDS died, representing 25 percent of the 16,316 persons with AIDS who died in the 50 states and the District of Columbia.

- From the beginning of the epidemic (1981) through 2005, women accounted for 182,822 diagnoses, a number that represents 19 percent of the 956,666 AIDS diagnoses in the 50 states and the District of Columbia during this period.

- From the beginning of the epidemic through 2005, an estimated 85,844 women with AIDS died, accounting for 16 percent of the 530,756 persons with AIDS who died in the 50 states and the District of Columbia.

- Women with AIDS made up an increasing part of the epidemic. In 1992, women accounted for an estimated 14 percent of adults and adolescents living with AIDS in the 50 states and the District of Columbia. By the end of 2005, this proportion had grown to 23 percent.

- Data from the 2005 census show that together, black and Hispanic women represent 24 percent of all U.S. women. However, women in these two groups accounted for 82 percent (9,641/11,710) of the estimated total of AIDS diagnoses for women in 2005.

Risk Factors and Barriers to Prevention

Younger Age

For women of all races and ethnicities, the largest number of HIV/AIDS diagnoses during recent years was for women aged 15–39. From 2001 through 2005, the number of HIV/AIDS diagnoses for women aged 15–39 decreased for white, black, and Hispanic women. There was an increase in the number of HIV/AIDS diagnoses during this period for Asian and Pacific Islander women and for American Indian and Alaska Native women aged 15–39.

Lack of Recognition of Partner's Risk Factors

Some women may be unaware of their male partner's risk factors for HIV infection (such as unprotected sex with multiple partners, sex with men, or injection drug use). Men who engage in sex both with men and women can acquire HIV from a male partner and then transmit the virus to female partners. In a 2003 report of a study of HIV-infected people (5,156 men and 3,139 women), 34 percent of black men who have sex with men (MSM), 26 percent of Hispanic MSM, and 13 percent of white MSM reported having had sex with women. However, their female partners may not have known of their male partner's bisexual activity: only 14 percent of white women, 6 percent of black women, and 6 percent of Hispanic women in this study acknowledged having a bisexual partner. In another CDC survey, 65 percent of the young men who had ever had sex with men also reported sex with women. Women who have sex only with women and who have no other risk factors, such as injection drug use, are at very low risk for HIV infection (CDC, unpublished data, 2006).

High-Risk Heterosexual Risk Factors

Most women are infected with HIV through high-risk heterosexual contact. Black and Hispanic women account for over 80 percent of the reported heterosexually acquired cases of HIV/AIDS. Lack of HIV knowledge, lower perception of risk, drug or alcohol use, and different interpretations of safer sex may contribute to this disproportion. Relationship dynamics also play a role. For example, some women may not insist on condom use because they fear that their partner will physically abuse them or leave them. Such sexual inequality is a major issue in relationships between young women and older men. In a CDC study of urban high schools, more than one-third of black and Hispanic women had their first sexual encounter with a male who was older (three or more years). These young women, compared with peers whose partners had been approximately their own age, had been younger at first sexual intercourse, less likely to have used a condom during first and most recently reported intercourse, or less likely to have used condoms consistently.

Biologic Vulnerability and Sexually Transmitted Diseases

A woman is significantly more likely than a man to contract HIV infection during vaginal intercourse. Additionally, the presence of some sexually transmitted diseases greatly increases the likelihood of acquiring or transmitting HIV infection. The rates of gonorrhea and syphilis are higher among women of color than among white women. These higher rates are especially marked at younger ages (15–24 years).

Substance Use

An estimated one in five new HIV diagnoses for women are related to injection drug use. Sharing injection equipment contaminated with HIV is not the only risk associated with substance use. Women who use crack cocaine or other noninjection drugs may also be at high risk for the sexual transmission of HIV if they sell or trade sex for drugs. Also, both casual and chronic substance users are more likely to engage in high-risk behaviors, such as unprotected sex, when they are under the influence of drugs or alcohol.

Socioeconomic Issues

Nearly one in four blacks and one in five Hispanics live in poverty.

Socioeconomic problems associated with poverty, including limited access to high-quality health care; the exchange of sex for drugs, money, or to meet other needs; and higher levels of substance use can directly or indirectly increase HIV risk factors. A study of HIV transmission among black women in North Carolina found that women with a diagnosis of HIV infection were significantly more likely than women who were not infected to be unemployed; to have had more sex partners; to use crack/cocaine; to exchange sex for money, shelter, or drugs; or to receive public assistance.

Racial/Ethnic Differences

The rates of HIV diagnosis and the risk factors for HIV infection differ for women of various races or ethnicities—a situation that must be considered when creating prevention programs. For example, even though the annual estimated rate of HIV diagnosis for black women decreased significantly—from 82.7 in 2001 to 61.4 in 2005—it remained 20 times the rate for white women. Overall, the rates of HIV diagnosis are much higher for black and Hispanic women than for white, Asian and Pacific Islander, or American Indian and Alaska Native women. The rates for black women are higher than the rates for all men except for black men.

Multiple Risk Factors

Some women infected with HIV report more than one risk factor, highlighting the overlap in risk factors such as inequality in relationships, socioeconomic stresses, substance abuse, and psychological issues. For example, in the North Carolina study of HIV infection in black women, the participants most commonly reported that that their reasons for risky behavior were financial dependence on male partners, feeling invincible, low self-esteem coupled with the need to feel loved by a male figure, and alcohol and drug use.

Prevention

In the United States, the annual number of new HIV infections has declined from a peak of more than 150,000 cases during the mid-1980s and has stabilized since the late 1990s at approximately 40,000. Populations of minority races/ethnicities are disproportionately affected by the HIV epidemic. To further reduce the incidence of HIV infection, CDC announced a new initiative, Advancing HIV Prevention, in 2003. This initiative comprises four strategies: making HIV testing a routine part of medical care, implementing new models for diagnosing HIV infections outside medical settings, preventing new infections by working with HIV-infected persons and their partners, and further decreasing perinatal HIV transmission.

In the United States, women, particularly women of color, are at risk for HIV infection. CDC, through the Department of Health and Human Services Minority AIDS Initiative, explores ways to reduce disparities in communities made up of persons of minority races/ethnicities who are at high risk for HIV infection. CDC is also conducting demonstration projects in which women's social networks are used to reach high-risk persons in communities of color; CDC is also conducting outreach and testing for partners of HIV-infected men. Additionally, CDC recognizes the importance of further incorporating culture- and gender-relevant material into current interventions.

CDC funds prevention programs in state and local health departments and community-based organizations.

CDC also funds research on interventions to reduce HIV-related risk behaviors or their outcomes.

CDC is actively involved in the promising area of microbicides—creams or gels that can be applied vaginally before sexual contact to prevent HIV transmission. The development of a safe, easy-to-use microbicide would be a milestone in the worldwide fight against HIV/AIDS. CDC is supporting the search for an effective microbicide agent through several lines of research:

- conducting laboratory and animal studies that can help evaluate the safety and the efficacy of microbicides before they are studied in humans

- supporting clinical trials to assess the safety of microbicides in humans in the United States, Asia, and Africa (Current human clinical studies include a Phase I safety trial of UC-781, which is being conducted among women in the United States and Thailand.)

To reduce mother-to-child HIV transmission in the United States, CDC has distributed approximately $10 million annually since 1999 to several national organizations and a number of states with high HIV/AIDS rates. These funds support perinatal HIV prevention programs, enhanced surveillance for HIV-infected mothers and babies, education, and capacity building among health care providers and public health practitioners.

94

Chapter 13

HIV, AIDS, and Older People

What is HIV? What is AIDS?

Like most people, you probably have heard a lot about HIV and AIDS. You may have thought that these diseases weren't your problem and that only younger people have to worry about them. But anyone at any age can get HIV/AIDS.

HIV (short for human immunodeficiency virus) is a virus that damages the immune system—the system your body uses to fight off diseases. HIV infection leads to a much more serious disease called AIDS (acquired immunodeficiency syndrome). When the HIV infection gets in your body, your immune system can weaken. This puts you in danger of getting other life-threatening diseases, infections, and cancers. When that happens, you have AIDS. AIDS is the last stage of HIV infection. If you think you may have HIV, it is very important to get tested. Today there are drugs that can help your body keep the HIV in check and fight against AIDS.

What are the symptoms of HIV/AIDS?

Many people have no symptoms when they first become infected with HIV. It can take as little as a few weeks for minor, flu-like symptoms to show up, or more than ten years for more serious symptoms to appear. Signs of HIV include headache, cough, diarrhea, swollen

"HIV, AIDS, and Older People," National Institute of Aging (http://www .niapublications.org), June 2004.

95

glands, lack of energy, loss of appetite and weight loss, fevers and sweats, repeated yeast infections, skin rashes, pelvic and abdominal cramps, sores in the mouth or on certain parts of the body, or short-term memory loss.

Getting Tested for HIV/AIDS

- It can take as long as three to six months after the infection for the virus to show up in your blood.

- Your health care provider can test your blood for HIV/AIDS. If you don't have a health care provider, check your local phone book for the phone number of a hospital or health center where you can get a list of test sites.

- Many health care providers who test for HIV also can provide counseling.

- In most states the tests are private, and you can choose to take the test without giving your name.

You can now also test your blood at home. The "Home Access Express HIV-1 Test System" is made by the Home Access Health Corporation. You can buy it at the drug store. It is the only HIV home test system approved by the Food and Drug Administration (FDA) and legally sold in the United States. Other HIV home test systems and kits you might see on the internet or in magazines or newspapers have not been approved by FDA and may not always give correct results.

How do people get HIV and AIDS?

Anyone, at any age, can get HIV and AIDS. HIV usually comes from having unprotected sex or sharing needles with an infected person, or through contact with HIV-infected blood. No matter your age, you may be at risk if the following apply to you:

- You are sexually active and do not use a latex or polyurethane condom. You can get HIV/AIDS from having sex with someone who has HIV. The virus passes from the infected person to his or her partner in blood, semen, and vaginal fluid. During sex, HIV can get into your body through any opening, such as a tear or cut in the lining of the vagina, vulva, penis, rectum, or mouth. Latex condoms can help prevent an infected person from transferring the HIV virus to you. (Natural condoms do not protect against HIV/AIDS as well as the latex and polyurethane types.)

- You do not know your partner's drug and sexual history. What you don't know can hurt you. Even though it may be hard to do, it's very important to ask your partner about his or her sexual history and drug use. Here are some questions to ask: Has your partner been tested for HIV/AIDS? Has he or she had a number of different sex partners? Has your partner ever had unprotected sex with someone who has shared needles? Has he or she injected drugs or shared needles with someone else? Drug users are not the only people who might share needles. For example, people with diabetes who inject insulin or draw blood to test glucose levels might share needles.

- You have had a blood transfusion or operation in a developing country at any time.

- You had a blood transfusion in the United States between 1978 and 1985.

Is HIV/AIDS different in older people?

A growing number of older people now have HIV/AIDS. About 19 percent of all people with HIV/AIDS in this country are age 50 and older. This is because doctors are finding HIV more often than ever before in older people, and because improved treatments are helping people with the disease live longer.

But there may even be many more cases than we know about. Why? One reason may be that doctors do not always test older people for HIV/AIDS and so may miss some cases during routine checkups. Another may be that older people often mistake signs of HIV/AIDS for the aches and pains of normal aging, so they are less likely than younger people to get tested for the disease. Also, they may be ashamed or afraid of being tested. People age 50 and older may have the virus for years before being tested. By the time they are diagnosed with HIV/AIDS, the virus may be in the late stages.

The number of HIV/AIDS cases among older people is growing every year because of the following factors:

- Older Americans know less about HIV/AIDS than younger people. They do not always know how it spreads or the importance of using condoms, not sharing needles, getting tested for HIV, and talking about it with their doctor.

- Health care workers and educators often do not talk with middle-age and older people about HIV/AIDS prevention.

97

- Older people are less likely than younger people to talk about their sex lives or drug use with their doctors.

- Doctors may not ask older patients about their sex lives or drug use, or talk to them about risky behaviors.

Facts about HIV/AIDS

You may have read or heard things that are not true about how you get HIV/AIDS. Here are the facts:

- You cannot get HIV through casual contact such as shaking hands or hugging a person with HIV/AIDS.

- You cannot get HIV from using a public telephone, drinking fountain, restroom, swimming pool, Jacuzzi, or hot tub.

- You cannot get HIV from sharing a drink.

- You cannot get HIV from being coughed or sneezed on by a person with HIV/AIDS.

- You cannot get HIV from giving blood.

- You cannot get HIV from a mosquito bite.

Anyone facing a serious disease like HIV/AIDS may become very depressed. This is a special problem for older people, who may have no strong network of friends or family who can help. At the same time, they also may be coping with other diseases common to aging such as high blood pressure, diabetes, or heart problems. As the HIV/AIDS gets worse, many will need help getting around and caring for themselves. Older people with HIV/AIDS need support and understanding from their doctors, family, and friends.

HIV/AIDS can affect older people in yet another way. Many younger people who are infected turn to their parents and grandparents for financial support and nursing care. Older people who are not themselves infected by the virus may find they have to care for their own children with HIV/AIDS and then sometimes for their orphaned or HIV-infected grandchildren. Taking care of others can be mentally, physically, and financially draining. This is especially true for older caregivers. The problem becomes even worse when older caregivers have AIDS or other serious health problems. Remember, it is important to get tested for HIV/AIDS early. Early treatment increases the chances of living longer.

Are cases of HIV/AIDS in people of color and women increasing?

The number of HIV/AIDS cases is rising in people of color across the country. About half of all people with HIV/AIDS are African American or Hispanic.

The number of cases of HIV/AIDS for women has also been growing over the past few years. The rise in the number of cases in women of color age 50 and older has been especially steep. Most got the virus from sex with infected partners. Many others got HIV through shared needles. Because women may live longer than men, and because of the rising divorce rate, many widowed, divorced, and separated women are dating these days. Like older men, many older women may be at risk because they do not know how HIV/AIDS is spread. Women who no longer worry about getting pregnant may be less likely to use a condom and to practice safe sex. Also, vaginal dryness and thinning often occurs as women age; when that happens, sexual activity can lead to small cuts and tears that raise the risk for HIV/AIDS.

What treatment and prevention options are available?

There is no cure for HIV/AIDS. But if you become infected, there are drugs that help keep the HIV virus in check and slow the spread of HIV in the body. Doctors are now using a combination of drugs called HAART (highly active antiretroviral therapy) to treat HIV/AIDS. Although it is not a cure, HAART is greatly reducing the number of deaths from AIDS in this country.

Prevention

Remember, there are things you can do to keep from getting HIV/AIDS. Practice the following steps to lower your risk:

- If you are having sex, make sure your partner has been tested and is free of HIV. Use male or female condoms (latex or polyurethane) during sexual intercourse.

- Do not share needles or any other equipment used to inject drugs.

- Get tested if you or your partner had a blood transfusion between 1978 and 1985.

- Get tested if you or your partner has had an operation or blood transfusion in a developing country at any time.

Chapter 14

Minorities and HIV/AIDS

Chapter Contents

Section 14.1

The Devastating Impact of HIV/AIDS on Minorities

This section contains text from "HIV/AIDS (Data and Statistics)," Office of Minority Health (http://www.omhrc.gov), U.S. Department of Health and Human Services, modified February 23, 2007; and "AIDS among Minorities," Office of Minority Health, modified December 29, 2006.

HIV/AIDS Data and Statistics

HIV/AIDS has had a devastating impact on minorities in the United States. Racial and ethnic minorities accounted for almost 68 percent of the newly diagnosed cases of HIV and AIDS in 2005. In 2005, 86 percent of babies born with HIV/AIDS belonged to minority groups.

In the African American community, HIV/AIDS has become an epidemic. African Americans accounted for 49 percent of all HIV/AIDS cases diagnosed in 2005. African American men are more than nine times more likely to die of AIDS than non-Hispanic white men. AIDS is the leading cause of death in African American women aged 25–34 and the third leading cause of death in African American men in the same age group.

HIV/AIDS is spreading at a rapid rate in the Hispanic community. Hispanics accounted for 18 percent of AIDS cases in 2005, despite making up only 14 percent of the U.S. population. Hispanics are 3.5 times more likely to be diagnosed with AIDS than non-Hispanic whites. Hispanic males were also almost three times more likely to die of AIDS than their non-Hispanic white counterparts in 2004.

Though the numbers are small, American Indians are also impacted disproportionately by HIV/AIDS. American Indians are 1.3 times more likely to have AIDS than non-Hispanic whites.

For Asians and Pacific Islanders, HIV/AIDS is the seventh leading cause of death in men aged 25 to 34 and the seventh leading cause of death for Asian/Pacific Islander women of the same age group.

Quick Facts

- African American males have more than eight times the AIDS rate as non-Hispanic white males.

- American Indian/Alaska Native women have twice the AIDS rate as non-Hispanic white women.

- One Asian/Pacific Islander child was diagnosed with AIDS in 2005.

- Hispanic females have more than five times the AIDS rate as non-Hispanic white females.

AIDS among Minorities

This year [2006] we reached a sad landmark: the 25th anniversary of the HIV/AIDS epidemic. On June 5, 1981, the U.S. Centers for Disease Control and Prevention (CDC) issued its first warning about a disease that would become known as AIDS. Twenty-five years later a new survey by the Kaiser Family Foundation finds that significant percentages of Americans still think HIV might be spread through kissing, sharing a drinking glass, and touching a toilet seat—37 percent, 22 percent, and 16 percent respectively.

Obviously, this is a renewed call for spreading information and for shouting from the rooftops: go get tested!

Nearly a decade ago, an AIDS diagnosis was a death sentence for anybody. Today, it doesn't have to be, but ethnic and racial minorities are still lagging behind on testing and treatment, therefore, they have disproportionately high morbidity and mortality rates.

Since the approval in 1995 of the first drug "cocktail" by the Food and Drug Administration for the treatment of HIV, deaths from AIDS have declined by more than 70 percent. However, minorities yet again have not shared equally on this decline, particularly in the last few years.

According to statistics from the CDC, the number of deaths among African Americans with AIDS declined by 7 percent between 2000 and 2004; compared to a 19 percent decline among whites over this period.

In the case of Latinos, the picture is mixed. Between 2000 and 2004, AIDS diagnoses among Latinos increased by 8.9 percent, compared to a 5.5 percent increase among whites. The number of estimated deaths among Latinos with AIDS increased by 16.9 percent between 2000 and 2003 compared to a 4.4 percent decline for whites. On a positive note, there was an 8.7 percent decrease in Latino deaths from 2003 to 2004.

"The problem is Latinos come late," said Dr. Octavio Vallejo, himself a long-term survivor of HIV. "Compared to other groups, we are lagging behind in receiving treatment for HIV for many reasons. But the reason number one is stigma." Dr. Vallejo is the HIV/AIDS trainer at the UCLA Center for Health Promotion and Disease Prevention and serves on the faculty of the UCLA/Pacific AIDS Education and Training Centers.

"Our people are afraid to be tested for HIV, in a great part because of the perception of the disease. There is a bit of fatalism: 'It was my fate; I'm going to die,' but they don't know that now nobody has to die from AIDS," said Dr. Vallejo.

Today there are an estimated 1.039 million to 1.185 million HIV-positive individuals living in the United States—the largest number ever according to the Centers for Disease Control and Prevention—and nearly 20 percent are Latino.

Of the overall number, between 252,000–315,000 people do not know they are infected, and thus are suffering from a lack of treatment, while at the same time, may be unknowingly spreading the virus.

"There is a lack of information, lack of health insurance; there is shame, and the strong homophobic sentiments in the Latino community, where many people still believe AIDS is a 'gay thing,'" said Dr. Vallejo, "And then, of course, the immigration issue. Many Latinos believe that they can't get treatment if they are not legal residents, or don't know that there are free clinics to treat people."

The assumed connection between HIV/AIDS and homosexuality, according to Dr. Vallejo, not only prevents people from getting tested, but also keeps alive the idea that heterosexual promiscuity is safe.

Dr. Vallejo used to work in Mexico in the treatment of HIV/AIDS, and he recalls the horror stories of the people he treated. "We had nothing to treat them with; they came pretty much to die in our hands."

He has continued to work in building bridges in HIV care between the U.S. and Mexico. In March 1994, he received a commendation letter from the White House for his work against AIDS in Mexico and the United States.

"What surprised me when I came was that I found here, among our Latino community, all the problems I saw in Mexico—the same lack of information, the same denial," recalls Dr. Vallejo.

Women's Passive Role Is Killing Them, Literally

"It would break my heart when I worked in Mexico and a woman, whose husband already died, came to the hospital with HIV and with children with the disease. First, she would not be treating herself, because whatever little money she had she used for her children. Second, she wouldn't even know how she got the virus," Dr. Vallejo said.

"If you told them, 'do you know your husband infected you?' they would swear that their husband could not have done that to them. That's still the situation for many here in our community. We have to empower them," he said.

According to Dr. Vallejo, the numbers show that Latino and African American women, who are in monogamous relationships, are bearing the burden of the new HIV infections.

"The chance of transmission from woman to man is lower, although possible. But the transmission from man to woman is twice as likely as is the transmission from man to man. Therefore, it's believed that the high rate of infection among heterosexual and married women is due in great part to their male partners having sex with other men," explained Dr. Vallejo.

Jay Blackwell, Director of the Capacity Development Team with the Office of Minority Health Resource Center (OMHRC), points out the huge impact drug use has in spreading the epidemics among women.

"Sometimes the impact of drug use, particularly in women of color, is overlooked," said Blackwell. "It's the number two cause of infections in heterosexual women. Often the mates of women are active drug users."

In fact, according to CDC, the primary mode of HIV transmission among African American women was heterosexual contact, followed by injection drug use.

CDC statistics also show that in 2002, 50 percent of the HIV/AIDS diagnoses among Latino men were due to sex with other men.

"Dr. Rafael Díaz did a study and found that the Latino gay population has the worst experiences of homophobia, so much so that around 67 percent report having adopted a heterosexual persona at least once in their lives. That's a recipe for HIV transmission," said Dr. Vallejo.

Dr. Vallejo comes across a fair amount of criticism for advocating informing women about the problem of homosexuality and bisexuality among men, because, some say, it risks bringing more blame and shame to the gay community.

"The real issue is that women sometimes don't know, and they need to know this is happening, so they can figure out how to stand up for themselves, and seek help," said Dr. Vallejo.

This is something close to Dr. Vallejo's heart because he says the great success story of the AIDS epidemic is the ability to prevent the transmission from mother to child; however, it still happens in the Latino and African American communities. Latinos account for over 20 percent of AIDS cases due to mother to child transmission, according to the CDC.

In fact, the survey from Kaiser Family Foundation shows that a majority of Americans does not know that a pregnant woman with HIV can take drugs to reduce the risk of her baby being infected (55 percent), or that having another sexually transmitted disease (STD) may increase a person's risk of getting HIV (56 percent).

"Many Latinas don't come to prenatal care because they are undocumented. Then, they don't even know they are HIV positive and don't get the preventive treatment that would avoid the transmission to the baby. The earlier the process begins the greater the success," said Dr. Vallejo.

According to Nelson Vergel in Houston, who has lived with HIV since 1983 in Houston and is a community educator and patient advocate, the problem of homophobia brings about the denial.

"Many Latinos learn they are HIV positive when they fall sick, but this makes no sense, because the retrovirals are there and everybody could have access to them. But Latinos don't get tested," said Vergel.

On the other hand, he is also sensitive to the issue of increasing infections in women, and he attributes that to a low use of condoms.

"Our women still see their men get insulted when the word *condom* is mentioned, but the men are not being faithful and are engaging in very risky behavior that endangers themselves and their partners," concluded Vergel.

—by Isabel M. Estrada Portales,
OMHRC Director of Communications

Section 14.2

HIV/AIDS Disproportionately Impacts Latinos

"Latinos and HIV/AIDS," (#6007-04), The Henry J. Kaiser Family Foundation, © December 2006. This information was reprinted with permission from The Henry J. Kaiser Family Foundation. The Kaiser Family Foundation, based in Menlo Park, California, is a nonprofit, private operating foundation focusing on the major health issues facing the nation and is not associated with Kaiser Permanente or Kaiser Industries.

Latinos in the United States continue to be affected by the HIV/AIDS epidemic, accounting for a greater proportion of AIDS cases than their representation in the U.S. population overall, and the second highest AIDS case rate in the nation, by race/ethnicity.[1] The epidemic has had a disproportionate impact on Latinas and young adults, and the impact of HIV/AIDS among Latinos varies across the country and by place of birth.[1,2] Moreover, studies have shown that Latinos with HIV/AIDS may face additional barriers to accessing care than their white counterparts.[3,4,5] Today, there are approximately 1.2 million

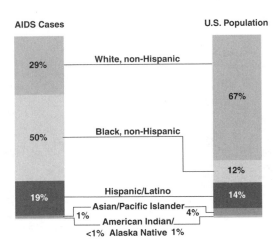

Figure 14.1. *Estimated AIDS diagnoses and U.S. population by race/ethnicity, 2005*[1,7,8]

people living with HIV/AIDS in the U.S., including about 200,000
Latinos.[6] As the largest and fastest growing ethnic minority group in
the U.S., addressing the impact of HIV/AIDS in the Latino community takes on increased importance in efforts to improve the nation's
health.

Snapshot of the Epidemic

- Although Latinos represent approximately 14 percent of the
  U.S. population,[8] they account for 19 percent of the AIDS cases
  diagnosed in 2005 and 16 percent of the AIDS cases diagnosed
  since the start of the epidemic (Figure 14.1).[1,7] Latinos account
  for 18 percent of HIV/AIDS cases diagnosed in 2005 in the 33
  states with confidential names-based reporting.[1,7]

- The AIDS case rate per 100,000 among Latino adults/adoles-
  cents was the second highest of any racial/ethnic group in the
  U.S. in 2005—3.5 times that of whites, but about one-third that
  of blacks (Figure 14.2).[1,9]

- HIV was the sixth leading cause of death for Latinos aged 25–
  34 in 2002, the same ranking as for whites. HIV was the third
  leading cause of death for blacks in this age group.[10] In 2003,
  HIV deaths rates per 100,000 population, aged 25–44, were
  higher among Latinos (10.3 for men and 3.8 for Latinas) compared to whites, although they were highest for blacks.[11]

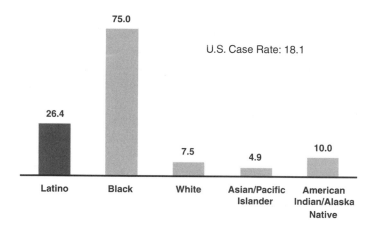

*Figure 14.2. AIDS case rate per 100,000 population by race/ethnicity for
adults/adolescents, 2005[1,9]*

Key Trends and Current Cases

- Latinos account for a growing share of AIDS diagnoses over time, rising from 15 percent in 1985 to 19 percent in 2005; in recent years, this share has remained relatively stable.[1,7,12]

- The number of Latinos living with AIDS has also increased over time, in part due to treatment advances but also to the epidemic's continued impact. Estimated AIDS prevalence among Latinos increased by 33 percent between 2001 and 2005, compared to a 21 percent increase among whites.[1]

- The number of deaths among Latinos with AIDS remained stable between 2001 and 2005, while both blacks and whites experienced slight decreases.[1]

Women and Young People

- Among women, Latinas account for 16 percent of new AIDS cases in 2005; black women account for 67 percent and white women account for 16 percent.[1,7,9]

- Latinas represent 22 percent of AIDS cases diagnosed among Latinos in 2005; by comparison, white women represent 14 percent of cases among whites, and black women represent 35 percent of cases diagnosed among blacks.[1,9]

- The AIDS case rate per 100,000 among Latinas (12.2) was nearly six times higher than the case rate for white women (2.1).[1,9]

- Latino teens, aged 13–19, accounted for 14 percent of AIDS cases among teens compared to 16 percent of all U.S. teens in 2004.[2]

- Latinos aged 20–24 accounted for 23 percent of new AIDS cases reported among young adults, but represented 18 percent of U.S. young adults, in 2004.[2]

Transmission

- HIV transmission patterns among Latino men vary from those of white men. Although both groups are most likely to be infected through sex with other men, white men are more likely to have been infected this way. Heterosexual transmission and injection drug use account for a greater share of infections among Latino men than white men.[1,13]

109

- Latinas are somewhat more likely to have been infected through heterosexual transmission than white women, although this is the most common transmission route for both groups and for women overall. White women are somewhat more likely to have been infected through injection drug use than Latinas.[1,13]

- Studies have found high HIV/AIDS prevalence among Latino men who have sex with men (MSM).[14] A study in five major U.S. cities found that 17 percent of Latino MSM in the study were infected with HIV. Prevalence among white MSM was 21 percent and among black MSM, 46 percent, the highest of any group.[15] Knowledge of HIV status among those already infected was also very low.[14]

Geography

Although AIDS cases among Latinos have been reported throughout the country, the impact of the epidemic is not uniformly distributed:

- AIDS case rates per 100,000 among Latinos are highest in the eastern part of the U.S., particularly in the Northeast.[16] The Northeast also has the greatest proportion of Latinos estimated to be living with AIDS (37 percent in 2005) and new AIDS cases among Latinos (33 percent).[16,17]

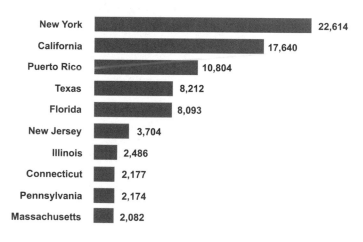

Figure 14.3. *Number of Latinos estimated to be living with AIDS: Top ten states/areas, 2005*[16]

- AIDS prevalence among Latinos is clustered in a handful of states, with ten states accounting for 89 percent of Latinos estimated to be living with AIDS in 2005. New York, California, and Puerto Rico top the list (Figure 14.3). Ten states also account for the majority of newly reported AIDS cases among Latinos (86 percent in 2005).[16,17]

- AIDS cases among Latinos vary by place of birth. Latinos born in the U.S. accounted for 41 percent of estimated AIDS cases among Latinos in 2005, followed by Latinos born in Puerto Rico (22 percent) and Mexico (22 percent).[1,18] HIV transmission patterns among Latinos also vary by place of birth.

Access to and Use of the Health Care System

The HIV Cost and Services Utilization Study (HCSUS), the only nationally representative study of people with HIV/AIDS receiving regular or ongoing medical care for HIV infection, found that Latinos fared more poorly on several important measures of access and quality, differences that diminished over time but were not completely eliminated.[3] In addition, HCSUS found that Latinos were more likely to report postponing medical care due to factors such as lack of transportation.[4] Latinos were also more likely than whites to delay care after an HIV diagnosis.[5]

Health Insurance

Having health insurance, either public or private, improves access to care. Insurance coverage of those with HIV/AIDS varies by race/ethnicity, as it does for the U.S. population overall.

- The HCSUS study found that Latinos with HIV/AIDS were more likely to be publicly insured or uninsured than their white counterparts, with half relying on Medicaid compared to 32 percent of whites. Approximately one-quarter of Latinos with HIV/AIDS (24 percent) were uninsured compared to 17 percent of whites. Latinos were also about half as likely to be privately insured as whites (23 percent compared to 44 percent).[19]

- Insurance status also varies at the time of HIV diagnosis. Analysis of data from 25 states between 1994 and 2000 found that Latinos were less likely than whites to have private coverage and more likely to be covered by Medicaid at the time of their HIV diagnosis. A third of Latinos were uninsured at the time of their diagnosis, higher than other groups.[20]

111

HIV Testing

- Among the U.S. population overall, Latinos are more likely than whites to report ever having ever been tested for HIV (54 percent compared to 45 percent). However, these self-reported testing rates may be overestimates, since 20 percent of Latinos assumed that the test was a routine part of an exam.[21]

- Among those who are HIV positive, CDC data indicate that more than one in four Latinos (43 percent) were tested for HIV late in their illness—that is, diagnosed with AIDS within one year of testing positive (in 33 areas with HIV reporting); by comparison, 40 percent of blacks and 37 percent of whites were tested late.[1]

Concern about HIV/AIDS[21]

- A recent survey found that Latinos express concern about HIV/AIDS. Nearly a quarter of Latinos named it as the most urgent health problem facing the nation, ranked second after cancer. More Latinos believe the U.S. is making progress on the domestic epidemic (39 percent) than losing ground (30 percent), as do whites; by contrast, black Americans are more likely to say the U.S. is losing ground.

- Almost half (46 percent) of Latinos say they think AIDS is a more urgent problem in their community than it was a few years ago compared to 15 percent of whites. Although 31 percent of Latinos say they are personally very concerned about becoming infected with HIV, this proportion has declined since the mid-1990s.

References

1. CDC, *HIV/AIDS Surveillance Report,* Volume 17; 2006.

2. CDC, *HIV/AIDS Surveillance in Adolescents and Young Adults* (through 2004).

3. Shapiro MF et al., "Variations in the Care of HIV-Infected Adults in the United States." *JAMA,* Volume 281, Number 24; 1999.

4. Cunningham WE et al., "The Impact of Competing Subsistence Needs and Barriers to Access to Medical Care for Persons with Human Immunodeficiency Virus Receiving Care in the United States." *Medical Care,* Volume 37, Number 12; 1999.

5. Turner BJ et al., "Delayed Medical Care after Diagnosis in a U.S. Probability Sample of Persons Infected with the Human Immunodeficiency Virus." *Archives of Internal Medicine,* Volume 160; 2000.

6. Kaiser Family Foundation calculations based on: Glynn MK and Rhodes P, "Estimated HIV Prevalence in the United States at the end of 2003." Presentation, National HIV Prevention Conference; June 2005.

7. Calculations based only on cases for which race/ethnicity data were provided.

8. U.S. Census Bureau, 2005 Population Estimates.

9. Includes reported cases among those 13 years of age and older. Estimates do not include cases from the U.S. dependencies, possessions, and associated nations, and cases of unknown residence.

10. NCHS, "Deaths: Leading Causes for 2002," *NVSR,* Volume 53, Number 17; 2005.

11. NCHS, *Health, United States, 2005.*

12. CDC data request; January 2006.

13. CDC, *HIV/AIDS Surveillance by Race/Ethnicity* (through 2004).

14. CDC, *Fact Sheet: HIV/AIDS among Men Who Have Sex with Men,* July 2005.

15. CDC, "HIV Prevalence, Unrecognized Infection, and HIV Testing Among Men Who Have Sex with Men—Five U.S. Cities, June 2004–April 2005," *MMWR,* Volume 54, Number 24; June 24, 2005.

16. Kaiser Family Foundation, www.statehealthfacts.org. Data Source: Centers for Disease Control and Prevention, Division of HIV/AIDS Prevention—Surveillance and Epidemiology, Special Data Request; November 2006.

17. Estimates include U.S. dependencies, possessions, and associated nations, and cases of unknown residence.

18 Calculations based only on cases for which data by place of birth were provided.

19. Fleishman JA. Personal Communication, Analysis of HCSUS Data; January 2002.

20. Kaiser Family Foundation analysis of CDC data.

21. KFF, *Survey of Americans on HIV/AIDS*; 2006.

Section 14.3

HIV/AIDS among African Americans

"HIV/AIDS among African Americans," Centers for Disease Control and Prevention (CDC), January 2007. This document, along with references and examples of prevention programs, is available online at http://www.cdc.gov/hiv/topics/aa/resources/factsheets/aa.htm.

In the United States, the HIV/AIDS epidemic is a health crisis for African Americans. At all stages of HIV/AIDS—from infection with HIV to death with AIDS—blacks (including African Americans) are disproportionately affected compared with members of other races and ethnicities.

Statistics

HIV/AIDS in 2005

- According to the 2000 census, blacks make up approximately 13 percent of the U.S. population. However, in 2005, blacks accounted for 18,510 (49 percent) of the estimated 38,096 new HIV/AIDS diagnoses in the United States in the 33 states with long-term, confidential name-based HIV reporting.

- Of all black men living with HIV/AIDS, the primary transmission category was sexual contact with other men, followed by injection drug use, and high-risk heterosexual contact.

- Of all black women living with HIV/AIDS, the primary transmission category was high-risk heterosexual contact, followed by injection drug use.

- Of the estimated 141 infants perinatally infected with HIV, 91 (65 percent) were black (CDC, HIV/AIDS Reporting System, unpublished data, December 2006).

- Of the estimated 18,849 people under the age of 25 whose diagnosis of HIV/AIDS was made during 2001–2004 in the 33 states with HIV reporting, 11,554 (61 percent) were black.

AIDS in 2005

- Blacks accounted for 22,030 (50 percent) of the estimated 44,198 AIDS cases diagnosed in the 50 states and the District of Columbia.

- The rate of AIDS diagnoses for black adults and adolescents was ten times the rate for whites and nearly three times the rate for Hispanics. The rate of AIDS diagnoses for black women was nearly 24 times the rate for white women. The rate of AIDS diagnoses for black men was eight times the rate for white men.

- The 188,077 blacks living with AIDS in the 50 states and the District of Columbia accounted for 44 percent of the 425,910 people in the United States living with AIDS.

- Of the 58 U.S. children (younger than 13 years of age) who had a new AIDS diagnosis, 39 were black.

- Since the beginning of the epidemic, blacks have accounted for 399,637 (42 percent) of the estimated 956,666 AIDS cases diagnosed in the 50 states and the District of Columbia.

- From the beginning of the epidemic through December 2005, an estimated 211,559 blacks with AIDS died.

- Of persons whose diagnosis of AIDS had been made during 1997–2004, a smaller proportion of blacks (66 percent) were alive after nine years compared with American Indians and Alaska Natives (67 percent), Hispanics (74 percent), whites (75 percent), and Asians and Pacific Islanders (81 percent).

Risk Factors and Barriers to Prevention

Race and ethnicity, by themselves, are not risk factors for HIV infection. Even though HIV testing rates are higher for blacks than for members of other races and ethnicities, rates of undetected or late diagnosis of HIV infection are higher for black men who have sex with men (MSM).

Blacks are also more likely to face challenges associated with risk factors for HIV infection, including the following:

Sexual Risk Factors

Black women are most likely to be infected with HIV as a result of sex with men who are infected with HIV. They may not be aware of their male partners' possible risk factors for HIV infection, such as unprotected sex with multiple partners, bisexuality, or injection drug use. Sexual contact is also the main risk factor for black men. Male-to-male sexual contact was the primary risk factor for 48 percent of black men with HIV/AIDS at the end of 2005, and high-risk heterosexual contact was the primary risk factor for 22 percent.

Substance Use

Injection drug use is the second leading cause of HIV infection both for black men and women. In addition to being at risk from sharing needles, casual and chronic substance users are more likely to engage in high-risk behaviors, such as unprotected sex, when they are under the influence of drugs or alcohol. Drug use can also affect treatment success. A recent study of HIV-infected women found that women who used drugs, compared with women who did not, were less likely to take their antiretroviral medicines exactly as prescribed.

Lack of Awareness of HIV Serostatus

Not knowing one's HIV serostatus is risky for black men and women. In a recent study of MSM in five cities participating in CDC's National HIV Behavioral Surveillance System, 46 percent of the black MSM were HIV positive, compared with 21 percent of the white MSM and 17 percent of the Hispanic MSM. The study also showed that of participating black MSM who tested positive for HIV, 67 percent were unaware of their infection; of participating Hispanic MSM who tested positive for HIV, 48 percent were unaware of their infection; of participating white MSM who tested positive for HIV, 18 percent were unaware of their infection; and of participating multiracial/other MSM who tested positive for HIV, 50 percent were unaware of their infection. Persons who are infected with HIV but don't know it cannot benefit from life-saving therapies or protect their partners from becoming infected with HIV.

Sexually Transmitted Diseases

The highest rates of sexually transmitted diseases (STDs) are those for blacks. In 2005, blacks were about 18 times as likely as whites to have gonorrhea and about five times as likely to have syphilis. Partly because of physical changes caused by STDs, including genital lesions that can serve as an entry point for HIV, the presence of certain STDs can increase one's chances of contracting HIV infection three- to five-fold. Similarly, a person who has both HIV infection and certain STDs has a greater chance of spreading HIV to others. A recent CDC literature review showed that high rates of HIV infection for black MSM may be partly attributable to a high prevalence of STDs that facilitate HIV transmission.

Homophobia and Concealment of Homosexual Behavior

Homophobia and stigma can cause some black MSM to identify themselves as heterosexual or not to disclose their sexual orientation. Indeed, black MSM are more likely than other MSM not to identify themselves as gay. The absence of self-identification or the absence of disclosure presents challenges to prevention programs. However, data suggest that these men are not at greater risk for HIV infection than are black MSM who identify themselves as gay. The findings of these studies do not mean that black MSM who do not identify themselves as gay or who do not disclose their sexual orientation do not engage in risky behaviors, but the findings do suggest that these men are not engaging in higher levels of risky behavior than are other black MSM.

Socioeconomic Issues

Socioeconomic issues and other social and structural influences affect the rates of HIV infection among blacks. In 1999, nearly one in four blacks was living in poverty. Studies have found an association between higher AIDS incidence and lower income. The socioeconomic problems associated with poverty, including limited access to high-quality health care, housing, and HIV prevention education, may directly or indirectly increase the risk factors for HIV infection.

Prevention

In the United States, the annual number of new HIV infections has decreased from a peak of more than 150,000 in the mid-1980s and has stabilized since the late 1990s at approximately 40,000. Populations of minority races and ethnicities are disproportionately affected by the HIV epidemic. To reduce further the incidence of HIV, CDC announced the Advancing HIV Prevention (AHP) initiative in 2003. This initiative comprises four strategies: making HIV testing a routine part of medical care, implementing new models for diagnosing

117

HIV infections outside medical settings, preventing new infections by working with HIV-infected persons and their partners, and further decreasing perinatal HIV transmission.

CDC has also established the African American HIV/AIDS Work Group to focus on the urgent issue of HIV/AIDS in African Americans. The work group developed a comprehensive response to guide CDC's efforts to increase and strengthen HIV/AIDS prevention and intervention activities directed toward African Americans. Already, CDC is engaged in a wide range of activities to involve community leaders in the African American community and to decrease the incidence of HIV/AIDS in blacks.

Section 14.4

Young African American Adults at High Risk for HIV Even in Absence of High-Risk Behavior

"Young African Americans at High Risk for HIV, STDs Even in Absence of High-Risk Behaviors," *NIH News,* National Institutes of Health (NIH), December 5, 2006.

Results of a new study supported by the National Institute on Drug Abuse (NIDA), National Institutes of Health, suggest that young African American adults—but not young white adults—are at high risk for HIV and other sexually transmitted diseases (STDs) even when their relative level of risky behaviors is low. The findings imply that the marked racial disparities in the prevalence of these diseases are not exclusively affected by individual risk behaviors. The paper can be viewed online in the *American Journal of Public Health.*

"Improving our understanding of the factors that contribute to the health disparities seen in HIV is one of our top priorities," says Dr. Elias Zerhouni, director of the National Institutes of Health. "Studies like this help define the problem, but further research may provide us with a greater understanding of why this population is at higher risk and how best to intervene."

Environmental, institutional, and contextual influences, such as differences in social and dating patterns, are among the many factors identified by the researchers that may play a role in one's risk for HIV. The authors recognize that research that seeks to address racial disparities in STD and HIV infection must proceed with sensitivity and involve dialogue and consensus among all community groups.

"NIDA has conducted many studies that link drug abuse and other risky behaviors to HIV infection," says NIDA Director Dr. Nora D. Volkow. "This study is particularly interesting because it suggests that given similar patterns of risk behaviors across racial groups, young African American adults are more likely to become infected. As a result, we need to look beyond strategies that target individual risk behaviors and focus on outreach and education for this population as a group."

"We found that the most normative category for young African American adults (almost 38 percent of participants) was one of the lowest-risk categories, characterized by having few sexual partners and low alcohol, tobacco, or drug abuse. Yet these same individuals were more than seven times as likely as young white adults in the same category to harbor an STD/HIV infection" says lead scientist Dr. Denise Hallfors of the Pacific Institute for Research and Evaluation in Chapel Hill, North Carolina.

The scientists stratified the participants into 15 behavioral patterns ranging in risk level from relatively low (e.g., having few sexual partners and low alcohol, tobacco, or drug use) to high (e.g., intravenous drug abusers). The researchers observed that the STD/HIV prevalence among young African American adults was high for all 15 defined behavior patterns regardless of risk level, whereas among young white adults, the STD/HIV infection prevalence was only high for the four most risky behavior patterns—exchanging sex for money, intravenous drug abuse, men having sex with men, and abusing marijuana and other drugs.

The study authors recommend continuing a proactive strategy to reach all African American young adults, including universal screening and expanding information, testing and treatment services to nontraditional venues, such as churches, beauty salons and barber shops, colleges, prisons, and jails.

The researchers analyzed 2001–2002 population-based data from 6,257 young white adults and 2,449 young African American adults nationwide 18 to 26 years old. They were participants in the National Longitudinal Study of Adolescent Health and had completed initial surveys when they were in seventh to twelfth grades in 1994–1995. In this assessment, participants used computer assisted self-interviewing technology to respond to sensitive questions about sexual and substance abuse history. Following the interview, participants were tested for STDs and HIV.

"These surprising new findings suggest that a more comprehensive research approach is needed to understand the factors that make young African American adults vulnerable to STD and HIV infection beyond the commonly known individual risk behaviors," says Dr. Volkow. "Most STDs can be cured, the health and lifespan of people infected with HIV can be significantly increased by available therapies, and prompt diagnosis and treatment may reduce the spread of these diseases."

Chapter 15

Sexual Orientation and the Risk of HIV Transmission

HIV/AIDS among Men Who Have Sex with Men

In the United States, HIV infection and AIDS have had a tremendous effect on men who have sex with men (MSM). MSM accounted for 72 percent of all HIV infections among male adults and adolescents in 2005 (based on data from 33 states with long-term, confidential name-based HIV reporting), even though only about 5 percent to 7 percent of male adults and adolescents in the United States identify themselves as MSM.

The number of HIV diagnoses for MSM decreased during the 1980s and 1990s, but recent surveillance data show an increase in HIV diagnoses for this group. Additionally, racial disparities exist with regard to HIV diagnoses within the MSM population. A recent study, conducted in five large U.S. cities, found that HIV prevalence among black MSM (46 percent) was more than twice that among white MSM (21 percent).

The recent overall increase in HIV diagnoses for MSM, coupled with racial disparities, strongly points to a continued need for appropriate prevention and education services tailored for specific subgroups of MSM, especially those who are members of minority races/ethnicities.

This chapter includes text from the following documents: "HIV/AIDS among Men Who Have Sex with Men," Centers for Disease Control and Prevention (CDC), May 17, 2007, references and examples of prevention programs are available online at http://www.cdc.gov/hiv/topics/msm/resources/factsheets/msm.htm;"Questions and Answers: Men on the Down Low," CDC, October 16, 2006, and, "Fact Sheet: HIV/AIDS among Women Who Have Sex with Women," CDC, October 17, 2006.

Figure 15.1. Transmission categories of male adults and adolescents with HIV/AIDS diagnosed during 2005. (Note: Based on data from 33 states with long-term, confidential name-based HIV reporting. Because of rounding, percentages may not equal 100.)

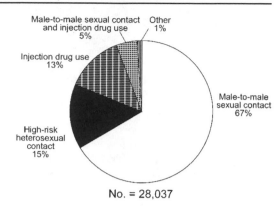

No. = 28,037

Figure 15.2. Race/ethnicity of MSM living with HIV/AIDS, 2005. (Note: Based on 33 states with long-term, confidential name-based HIV reporting.)

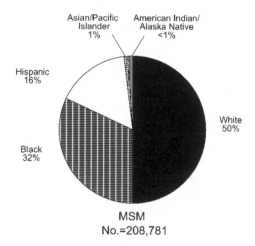

MSM
No.=208,781

Figure 15.3. Race/ethnicity of MSM living with AIDS who inject drugs, 2005. (Note: Based on 33 states with long-term, confidential name-based HIV reporting.)

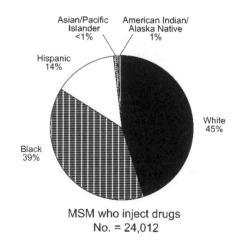

MSM who inject drugs
No. = 24,012

Statistics: HIV/AIDS in 2005

The following bullets refer to the 33 states with long-term, confidential name-based HIV reporting.

- In the 33 states with long-term, confidential name-based HIV reporting, an estimated 20,058 MSM (18,722 MSM and 1,336 MSM who inject drugs) received a diagnosis of HIV/AIDS, accounting for 72 percent of male adults and adolescents and 53 percent of all people receiving an HIV/AIDS diagnosis that year.

- The number of HIV/AIDS diagnoses among MSM (including MSM who inject drugs) increased 13 percent from 2001 through 2005. It is not known whether this increase is due to an increase in the testing of persons with risk factors, which results in more HIV diagnoses, or due to an increase in cases of HIV infection.

- An estimated 232,793 MSM (208,781 MSM and 24,012 MSM who inject drugs) were living with HIV/AIDS.

Statistics: AIDS in 2005

- An estimated 21,129 MSM (18,939 MSM and 2,190 MSM who inject drugs) received a diagnosis of AIDS, accounting for 65 percent of male adults and adolescents and 48 percent of all people who received a diagnosis of AIDS.

- An estimated 7,293 MSM (5,929 MSM and 1,364 MSM who inject drugs) with AIDS died, accounting for 60 percent of all men and 45 percent of all people with AIDS who died.

- Since the beginning of the epidemic, an estimated 520,187 MSM (454,106 MSM and 66,081 MSM who inject drugs) had received a diagnosis of AIDS, accounting for 68 percent of male adults and adolescents who received a diagnosis of AIDS and 54 percent of all people who received a diagnosis of AIDS.

- Since the beginning of the epidemic, an estimated 300,669 MSM (260,749 MSM and 39,920 MSM who inject drugs) with AIDS had died, accounting for 68 percent of male adults and adolescents with AIDS who had died and 57 percent of all people with AIDS who had died.

- At the end of 2005, an estimated 219,517 MSM (193,357 MSM and 26,160 MSM who inject drugs) were living with AIDS, representing 68 percent of male adults and adolescents living with AIDS and 52 percent of all people living with AIDS.

Risk Factors and Barriers to Prevention

Sexual risk factors: Sexual risk factors account for most HIV infections in MSM. These factors include unprotected sex and sexually transmitted diseases (STDs).

- Having anal sex without a condom continues to be a significant threat to the health of MSM. Unprotected anal sex (barebacking) with casual partners is an increasing concern. Not all the reasons for an apparent increase in unprotected anal intercourse are known, but research points to the following factors: optimism about improved HIV treatment, substance use, complex sexual decision making, seeking sex partners on the internet, and failure to practice safer sex. Some of these men may be serosorting, or only having sex (or unprotected sex) with a partner whose HIV serostatus, they believe, is the same as their own. Although serosorting between MSM who have tested HIV positive is likely to prevent new HIV transmission to persons who are not infected, the effectiveness of serosorting between men who have tested HIV negative has not been established. Serosorting with condom use may further reduce the risk of HIV transmission. However, for men with casual partners, serosorting alone is likely to be less effective than always using condoms because some men do not know or disclose their HIV serostatus.

- STDs, which increase the risk for HIV infection, remain an important health issue for MSM. According to the Gonococcal Isolate Surveillance Project, the proportion of gonorrhea-positive test results among MSM increased from 4 percent in 1988 to 20.2 percent in 2004. Rates of syphilis among MSM have increased in some urban areas, including Chicago, New York, San Francisco, and Seattle. In the nine U.S. cities participating in the MSM Prevalence Monitoring Project, the rates of STDs and HIV positivity varied by race and ethnicity but tended to be highest among black and Hispanic MSM. In addition to increasing susceptibility to HIV, STDs are markers for high-risk sexual practices, through which HIV infection can be transmitted.

Unknown HIV serostatus: Approximately 25 percent of people in the United States who are infected with HIV do not know they are infected.

- Through its National HIV Behavioral Surveillance system, the Centers for Disease Control and Prevention (CDC) found that 25 percent of the MSM surveyed in five large U.S. cities were infected with HIV and 48 percent of those infected were unaware of their infections.

- In a recent CDC study of young MSM, 77 percent of those who tested HIV positive mistakenly believed that they were not infected. Young black MSM in this study were more likely to be unaware of their infection—approximately nine of ten young black MSM compared with six of ten young white MSM. Of the men who tested positive, most (74 percent) had previously tested negative for HIV infection, and 59 percent believed that they were at low or very low risk.

Research has shown that many people who learn that they are infected with HIV alter their behaviors to reduce their risk of transmitting the virus. Therefore, increasing the proportion of people who know their HIV serostatus can help decrease HIV transmission.

Substance use: The use of alcohol and illegal drugs continues to be prevalent among some MSM and is linked to risk factors for HIV infection and other STDs. Substance use can increase the risk for HIV transmission through the tendency toward risky sexual behaviors while under the influence and through sharing needles or other injection equipment. Reports of increased use of the stimulant drug methamphetamine are also a concern because methamphetamine use has been associated both with risky sexual behaviors for HIV infection and other STDs and with the sharing of injection equipment when the drug is injected. Methamphetamine and other "party" drugs (such as ecstasy, ketamine, and GHB [gamma hydroxybutyrate]) may be used to decrease social inhibitions and enhance sexual experiences. These drugs, along with alcohol and nitrate inhalants ("poppers"), have been strongly associated with risky sexual practices among MSM.

Complacency about risk: More than 25 years into the HIV epidemic, there is evidence of an underestimation of risk, of difficulty in maintaining safer sex practices, and of a need to sustain prevention efforts for all gay and bisexual men.

- The success of highly active antiretroviral therapy (HAART) may have had the unintended consequence of increasing the risk behaviors of some MSM.

  - Some research suggests that the perceptions of the negative aspects of HIV infection have been minimized since the introduction of HAART, which has led to a false understanding of what living with HIV means and thus to an increase in risky sexual behaviors. For example, some MSM may mistakenly believe that they or their partners are not infectious when they take antiretroviral medication or when they have low or undetectable viral loads.

- Optimism about HIV treatments is associated with a greater willingness to have unprotected anal intercourse.

- Long-term efforts to practice safer sex present a significant challenge. A four-city study indicates that years of exposure to prevention messages and long-term efforts to practice safer sex may play a role in the decision of HIV-positive MSM to engage in unprotected anal intercourse.

- The rates of risky behaviors are higher among young MSM than among older MSM. Not having seen firsthand the toll of AIDS in the early years of the epidemic, young MSM may be less motivated to practice safer sex.

MSM who are HIV positive: HAART has enabled HIV-infected MSM to live longer. However, HAART's success means there are more MSM living with HIV who have the potential to transmit the virus to their sex partners. This emphasizes the importance of focusing prevention efforts on those who are living with HIV.

Although many MSM reduce their risk behaviors after learning that they have HIV, most remain sexually active. Most HIV-infected MSM believe that they have a personal responsibility to protect others from HIV, but some engage in risky sexual behaviors that may result in others contracting HIV. Interventions to reduce the risk for transmission, some of which were tested with MSM, are available for persons living with HIV.

The internet: During the past decade, the internet has created new opportunities for MSM to meet sex partners. Internet users can anonymously find partners with similar sexual interests without having to leave their residence or having to risk face-to-face rejection if the behaviors they seek are not consistent with safer sex. The internet may also normalize certain risky behaviors by making others aware of these behaviors and creating new connections between those who engage in them. At the same time, however, the internet has the potential to be a powerful tool for use with HIV prevention interventions.

Social discrimination and cultural issues: MSM are members of all communities, all races and ethnicities, and all strata of society. To reduce the rate of HIV infection, prevention efforts must be designed with respect for the many differences among MSM and with recognition of the discrimination against MSM and other persons infected with HIV in many parts of the country.

- Social and economic factors, including racism, homophobia, poverty, and lack of access to health care are barriers to HIV prevention services, particularly for MSM of minority races or ethnicities. Black and Hispanic men are more likely than white men to be given a diagnosis of HIV infection in the late stages of infection, often when they already have AIDS, suggesting that they are not accessing testing or health care services through which HIV infection could be diagnosed at an earlier stage.

- The stigma associated with homosexuality may inhibit some men from identifying themselves as gay or bisexual, even though they have sex with other men. Some men who have sex with men and with women don't identify themselves as gay or bisexual. Research among black men has shown that even if these men do not identify themselves as gay or bisexual, they do not engage in risky behavior more often than the men who do identify themselves as gay or bisexual. This research suggests that elevated rates of STDs and undetected or late diagnosis of HIV infection may contribute to higher rates of HIV infection among black MSM.

- Black and Hispanic MSM are less likely than white MSM to live in gay-identified neighborhoods. Therefore, prevention programs directed to gay-identified neighborhoods may not reach these MSM.

- For Hispanic MSM, unique cultural factors may discourage openness about homosexuality: *machismo*, the high value placed on masculinity; *simpatia*, the importance of smooth, nonconfrontational relationships; and *familismo*, the importance of a close relationship with one's family.

- Although Asians/Pacific Islanders and American Indians/Alaska Natives accounted for less than 2 percent of the AIDS cases in MSM reported nationally during 1989–1998, these groups accounted for noteworthy proportions of cases in certain metropolitan areas. Also, HIV infection among American Indians and Alaska Natives may be underestimated because not all surveillance systems recognize American Indian or Alaska Native as a race/ethnicity.

Combinations of risk factors: There is growing recognition that combinations of individual, sociocultural, and biomedical factors affect HIV risk behavior among MSM. Childhood sexual abuse, substance use, depression, and partner violence have been shown to increase the practice of risky sexual behaviors. Further research has shown that the combined effects of these problems may be greater than their individual effects. Therefore, MSM with more than one of these problems may have additional risk factors for HIV infection. The expansion and wider awareness of this type of research, which shows the additive effect of various psychosocial problems, will result in more precise prevention efforts.

Differences within the MSM population: Even though MSM constitute a group at risk for HIV, not all MSM are at risk for HIV. Analyzing the context within which individuals of the larger MSM community live and socialize may be a promising method for developing and focusing HIV interventions. A recent large-scale HIV vaccine efficacy trial looked at combinations of demographic characteristics and risk behaviors to help identify MSM at greatest risk. This study of more than 5,000 HIV-negative MSM found that older men with large numbers of sex partners, young men who used "party" drugs, and older men who used nitrate inhalants were most likely to contract HIV.

The appreciation of differences within the MSM community will aid in the development of successful HIV prevention interventions.

Prevention

To reduce the incidence of HIV, CDC released the Revised Recommendations for HIV Testing of Adults, Adolescents, and Pregnant Women in Health-Care Settings in 2006. These recommendations include the routine HIV screening of adults, adolescents, and pregnant women in health care settings in the United States. They also include reducing barriers to HIV testing. In 2003, CDC announced Advancing HIV Prevention. This initiative comprises four strategies: making HIV testing a routine part of medical care, implementing new models for diagnosing HIV infections outside medical settings, preventing new infections by working with HIV-infected persons and their partners, and further decreasing perinatal HIV transmission.

Given that a large number of HIV-infected MSM are unaware of their infection, HIV testing is an important strategy for this population. Many of these men have previously tested HIV-negative, so CDC recommends that all sexually active MSM be tested for HIV at least once a year. MSM who engage in high-risk behaviors (e.g., unprotected anal sex with casual partners) should be tested more frequently.

MSM as a group continues to be the population most affected by HIV infection and AIDS. However, research shows that HIV prevention efforts can reduce sexual risk factors: one review found that among men who received an HIV prevention intervention, the proportion who engaged in unprotected sex decreased, on average, 26 percent.

CDC offers effective interventions for MSM (http://www.effective interventions.org). These interventions can be tailored to various audiences, such as African American or Hispanic MSM.

In 2006, CDC provided 54 awards to community-based organizations that focus primarily on MSM. CDC also provides funding through state, territorial, and local health departments. Of these 54 awards, 63 percent focus on African Americans, 43 percent on Hispanics, 13 percent on Asians and Pacific Islanders, and 20 percent on whites (the percentages do not add to 100 percent because some of the organizations focus on more than one racial/ethnic group).

Questions and Answers: Men on the Down Low

What are the origins of the term down low and what does it refer to?

The most generic definition of the term *down low,* or *DL,* is "to keep something private," whether that refers to information or activity.

The term is often used to describe the behavior of men who have sex with other men as well as women and who do not identify as gay or bisexual. These men may refer to themselves as being "on the down low," "on the DL," or "on the low low." The term has most often been associated with African American men. Although the term originated in the African American community, the behaviors associated with the term are not new and not specific to black men who have sex with men.

What are the sexual risk factors associated with being on the down low?

Much of the media attention about men on the down low and HIV/AIDS has focused on the concept of a transmission bridge between bisexual men and heterosexual women. Some women have become infected through sexual contact with bisexual men. However, many questions, like the following, have not yet been answered.

129

- Do bisexually active men account for more cases of HIV infection in women than do men who inject drugs?

- Are bisexually active men more likely than other groups of men to be HIV infected?

- What proportion of HIV-infected men who have sex with male and female partners identify with the down low?

- Do men on the down low engage in fewer or more sexual risk behaviors than men who are not on the down low?

- Do people other than bisexually active men who do not disclose their behavior to sex partners identify with the down low?

What are the implications for HIV prevention?

The phenomenon of men on the down low has gained much attention in recent years; however, there are no data to confirm or refute publicized accounts of HIV risk behavior associated with these men. What is clear is that women, men, and children of minority races and ethnicities are disproportionately affected by HIV and AIDS and that all persons need to protect themselves and others from getting or transmitting HIV.

What steps is CDC taking to address the down low?

CDC and its many research partners have several projects in the field that are exploring the HIV-related sexual risks of men, including men who use the term *down low* to refer to themselves. The results of these studies will be published in medical journals and circulated through press releases in the next few years as each study is concluded and the data analyzed. CDC has also funded several projects that provide HIV education, counseling, and testing in minority racial and ethnic communities. CDC's research and on-the-ground HIV prevention efforts will continue as more information about the demographics and HIV risk behaviors of men who do and men who do not identify with the down low becomes available.

HIV/AIDS among Women Who Have Sex with Women

To date, there are no confirmed cases of female-to-female sexual transmission of HIV in the United States database (K. McDavid, CDC, oral communication, March 2005). However, case reports of female-to-female transmission of HIV and the well-documented risk of female-to-male transmission indicate that vaginal secretions and menstrual blood are potentially infectious and that mucous membrane (for example, oral, vaginal) exposure to these secretions has the potential to lead to HIV infection.

Statistics

The following information comes from CDC unpublished data.

- Through December 2004, a total of 246,461 women were reported as HIV infected. Of these, 7,381 were reported to have had sex with women; however, most had other risk factors (such as injection drug use, sex with men who are infected or who have risk factors for infection, or, more rarely, receipt of blood or blood products).

- Of the 534 (of 7,381) women who were reported to have had sex only with women, 91 percent also had another risk factor—typically, injection drug use.

- HIV-infected women whose only initially reported risk factor is sex with women are given high priority for follow-up investigation. As of December 2004, none of these investigations had confirmed female-to-female HIV transmission, either because other risk factors were later identified or because some women declined to be interviewed.

- A study of more than 1 million female blood donors found no HIV-infected women whose only risk factor was sex with women. Despite the absence of confirmed cases of female-to-female transmission of HIV, the findings do not negate the possibility. Information on whether a woman had sex with women is missing in more than 60 percent of the 246,461 case reports—possibly because the physician did not ask or the woman did not volunteer the information.

Risk Factors and Barriers to Prevention

Surveys of behavioral risk factors have been conducted in groups of women who have sex with women (WSW). These surveys generally have been of WSW samples that differ in criteria for participation, location for recruitment, and definition of WSW. As a result, the findings of these surveys cannot be generalized to all WSW. The findings have, however, suggested that some WSW have other behavioral risk factors, such as injection drug use and unprotected vaginal sex with men who have sex with men (MSM) or men who inject drugs.

Prevention

Although there are no confirmed cases of female-to-female transmission of HIV, female sexual contact should be considered a possible means of transmission among WSW. These women need to know the following:

- **Their own and their partner's HIV serostatus:** This knowledge can help women who are not infected to change their behaviors and thus reduce their risk of becoming infected. For women who are infected, this knowledge can help them get early treatment and avoid infecting others.

- **The risk for exposure through a mucous membrane:** Potentially, HIV can be transmitted through the exposure of a mucous membrane (in the mouth, for example), especially if the tissue is cut or torn, to vaginal secretions and menstrual blood. The potential for transmission is greater during early and late-stage HIV infection, when the amount of virus in the blood is expected to be highest.

- **The potential benefits of using condoms:** Condoms should be used consistently and correctly during every sexual contact with men or when using sex toys. Sex toys should not be shared. No barrier methods for use during oral sex have been evaluated as effective by the Food and Drug Administration. However, natural rubber latex sheets, dental dams, condoms that have been cut and spread open, or plastic wrap may offer some protection from contact with body fluids during oral sex and thus may reduce the possibility of HIV transmission.

Health care providers need to remember that sexual identity does not necessarily predict behavior and that some women who identify themselves as WSW or lesbian may be at risk for HIV infection through unprotected sex with men.

Chapter 16

HIV/AIDS among Prison Populations

Background

Caring for the HIV-infected incarcerated patient is complex and challenging. For many of these patients, the prison health service provides their first opportunity for access to health care. HIV seroprevalence rates among inmates in the United States are five times higher than in the nonincarcerated population. Within the prison system in the United States, mortality due to AIDS has dropped dramatically since the advent of effective combination antiretroviral therapy (ART), with the number of AIDS-related deaths decreasing by 72 percent in state prisons between 1995 and 2002.

Often, behaviors that lead to incarceration also put inmates at high risk for becoming infected with HIV, hepatitis C virus (HCV), and other infectious diseases. These risk factors may include unsafe substance use behaviors, such as sharing syringes and other injection equipment, and high-risk sexual practices, such as having multiple sex partners or unprotected sex. Many inmates also may have conditions that increase the risk of HIV transmission or acquisition, such as untreated sexually transmitted diseases (STDs).

"Correctional Settings," pp. 388–391, excerpted from *Clinical Manual for Management of the HIV-Infected Adult,* © 2006 AIDS Education and Training Centers National Resource Center. All rights reserved. Reprinted with permission. The complete document, including references, is available online at http://aidsetc.org/aetc/pdf/AETC-CM_092206.pdf.

133

Of the approximately 1.8 million inmates in the United States, 30–40 percent are infected with HCV. The incidence is ten times higher among inmates than among noninmates and is 33 percent higher in women than in men. Chronic hepatitis B virus (HBV) infection and tuberculosis are substantially more common in the incarcerated population than in the general public. The presence of any of these conditions should prompt HIV testing.

Incarcerated Women

Women represent 5–10 percent of the prison population in the United States. The HIV epidemic in the United States increasingly affects women of color, and this trend is reflected in HIV rates among the incarcerated. Incarcerated women have higher HIV seroprevalence rates than incarcerated men (3 percent versus 1.9 percent). Several risk factors for HIV are present in abundance among female inmates, including the following:

• history of childhood sexual abuse and neglect

• history of sex work, with increased frequency of forced, unprotected sex

• high rates of STDs

• high rates of mental illness

• history of injection drug use (IDU) and/or sex partners with IDU history

• poverty

Among all women entering a correctional facility, 10 percent are pregnant. These women should be offered HIV testing, and HIV-infected pregnant women should be offered ART immediately to prevent perinatal HIV transmission. Many incarcerated women will receive their first gynecologic care in prison. Because the incidence of cervical cancer is higher in women with HIV, referrals for colposcopy should be made for any HIV-infected woman with an abnormal Papanicolaou [Pap] test.

Testing and Prevention

The correctional facility is an ideal location for identifying those already infected with HIV, HCV, and/or HBV, and for preventing infection among those at highest risk for these diseases. The corrections setting is often the first site at which an HIV-infected person interacts with the health care system, making it an important avenue for HIV testing. HIV testing policies in correctional facilities vary from state to state and among local, state, and federal penal institutions. Depending on the setting, policies may require testing of inmates upon entry, upon release, or both. Testing may be based on clinical indication or risk exposure during incarceration, and may be voluntary or mandatory. The U.S. Centers for Disease Control and Prevention (CDC) recommends routine counseling and testing in settings with an HIV prevalence of 1 percent or higher. In high-risk settings such as correctional facilities, routine, voluntary HIV testing has been shown to be cost-effective and clinically advantageous.

Testing and treatment of HIV-infected inmates prior to release is critical. Given the high HIV seroprevalence rates among inmates, the reentry of inmates into the community presents the danger of spreading HIV and other infectious diseases, and thus is a public health concern. Inmates need adequate HIV prevention counseling before release both to protect themselves and to decrease transmission of HIV to others in their communities.

Health care providers in correctional settings are in a key position to evaluate inmates for HIV risk factors, to offer HIV testing, and to educate and counsel this high-risk group about HIV. Inmates often are hesitant to be tested for HIV because of fear of a positive diagnosis and because of the potential stigma involved. Often, they lack accurate information about HIV, including awareness of behaviors that may have put them at risk and knowledge of means for protecting themselves from becoming infected.

The World Health Organization (WHO) has stated: "All inmates and correctional staff and officers should be provided with education concerning transmission, prevention, treatment, and management of HIV infection. For inmates, this information should be provided at intake and updated regularly thereafter." (See: http://www.who.int/en.) Risk reduction counseling addresses specific ways the inmate can reduce the risk of becoming infected with HIV. If already HIV infected, the goal of counseling is to reduce the risk of infecting others or becoming infected with a drug-resistant strain of HIV. Education should focus on the use of latex barriers with all sexual activity. Although condoms and dental dams are not available in most prisons and jails, the inmate should receive education regarding their proper use.

Inmates with a history of IDU should be educated that needle sharing conveys a high risk of transmitting HIV, HCV, and HBV. Substance abuse treatment should be provided when appropriate.

Recovery from addiction often is a chronic process and relapses are common. In addition to treatment, risk reduction strategies should include planning for support after release. For example, prior to release, inmates should be provided with information about needle exchange or clean needle access programs in their communities. These programs have proved to be quite effective in decreasing the rate of parenteral HIV transmission. [See the section on Syringe Exchange Programs in Chapter 24 for more information.]

Antiretroviral Therapy in Correctional Facilities

In correctional facilities, as in any setting, a consideration of HIV treatment must begin with educating the patient about the risks and benefits of treatment and the need to fully adhere to the entire regimen, as well as with an assessment of the patient's motivation to take ART.

Correctional facilities have two medical policies for dispensing medications. Each has advantages and disadvantages that can impact treatment adherence.

Directly Observed Therapy

Directly Observed Therapy (DOT) is the system in which the inmate goes directly to the medical unit or pharmacy for all medication doses. This system offers the advantage of more frequent interaction between the patient and the health care team, allowing for earlier identification of side effects and other issues. In general, patients have better medication adherence in this system, resulting in better control of HIV. For some inmates, however, the need for frequent visits to the medical unit or pharmacy may be a barrier to treatment, particularly if they are housed at a distance from the unit. Another disadvantage of DOT is the potential loss of confidentiality, as many inmates feel that the frequency of treatment and the large number of pills they must take will reveal clues that they are HIV infected. In addition, this system puts the inmate in a passive role in terms of medication treatment and does not foster self-sufficiency.

Keep on Person

Keep on Person (KOP) is the system that allows the inmates to keep their medications in their cells and take them independently. Monthly supplies are obtained at the medical unit or pharmacy. This system offers greater privacy and confidentiality regarding HIV status. It also allows the inmate to develop self-sufficiency in managing medications, which may facilitate improved adherence upon release. However, as the KOP system involves less interaction with medical staff, problems with adherence can be more difficult to identify.

In a study comparing DOT in HIV-infected inmates with KOP in nonincarcerated HIV-infected patients receiving ART as part of a clinical trial, a higher percentage of DOT patients achieved undetectable viral loads compared with the KOP patients (85 percent versus 50 percent) over a 48-week period.

Adherence

Adherence is one of the most important factors in determining success of ART. For the HIV-infected inmate starting ART, a number of issues can affect medication adherence. These include patient-related factors, factors related to systems of care (including the medication dispensing systems described above), and medication-related factors. The following are suggestions for supporting adherence to ART.

Patient-Related Factors

- Provide alcohol and substance abuse treatment prior to initiating ART. Without appropriate treatment during incarceration, linkages to supports, and follow-up treatment upon discharge, the inmate is at risk for returning to high-risk behaviors that may interfere with adherence to ART.

- Utilize mental health consultation to identify inmates with psychiatric needs. Treatment for underlying mental health disorders should precede or occur simultaneously with the initiation of ART to ensure successful adherence. Depression and other psychiatric illnesses are more prevalent among inmates than among the general population.

- Correct misconceptions about HIV and ART that are common among inmates and could affect adherence adversely. The inmate should be educated about the disease process and the role of the medications, along with the potential risks and benefits of taking ART.

- Encourage participation in peer support groups. These can be effective ways to foster self-esteem, empower inmates to come to terms with a positive diagnosis, allay fears and correct misconceptions about HIV disease, and aid adherence. Upon release, telephone hotlines may be available to provide follow-up support and linkages to community services. To the extent possible, family and friends should be included in the education process.

- Use teaching tools that are appropriate in terms of language and reading level. Illiteracy and low-level reading ability are common among inmates. Diagrams and videos may be more effective than reading-intensive material in some cases. Basic HIV education prior to initiation of ART should include the following:
  - how the medications work
  - consequences of nonadherence
  - names and dosages of all medications
  - potential side effects with strategies to manage them

Factors Related to Systems of Care

- Educate security staff about the importance of timely medication dosing, and communicate with other facilities in advance of a transfer; this can eliminate or limit missed doses.

- Schedule frequent follow-up medical visits in the early weeks after ART is initiated; these can make the difference in whether or not patients "stay the course."

- Consult with an HIV specialist, if possible. If a facility's medical provider lacks experience in treating patients with HIV, the results may be undertreatment of side effects, or ART prescribing errors. Because caring for HIV patients is complicated, HIV specialists can provide assurance that patients are receiving proper care. Of particular concern are patients whose current ART regimens are failing, those who are declining clinically, and those who are co-infected with other infectious diseases such as tuberculosis, HCV, and HBV.

Medication-Related Factors

Any consideration of HIV treatment must begin with educating the patient about the risks and benefits of treatment and the need to fully adhere to the entire regimen, as well as with assessing the patient's motivation to take ART.

- Aggressively monitor and treat side effects. The most common barrier to adherence to ART is side effects from the medications.

The inmate should be educated in advance about potential adverse events to observe and report. In the first weeks after starting a new ART regimen, patients should be assessed frequently for side effects. For treating gastrointestinal toxicities, antiemetics [for vomiting] and antidiarrheals [for diarrhea] should be available on an as-needed basis. As with all patients on ART, inmates should have appropriate laboratory monitoring.

- Be aware of food requirements. Various food requirements must be considered carefully when administering ART. This can be especially challenging in the correctional environment, particularly if the facility does not allow inmates to self-administer medications. Make arrangements with prison authorities to provide food when inmates are taking medications that require administration with food.

- Avoid complex regimens and regimens with large pill burdens, if possible. Simple regimens with few pills appear to help improve adherence.

- Avoid drug-drug interactions. Some antiretroviral medications have clinically significant interactions with other drugs (e.g., methadone, oral contraceptives, cardiac medications, antacids). These interactions may cause failure of either the antiretroviral drug or the other medication, or may cause additional toxicity. Consult an HIV specialist or pharmacologist for information on drug interactions.

- The patient should be questioned about medication adherence at each appointment.

- ART regimens need to fit into each patient's schedule and lifestyle. This becomes a bigger issue when the inmate is close to release. Education about HIV management, including ART adherence, should begin well before the inmate is discharged back to the community. At the time of discharge from the correctional facility, all HIV-infected inmates should have a discharge plan that addresses the following:
  - housing
  - health insurance
  - 30-day supply of HIV medications
  - follow-up appointments for medical care and, if necessary, psychiatric and substance abuse care

139

A number of HIV education resources for inmates and correctional health care providers are cited on Albany Medical College's website at http://www.amc.edu/patient/hiv/index.htm (go to the section on correctional education).

—by Minda Hubbard, ANP-C, Research Nurse Practitioner; Douglas G. Fish, MD, Medical Director; Sarah Walker, MS, Correctional Education Coordinator; and Abigail V. Gallucci, Director of HIV Education—Albany Medical College's Division of HIV Medicine

Chapter 17

HIV/AIDS and Homelessness

Lack of affordable housing is a critical problem facing a growing number of people living with acquired immunodeficiency syndrome (AIDS) and other illnesses caused by the human immunodeficiency virus (HIV). People with HIV/AIDS may lose their jobs because of discrimination or because of the fatigue and periodic hospitalization caused by HIV-related illnesses. They may also find their incomes drained by the costs of health care.

Tragically, individuals with HIV/AIDS may die before they are able to receive housing assistance. Efforts to build HIV/AIDS housing often encounter chronic funding shortfalls, bureaucratic indifference, and the stigma and fear of AIDS. Projects to create HIV/AIDS housing may fail because of local opposition by neighborhood or community groups.

Prevalence

- Studies indicate that the prevalence of HIV among homeless people is between 3 percent and 20 percent, with some subgroups having much higher burdens of disease.

- In general, people who are homeless have higher rates of chronic diseases than people who are housed, due in part to the effects

"HIV/AIDS and Homelessness," © 2006 National Coalition for the Homeless. Reprinted with permission. The complete document, including a list of resources, is available online at http://www.nationalhomeless.org/publications/facts/HIV.pdf.

141

of lifestyle factors (such as drug, alcohol, or tobacco use), exposure to extreme weather, nutritional deficiencies, and being victimized by violence.

- An estimated 3.5 million people are homeless in the United States every year.

- People living with HIV/AIDS are at higher risk of becoming homeless. A Los Angeles study found that 50 percent of domiciled people living with HIV/AIDS felt they were at risk of becoming homeless, while a Philadelphia study found that 44 percent of persons living with HIV/AIDS were unable to afford their housing, a risk factor for homelessness.

- Of nearly 12,000 people living with HIV/AIDS surveyed by AIDS Housing of Washington, 40 percent report having been homeless at least once in the past.

- The homeless population has a median rate of HIV prevalence at least three times higher—3.4 percent versus 1 percent—than the general population. Even higher rates (8.5 to 62 percent) have been found in various subpopulations.

- A 1995 survey of homeless adults found that 69 percent were at risk for HIV infection from unprotected sex with multiple partners, injection drug use (IDU), sex with IDU partners, or exchanging unprotected sex for money or drugs.

- Homeless women and adolescents are particularly at risk. Single homeless women are more likely to be victims of domestic violence and sexual abuse, both of which have been linked to HIV infection. Homeless adolescents are at risk due to higher rates of sexual abuse and exploitation. It has been estimated that 70 to 85 percent of homeless adolescents abuse substances.

- Homeless women have special barriers to health care. Homeless mothers, in particular, have been found to subordinate their own health care needs for the needs of their children.

- Many homeless adolescents find that exchanging sex for food, clothing, and shelter is their only chance of survival on the streets. In turn, homeless youth are at a greater risk of contracting AIDS or HIV-related illnesses. HIV prevalence studies anonymously performed in four cities found a median HIV-positive rate of 2.3 percent for homeless persons under age 25.

Issues

To address the special considerations and challenges that primary care providers may face in caring for homeless individuals with HIV, the Health Care for the Homeless Clinicians' Network is undertaking a project focusing on HIV and homelessness. The following information is taken from the Network's September 1999 newsletter, *Healing Hands*.

HIV infection exacerbated by homelessness deserves special attention for the following reasons:

High morbidity and mortality: HIV-infected homeless persons are believed to be sicker than their domiciled counterparts. For example, they tend to have higher rates and more advanced forms of tuberculosis (TB), and higher incidence of other illnesses such as Bartonella. Another study has demonstrated that more homeless people die of AIDS than other HIV-infected populations.

Barriers to care: Homeless people with HIV may face many barriers to optimal care. Injection drug use and lack of insurance, common among homeless people, have been shown to negatively affect health care utilization, level of medical care, and health status.

Challenges to adherence: Adherence to complex medical regimens may be more difficult if one does not have stable housing or access to basic subsistence needs such as food. As it is believed that decreased adherence is the single best predictor of protease inhibitor failure and the primary cause of medication resistance, this problem has grave personal and public health implications.

Policy Recommendations

Homeless persons with HIV/AIDS need safe, affordable housing and supportive, appropriate health care. Emergency housing grants should be available for persons with HIV-related illnesses who are in danger of losing their homes, and housing assistance should be available for those already on the streets. Federal assistance must be provided through adequate funding of targeted housing and health programs, and through the enforcement of anti-discrimination laws.

Chapter 18

Alcohol and HIV/AIDS

People with alcohol use disorders are more likely than the general population to contract HIV (human immunodeficiency virus). HIV is the virus that causes acquired immunodeficiency syndrome (AIDS). Similarly, people with HIV are more likely to abuse alcohol at some time during their lives. Alcohol use is associated with high-risk sexual behaviors and injection drug use, two major modes of HIV transmission. Concerns about HIV have increased as recent trends suggest a resurgence of the epidemic among "men who have sex with men" (this phrase refers to any male who has ever had sexual contact with another male, regardless of primary sexual orientation or gender role identification), as well as dramatic increases in the proportion of cases transmitted heterosexually. In persons already infected, the combination of heavy drinking and HIV has been associated with increased medical and psychiatric complications, delays in seeking treatment, difficulties with HIV medication compliance, and poorer HIV treatment outcomes. Decreasing alcohol use in people who have HIV or who are at risk for becoming infected reduces the spread of HIV and the diseases associated with it.

This text briefly examines the changing patterns of HIV transmission in the United States; the role of alcohol in the transmission of HIV within, and potentially beyond, high-risk populations; the potential

"Alcohol Alert #57—Alcohol and HIV/AIDS," National Institute on Alcohol Abuse and Alcoholism (NIAAA), National Institutes of Health (NIH), September 2002. Revised by David A. Cooke, MD, Diplomate, American Board of Internal Medicine, April 2007. References are available online at http://pubs.niaaa.nih.gov/publications/aa57.htm.

influence of alcohol abuse on the progression and treatment of HIV-related illness; and the benefits of making alcoholism treatment an integral part of HIV prevention programs.

Trends in HIV Transmission in the United States

HIV is most commonly transmitted by sexual contact and the sharing of contaminated needles by injection drug users. By the end of 2003, an estimated 1,039,000 to 1,185,000 Americans were living with HIV. Approximately 40,000 new cases of active AIDS disease are diagnosed annually. Historically, HIV has been most prevalent among men who have sex with men whereas most new HIV infections are reported among men who have sex with men and among injection drug users. Recently, however, the proportion of HIV cases acquired through heterosexual contact has increased and almost equals the proportion of cases attributable to injection drug use. The proportion of all AIDS cases reported among women has tripled since the mid-1980s, primarily as a result of heterosexual exposure and secondarily through injection drug use. Minority groups are the most heavily affected by HIV associated with drug injection, and blacks and Hispanics now account for an estimated 70 percent of all new AIDS cases.

Alcohol and HIV Transmission

People who abuse alcohol are more likely to engage in behaviors that place them at risk for contracting HIV. For example, rates of injection drug use are high among alcoholics in treatment, and increasing levels of alcohol ingestion are associated with greater injection drug-related risk behaviors, including needle sharing.

A history of heavy alcohol use has been correlated with a lifetime tendency toward high-risk sexual behaviors, including multiple sex partners, unprotected intercourse, sex with high-risk partners (e.g., injection drug users, prostitutes), and the exchange of sex for money or drugs. There may be many reasons for this association. For example, alcohol can act directly on the brain to reduce inhibitions and diminish risk perception. However, expectations about alcohol's effects may exert a more powerful influence on alcohol-involved sexual behavior. Studies consistently demonstrate that people who strongly believe that alcohol enhances sexual arousal and performance are more likely to practice risky sex after drinking.

Some people report deliberately using alcohol during sexual encounters to provide an excuse for socially unacceptable behavior or to reduce their conscious awareness of risk. This practice may be especially common among men who have sex with men. This finding is consistent with the observation that men who drink prior to or during homosexual contact are more likely than heterosexuals to engage in high-risk sexual practices.

Finally, the association between drinking levels and high-risk sexual behavior does not imply that alcohol necessarily plays a direct role in such behavior or that it causes high-risk behavior on every occasion. For example, bars and drinking parties serve as convenient social settings for meeting potential sexual partners. In addition, alcohol abuse occurs frequently among people whose lifestyle or personality predisposes them to high-risk behaviors in general.

Alcohol and Medical Aspects of AIDS

Alcohol increases susceptibility to some infections that can occur as complications of AIDS. Infections associated with both alcohol and AIDS include tuberculosis; pneumonia caused by the bacterium *Streptococcus pneumoniae;* and the viral disease hepatitis C, a leading cause of death among people with HIV. Alcohol may also increase the severity of AIDS-related brain damage, which is characterized in its severest form by profound dementia and a high death rate.

The progression of HIV and the development of AIDS-associated infections may be controlled by highly active antiretroviral therapy (HAART), a combination of powerful antiviral medications. Despite markedly increased survival rates, HAART is associated with several disadvantages, including the emergence of medication-resistant HIV strains and the occurrence of adverse interactions with other medications, some of which are prescribed for AIDS-related infections. In addition, many patients fail to comply with the complex medication regimen. Studies have associated heavy alcohol use with decreased medication compliance as well as with poorer response to HIV therapy in general. The outcome of HIV therapy improved significantly among alcoholics who stopped drinking.

Alcoholism Treatment as HIV Prevention

Studies show that decreasing alcohol use among HIV patients not only reduces the medical and psychiatric consequences associated with alcohol consumption, but also decreases other drug use and HIV transmission. Thus, alcohol and other drug abuse treatment can be considered primary HIV prevention as well. For example, studies have

147

found a 58 percent reduction in injection drug use, with similar decreases in high-risk sexual behaviors, among heterosexual patients one year after treatment. Participants who remained abstinent showed substantially greater improvement in both outcomes compared with those who continued to drink.

It has been suggested that for heterosexual alcoholics, the focus of screening and prevention for HIV risk factors should be on people with more severe alcohol dependence. For male alcoholics who have sex with men, the focus should be on those who socialize primarily in bars.

Alcoholism prevention among youth is of particular importance. AIDS is a leading cause of death among people ages 15 to 24, and new injection drug users who contract HIV or viral hepatitis often become infected within two years after beginning to inject drugs. Researchers have found the following:

- The prevalence of current, binge, and heavy drinking peaks between the ages of 18 and 24, which is a high-risk period for initiating injection drug use.

- Drug injection is usually associated with prior use of alcohol in conjunction with non-injection drugs, especially among adolescents with alcohol use disorders.

- High rates of risky sexual practices have been reported among adolescents and may be correlated with alcohol consumption.

Therefore, it has been suggested that HIV prevention programs for youth should target alcohol consumption in addition to injection drug use and sexual risk reduction.

Treatment Access and Integration

Analyses of HIV surveillance data collected by the National Centers for Disease Control and Prevention, urban and rural health departments, and health maintenance organizations revealed that blacks, Hispanics, women, the chronically mentally ill, and the poor are less likely to obtain appropriate HIV therapy compared with the general population. HIV-infected people in rural areas report reduced access to medical and mental health care services relative to their urban counterparts.

Timeliness is an essential aspect of effective HIV treatment and prevention. Early detection of HIV infection facilitates the prompt initiation of behavioral changes aimed at reducing transmission and also may enhance treatment effectiveness. Unfortunately, many facilities for the treatment of alcohol or other drug use disorders do not routinely or consistently screen their patients for HIV. In addition, many people who test positive for HIV fail to seek medical care until the disease has reached an advanced stage. Alcohol abuse has been associated with longer delays in seeking treatment.

Some evidence suggests that such problems may be ameliorated in part by designing programs that link primary medical care with treatment for abuse of alcohol and other drugs, HIV risk-reduction education, and psychiatric care when appropriate. In drug treatment programs, for example, both patients and clinicians may focus on what is perceived as the main problem (typically heroin or cocaine use), and neglect or minimize the use of other drugs, including alcohol. Yet in one study, a large proportion of patients in a residential drug treatment program reported daily consumption of large quantities of alcohol.

A randomized controlled trial, demonstrated the feasibility of incorporating a multidisciplinary medical clinic within a detoxification unit designed to treat alcohol, heroin, and cocaine dependence. Because the integration of different services at a single site can be expensive, the researchers recommended that efforts be made to facilitate information transfer or patient transportation among programs based at multiple locations.

Alcohol and AIDS

A Commentary by Raynard Kington, MD, PhD

Research findings clearly show that the use of alcohol and other substances of abuse is a factor in the spread of HIV and can complicate the long-term health outcomes of HIV-positive individuals. Therefore it is important that health care providers screen their HIV patients for alcohol use problems and that patients being treated for alcohol and other substance use be screened for HIV infection. In both cases, steps should be taken to ensure that HIV-positive patients have access to appropriate care.

Health care providers should monitor their HIV-positive patients' alcohol use and initiate interventions to reduce alcohol-related problems when necessary. To begin this process, health care providers should establish good relationships with their patients to encourage open discussions about substance use. Those discussions can form the basis for reducing drinking problems, increasing adherence to HIV medication regimens, and decreasing sexually risky behaviors. Many health care providers believe that, whenever possible, stabilizing the substance user's social life prior to initiating HIV therapy will increase his or her likelihood of sustaining treatment.

Researchers continue to discover and test appropriate interventions for the behavioral, social, and biomedical problems encountered by HIV-positive individuals with alcohol problems. This research can be implemented effectively only when both HIV and substance abuse problems are addressed within a medical system capable of providing the appropriately integrated services.

Chapter 19

Drug Abuse and the Link to HIV/AIDS and Other Infectious Diseases

Behavior associated with drug abuse, such as sharing needle injection equipment and/or risky sexual behavior after drug or alcohol intoxication whether or not injection equipment is used, has been central to the spread of HIV/AIDS since the pandemic began more than 25 years ago.

HIV, the human immunodeficiency virus, which causes acquired immunodeficiency syndrome (AIDS), is a virus that lives and multiplies primarily in white blood cells (CD4+ lymphocytes), which are part of the immune system. HIV ultimately causes severe depletion of these cells. An HIV-infected person may look and feel fine for many years and may therefore be unaware of the infection. However, as the immune system weakens, the individual becomes more vulnerable to illnesses and common infections.

Over time, a person with untreated HIV is likely to succumb to multiple, concurrent illnesses and to develop AIDS. Because HIV/AIDS is a condition characterized by a defect in the body's natural immunity to diseases, infected individuals are at risk for severe illnesses that are not usually a threat to anyone whose immune system is working properly.

As yet, there is no cure for AIDS, and there is no vaccine to prevent a person from acquiring HIV.

National Institute on Drug Abuse (http://www.nida.nih.gov), National Institutes of Health (NIH), December 2006.

How HIV/AIDS Is Spread

HIV can be transmitted by contact with the blood or other body fluids of an infected person. In addition, infected pregnant women can pass HIV to their infants during pregnancy, delivery, and breastfeeding.

Among drug abusers, HIV transmission can occur through sharing needles and other injection paraphernalia such as cotton swabs, rinse water, and cookers. However, another way people may be at risk for HIV is simply by using drugs—regardless of whether a needle and syringe are involved. Research sponsored by the National Institute on Drug Abuse (NIDA) and the National Institute on Alcohol Abuse and Alcoholism has shown that drugs and alcohol use can interfere with judgment and can lead to risky sexual behaviors that put people in danger of contracting or transmitting HIV.

Preventing the Spread of HIV/AIDS

Early detection of HIV can help prevent HIV transmission. Research indicates that routine HIV screening in health care settings among populations with a prevalence rate as low as 1 percent is as cost effective as screening for other conditions such as breast cancer and high blood pressure. These findings suggest that HIV screening can lower health care costs by preventing high-risk practices and decreasing virus transmission.

Cumulative research has shown that comprehensive HIV prevention—drug abuse treatment, community-based outreach, testing, and counseling for HIV and other infections, and HIV treatment— is the most effective way to reduce the risk of bloodborne infections.

Combined pharmacological and behavioral treatments for drug abuse have a demonstrated impact on HIV risk behaviors and incidence of HIV infection. For example, recent research showed that when behavioral therapies were combined with methadone treatment, about half of study participants who reported injection drug use at intake reported no such use at study exit, and over 90 percent of all participants reported no needle sharing at study exit. While these findings show great promise for achieving reductions in HIV risk behaviors, studies are now needed to improve the long-term effectiveness of such interventions.

Behavioral treatments for drug abuse have also shown promise for enhancing patient adherence to HAART. Interventions aimed at increasing HIV treatment adherence are crucial to treatment success, but usually require dramatic lifestyle changes to counter the often irregular lifestyle created by drug abuse and addiction. Adequate medical care for HIV/AIDS and related illnesses is also critical to reducing and preventing the spread of new infections.

Other Infectious Diseases

Besides increasing their risk of HIV infection, individuals who take drugs or engage in high-risk behaviors associated with drug use also put themselves and others at risk for contracting or transmitting hepatitis C (HCV), hepatitis B (HBV), tuberculosis (TB), as well as a number of other sexually transmitted diseases, including syphilis, chlamydia, trichomoniasis, gonorrhea, and genital herpes. Injecting drug users (IDUs) are also commonly susceptible to skin infections at the site of injection and to bacterial and viral infections, such as bacterial pneumonia and endocarditis, which, if left untreated, can lead to serious health problems.

HCV, HBV, and HIV/AIDS

HCV, the leading cause of liver disease, is highly prevalent among IDUs and often co-occurs with HIV; HBV is also common among drug abusers. These are two of several viruses which can cause an inflammation of the liver. Chronic infection with HCV or HBV can result in cirrhosis (liver scarring) or primary liver cancer. While a vaccine does not yet exist for HCV, HBV infection can be prevented by an effective vaccine.

HCV is highly transmissible through bloodborne exposure. NIDA-funded studies have found that, within three years of beginning injection drug use, most IDUs contract HCV—and up to 90 percent of HIV-infected IDUs may also be infected with HCV. Chronic HCV and HIV co-infection results in an accelerated progression to end-stage liver disease and death when compared with individuals infected with HCV alone.

While the treatment of co-occurring HIV and HCV presents certain challenges, treatment during the acute phase of HCV infection (i.e., within six to twelve months of detection) can be very effective in controlling the virus. Treatment for chronic HCV can significantly improve quality of life.

TB and HIV/AIDS

TB is a chronic and infectious lung disease. Through major public health detection and treatment initiatives, its prevalence declined in the U.S. for several years, with the 2005 report of 14,000 cases being the lowest since surveillance began in 1953. However, the decline of TB prevalence has slowed by half in recent years, and TB infection remains intertwined with HIV/AIDS and drug abuse.

People with latent TB infection do not have symptoms, may not develop active disease, and cannot spread TB. However, if such individuals do not receive preventive therapy, they may develop active TB, which is contagious. NIDA research has shown that IDUs have high rates of latent TB infection. Because HIV infection severely weakens the immune system, people infected with both HIV and latent TB are at increased risk of developing active TB disease and becoming highly infectious, thereby increasing the risk of further TB transmission. Effective treatment for HIV and TB can reduce TB/HIV-associated disease and the risk of transmission to others.

For More Information

To learn more about the link between drug abuse and HIV/AIDS, visit http://www.nida.nih.gov/DrugPages/HIV.html. To learn more about resources for HIV/AIDS, HCV, and TB information, or for testing and referral in your geographic area, visit http://www.cdc.gov/hiv or http://www.cdc.gov/ncidod/diseases/hepatitis. To find publicly-funded treatment services for drug abuse and addiction in your state, visit http://www.findtreatment.samhsa.gov.

Chapter 20

The Link between HIV/AIDS and Other Sexually Transmitted Diseases

The interconnectedness of HIV/AIDS, other sexually transmitted diseases (STDs), tuberculosis (TB), and viral hepatitis grows increasingly apparent as biomedical and behavioral scientists learn more about people's susceptibility and risks. The Centers for Disease Control and Prevention (CDC) is applying new research to the elimination of TB and the prevention of all major STDs, including HIV infection, and viral hepatitis.

HIV/AIDS and STDs

Having an STD does not necessarily mean that the infected person also has HIV infection. However, continuing the risky behavior that led to STD infection may increase the likelihood of eventually becoming infected with HIV.

HIV infection and other STDs are linked not only by common behaviors, but also by biological mechanisms. Other STDs increase both HIV infectiousness and susceptibility. The following are examples:

- Syphilis, genital herpes type 2, chancroid, and other infections that cause genital or rectal ulcers may increase the risk of HIV transmission per sexual exposure 10 to 50 times for male-to-female transmission and 50 to 300 times for female-to-male exposure.

"HIV/AIDS: Making the Connection," National Prevention Information Network (NPIN), Centers for Disease Control and Prevention (CDC), 2006. References are available online at http://www.cdcnpin.org/scripts/hiv/connect.asp.

- Nonulcerative STDs (e.g., chlamydia and gonorrhea) have been shown to increase the risk of HIV transmission by two-fold to five-fold.

- Treatment of gonorrhea in HIV-infected men reduces the prevalence of HIV shedding in urethral secretions by approximately 50 percent.

These relationships between HIV/AIDS and STDs illustrate why STD prevention is a key HIV prevention strategy. Integrating HIV and STD prevention efforts is vital to the success of both endeavors.

HIV/AIDS and TB

HIV weakens the immune system; TB thrives in a weakened immune system. Thus, each disease speeds the other's progress:

- Someone who is HIV positive and infected with TB is many times more likely to become sick with TB than someone who is HIV-negative and infected with TB.

- HIV is the most powerful known risk factor for reactivation of latent TB infection to active disease.

- TB is a leading cause of death among people who are HIV positive.

About one-third of the 36 million HIV-positive people worldwide are co-infected with TB, and it accounts for about 11 percent of AIDS deaths worldwide. In Africa, HIV is the single most important factor determining the increased incidence of TB in the past ten years.

HIV/AIDS and Hepatitis C

The hepatitis C virus (HCV) is transmitted primarily by large or repeated direct exposures to contaminated blood via skin puncture. About one-quarter of HIV-infected persons in the United States are also infected with hepatitis C virus (HCV). Co-infection rates vary by type of exposure:

- Co-infection with HIV and HCV is common among HIV-infected injection drug users (IDUs), between 50 percent–90 percent.

- Co-infection is also common among persons with hemophilia who received clotting factor concentrates before 1987, when concentrates were treated to inactivate both viruses.

156

- The risk for acquiring infection through perinatal or sexual exposures is much lower for HCV than for HIV. For persons infected with HIV through sexual exposure (e.g., male-to-male sexual activity), co-infection with HCV is no more common than among similarly aged adults in the general population (3 percent–5 percent).

HIV-HCV co-infection has been associated with higher titers of HCV, more rapid progression to HCV-related liver disease, and an increased risk for HCV-related cirrhosis of the liver. Because of this, HCV infection has been viewed as an opportunistic infection in HIV-infected persons. It is not considered an AIDS-defining illness. The effects of HCV co-infection on HIV disease progression are less certain. Since co-infected patients are living longer on highly active antiretroviral therapy (HAART), more data is needed to determine if HCV infection influences the long-term natural history of HIV infection.

Chapter 21

Questions and Answers about HIV Risk

Chapter Contents

Section 21.1

What Activities Increase HIV Transmission Risk?

"How Risky Is It?" Fact Sheet 152, © 2007 AIDS InfoNet.
Reprinted with permission. Fact sheets are regularly updated. Check
http://www.aidsinfonet.org for the most recent information.

What's My Risk of Getting Infected with HIV?

Most people know how HIV is transmitted. They also know about safer sex guidelines. However, they may still be exposed to HIV. This can be by accident or because they take part in some risky behavior. They always want to know how likely it is that they got infected with HIV.

There Are No Guarantees

You can't be sure that you're not infected with HIV unless you are 100 percent certain that you did not engage in any risky behavior and that you were not exposed to any HIV-infected fluids.

The only way to know for sure whether you have been infected is to get tested. You should wait for two or three months after a possible exposure. Then get an HIV blood test.

You might know that you were exposed to HIV by sharing needles, a work-related accident, or unsafe sexual activity. In these cases, talk to your health care provider immediately. Ask whether you can use HIV treatments to prevent infection.

What Do the Numbers Mean?

Studies of HIV transmission have calculated the risks of infection. The studies came up with very different rates. For example, one study reported the risk for infection from one episode of unprotected receptive anal intercourse with an HIV-infected partner at one in 3,333. Another study said one in 50 episodes.

For regular partners who were active in anal sex, the risk for transmission was one in ten. The risk for the insertive partner (the "top") is believed to be about ten times less than for the receptive partner (the "bottom").

The risk of HIV infection during vaginal intercourse is believed to be much less. One estimate was one in 200,000 for transmission from infected women to men and one in 100,000 for transmission from infected men to women.

These calculations only give a general idea of risk. They can tell you which activities carry a higher or lower risk. They cannot tell you if you have been infected. If the risk is one in 100, for example, it doesn't mean that you can engage in that activity 99 times without any risk of becoming infected. You might become infected with HIV after a single exposure. That can happen the first time you engage in a risky activity.

What Activities Are Riskiest?

The highest risk of becoming infected with HIV is from sharing needles to inject drugs with someone who is infected with HIV. When you share needles, there is a very high probability that someone else's blood will be injected into your bloodstream. Hepatitis can also be transmitted by sharing needles.

The next greatest risk for HIV infection is from unprotected sexual intercourse. Receptive anal intercourse carries the highest risk. The lining of the rectum is very thin. It is damaged very easily during sexual activity. This makes it easier for HIV to enter the body.

Vaginal intercourse has the next highest risk. The lining of the vagina is stronger than in the rectum, but it can still be damaged by sexual activity. All it takes is a tiny scrape that can be too small to see. The risk of infection is increased if there is any inflammation or infection in the vagina.

There is some risk for the active partner in anal or vaginal sex. It's possible for HIV to enter the penis through any open sores, or through the moist lining of the opening of the penis.

What about Oral Sex?

There have been many studies of HIV transmission through oral sex. They have come to different conclusions. However, the following points are clear:

- It is possible to get infected with HIV through oral sex. The risk is not zero.

- The risk of HIV infection through oral sex is extremely low. It is much lower than for other types of unprotected sexual activity. However, other diseases such as syphilis can be transmitted through oral sex.

What Increases the Risk of HIV Infection?

Syphilis can increase the risk of transmitting HIV. Rates of syphilis are increasing in many parts of the U.S. People with syphilis probably have unprotected sex, so they have a higher than average chance of being infected with HIV. Also, syphilis causes large, painless sores. It is easy for someone to be infected with HIV through syphilis sores. An active case of syphilis increases the amount of HIV in someone's system and can make it easier for them to pass it on to another person.

Several other factors increase the risk of transmitting HIV, or becoming infected. These factors apply to just about every possible way HIV can be transmitted.

- When the HIV-infected person is in the "acute infection" phase, the amount of virus in their blood is very high. This increases the chance that they can pass on the infection. Unfortunately, almost no one knows when they are in this phase of HIV infection. There's no way to tell by looking at them.

- When either person has a weakened immune system. This could be because of a long-term illness or an active infection like a herpes outbreak, syphilis, or the flu.

- When either person has open sores that get exposed to infected fluids. These could be cold sores, genital herpes, mouth ulcers, syphilis sores, or other cuts or breaks in the skin.

- When there is blood present.

The Bottom Line

Researchers have developed estimates of the risk of transmission of HIV. These estimates can give you a general idea of which activities are more or less risky. They cannot tell you that any activity is safe, or how many times you can do them without getting infected.

Section 21.2

Can Mosquitoes Transmit HIV?

"Can I Get HIV from Mosquitoes?" Centers for Disease Control and Prevention (http://www.cdc.gov), reviewed October 16, 2006.

Can I Get HIV from Mosquitoes?

No. From the start of the HIV epidemic there has been concern about HIV transmission from biting and bloodsucking insects, such as mosquitoes. However, studies conducted by the Centers for Disease Control and Prevention (CDC) and elsewhere have shown no evidence of HIV transmission from mosquitoes or any other insects—even in areas where there are many cases of AIDS and large populations of mosquitoes. Lack of such outbreaks, despite intense efforts to detect them, supports the conclusion that HIV is not transmitted by insects.

The results of experiments and observations of insect biting behavior indicate that when an insect bites a person, it does not inject its own or a previously bitten person's or animal's blood into the next person bitten. Rather, it injects saliva, which acts as a lubricant so the insect can feed efficiently. Diseases such as yellow fever and malaria are transmitted through the saliva of specific species of mosquitoes. However, HIV lives for only a short time inside an insect and, unlike organisms that are transmitted via insect bites, HIV does not reproduce (and does not survive) in insects. Thus, even if the virus enters a mosquito or another insect, the insect does not become infected and cannot transmit HIV to the next human it bites.

There also is no reason to fear that a mosquito or other insect could transmit HIV from one person to another through HIV-infected blood left on its mouth parts. Several reasons help explain why this is so. First, infected people do not have constantly high levels of HIV in their blood streams. Second, insect mouth parts retain only very small amounts of blood on their surfaces. Finally, scientists who study insects have determined that biting insects normally do not travel from one person to the next immediately after ingesting blood. Rather, they fly to a resting place to digest the blood meal.

Section 21.3

Can I Get HIV from a Tattoo or through Body Piercing?

"Can I Get HIV from Getting a Tattoo or through Body Piercing?"
Centers for Disease Control and Prevention (http://www.cdc.gov),
reviewed October 16, 2006.

A risk of HIV transmission does exist if instruments contaminated with blood are either not sterilized or disinfected or are used inappropriately between clients. The Centers for Disease Control and Prevention (CDC) recommends that single-use instruments intended to penetrate the skin be used once, then disposed of. Reusable instruments or devices that penetrate the skin and/or contact a client's blood should be thoroughly cleaned and sterilized between clients. A fact sheet on the sterilization of patient-care equipment and HIV is available from the CDC Division of Healthcare Quality Promotion website at http://www.cdc.gov/ncidod/dhqp/bp_sterilization_patient_care.html.

Personal service workers who do tattooing or body piercing should be educated about how HIV is transmitted and take precautions to prevent transmission of HIV and other bloodborne infections in their settings.

If you are considering getting a tattoo or having your body pierced, ask staff at the establishment what procedures they use to prevent the spread of HIV and other blood-borne infections, such as the hepatitis B virus. You also may call the local health department to find out what sterilization procedures are in place in the local area for these types of establishments. For links to the 50 U.S. state health departments, visit the CDC website at http://www.cdc.gov.

Part Three

Strategies for Preventing HIV Transmission

Chapter 22

Stopping the Spread of HIV

How do you get infected with HIV?

The human immunodeficiency virus (HIV) is not spread easily. You can only get HIV if you get infected blood or sexual fluids into your system. You can't get it from mosquito bites, coughing or sneezing, sharing household items, or swimming in the same pool as someone with HIV.

Some people talk about "shared body fluids" being risky for HIV, but no documented cases of HIV have been caused by sweat, saliva, or tears. However, even small amounts of blood in your mouth might transmit HIV during kissing or oral sex. Blood can come from flossing your teeth, or from sores caused by gum disease, or by eating very hot or sharp, pointed food.

To infect someone, the virus has to get past the body's defenses. These include skin and saliva. If your skin is not broken or cut, it protects you against infection from blood or sexual fluids. Saliva contains chemicals that can help kill HIV in your mouth.

If HIV-infected blood or sexual fluid gets inside your body, you can get infected. This can happen through an open sore or wound, during sexual activity, or if you share equipment to inject drugs.

HIV can also be spread from a mother to her child during pregnancy or delivery. This is called "vertical transmission." A baby can also be infected by drinking an infected woman's breast milk. Adults exposed to breast milk of an HIV-infected woman may also be exposed to HIV.

How can you protect yourself and others?

Unless you are 100 percent sure that you and the people you are with do not have HIV infection, you should take steps to prevent getting infected. People recently infected (within the past two or three months) are most likely to transmit HIV to others. This is when their viral load is the highest. In general, the risk of transmission is higher with higher viral loads.

This text provides an overview of HIV prevention. [Other fact sheets for more details on specific topics are available online at www.aidsinfonet.org.]

Sexual activity: You can avoid any risk of HIV if you practice abstinence (not having sex). You also won't get infected if your penis, mouth, vagina, or rectum doesn't touch anyone else's penis, mouth, vagina, or rectum. Safe activities include kissing, erotic massage, masturbation, or hand jobs (mutual masturbation). There are no documented cases of HIV transmission through wet clothing.

Having sex in a monogamous (faithful) relationship is safe if:

- both of you are uninfected (HIV-negative).

- you both have sex only with your partner.

- neither one of you gets exposed to HIV through drug use or other activities.

Oral sex has a lower risk of infection than anal or vaginal sex, especially if there are no open sores or blood in the mouth.

You can reduce the risk of infection with HIV and other sexually transmitted diseases by using barriers like condoms. Traditional condoms go on the penis, and a new type of condom goes in the vagina or in the rectum.

Some chemicals called spermicides can prevent pregnancy but they don't prevent HIV. They might even increase your risk of getting infected if they cause irritation or swelling.

Drug use: If you're high on drugs, you might forget to use protection during sex. If you use someone else's equipment (needles, syringes, cookers, cotton, or rinse water) you can get infected by tiny amounts of blood. The best way to avoid infection is to not use drugs.

If you use drugs, you can prevent infection by not injecting them. If you do inject, don't share equipment. If you must share, clean equipment with bleach and water before every use.

Some communities have started exchange programs that give free, clean syringes to people so they won't need to share.

Vertical transmission: With no treatment, about 25 percent of the babies of HIV-infected women would be born infected. The risk drops to about 4 percent if a woman takes AZT during pregnancy and delivery, and her newborn is given AZT. The risk is 2 percent or less if the mother is taking combination antiretroviral therapy (ART). Caesarean section deliveries probably don't reduce transmission risk if the mother's viral load is below 1000.

Babies can get infected if they drink breast milk from an HIV-infected woman. Women with HIV should use baby formulas or breast milk from a woman who is not infected to feed their babies.

Contact with blood: HIV is one of many diseases that can be transmitted by blood. Be careful if you are helping someone who is bleeding. If your work exposes you to blood, be sure to protect any cuts or open sores on your skin, as well as your eyes and mouth. Your employer should provide gloves, facemasks, and other protective equipment, plus training about how to avoid diseases that are spread by blood.

What if I've been exposed?

If you think you have been exposed to HIV, talk to your health care provider or the public health department, and get tested.

If you are sure that you have been exposed, call your health care provider immediately to discuss whether you should start taking antiretroviral drugs (ARVs). This is called "post-exposure prophylaxis" or PEP. You would take two or three medications for several weeks. These drugs can decrease the risk of infection, but they have some serious side effects.

The Bottom Line

HIV does not spread easily from person to person. To get infected with HIV, infected blood, sexual fluid, or mother's milk has to get into your body. HIV-infected pregnant women can pass the infection to their new babies.

To decrease the risk of spreading HIV:

- use condoms during sexual activity.
- do not share drug injection equipment.
- if you are HIV-infected and pregnant, talk with your health care provider about taking ARVs.
- if you are an HIV-infected woman, don't breastfeed any baby.
- protect cuts, open sores, and your eyes and mouth from contact with blood.

If you think you've been exposed to HIV, get tested and ask your health care provider about taking ARVs.

Chapter 23

How to Reduce Your Risk of HIV Infection

What is AIDS?

AIDS (acquired immunodeficiency syndrome) is a disease caused by a virus called HIV (human immunodeficiency virus). HIV attacks the body's immune system. A healthy immune system is what keeps you from getting sick.

When people have AIDS, their bodies can't fight disease. They get sick easily and have trouble getting well. They usually die of an infection or cancer.

How do people get HIV?

HIV can only be passed from person to person through body fluids, like blood, semen, and vaginal fluid. The most common ways HIV is passed are as follows:

- by having unprotected anal, vaginal or oral sex with an infected person

- by sharing needles and syringes for injecting drugs with an infected person

You may be at risk of getting HIV if you have any of the risk factors listed below. Children born to infected mothers can also become infected during pregnancy.

What are possible risk factors for HIV infection?

You should be tested for HIV if the following apply:

- You have had unprotected sex with many sex partners.
- You have a sexually transmitted disease (STD).
- You use illegal injected drugs.
- You had blood transfusions or received blood products before 1985.
- You have a sex partner with any of the above risk factors.

What contact is safe?

HIV can't live very long outside the body, so you can't get it through casual contact. You can't get the virus by touching, shaking hands, hugging, swimming in a public pool, giving blood, or using hot tubs, public toilets, telephones, doorknobs, or water fountains. You also can't get it from food, mosquitoes, or other insects.

Should I be tested for HIV?

You should think about getting tested for HIV infection if you think you're at risk. Most HIV antibody tests done by your doctor are accurate if they are done three to six months or longer after you think you may have been infected. It takes this long for the antibodies to show up in the blood.

Are there HIV tests I can do at home?

You can buy home HIV test kits at drug stores and pharmacies. Home tests offer the advantage of privacy and anonymity. However, they are expensive and may not be covered by most health insurance plans. [See section on Home Blood Tests in Chapter 31.]

Should I use a home test or see my doctor?

Your doctor is concerned about you, your health, and your privacy. If your lifestyle leads you to believe that you have HIV, you should see your doctor. He or she will help you decide if you should be tested and will give you the support you need before and after the test. You don't get this type of support with home tests.

However, if you are afraid to talk with your doctor about HIV or be tested even though you may be at risk, then a home test may be a good idea. If the test result is positive, you should see your doctor right away.

Remember, one negative test is not a guarantee that you don't have HIV or won't get it in the future. You should talk to your doctor and learn about ways to protect yourself from getting infected.

How can I avoid getting HIV?

The best ways to protect yourself from getting infected with HIV are to do the following:

- not have sex with a person who is infected or is having sex with others
- practice "safer" sex if you do have sex
- not share needles and syringes

You can't tell who's infected with HIV by how they look. It takes an average of eight years for symptoms of AIDS to develop after a person is infected with HIV. So even people who don't look or feel sick can give you AIDS.

What is "safer" sex?

The "safest" sex is no sex. If you are having sex, "safer" sex is sex between two people who don't have HIV infection, only have sex with each other and don't abuse injectable drugs.

Safer sex also means using condoms if you have any doubts about whether your partner is infected or whether he or she is having sex with someone else. Use male latex condoms every time you have sex.

If a man doesn't want to use a male condom, use a female condom. Female condoms may not be as effective as male condoms, but they offer some protection.

Never let someone else's blood, semen, urine, vaginal fluid, or feces get into your anus, vagina, or mouth.

What's the right way to use condoms?

Using condoms the right way is important to make sure you are protected. Latex condoms should be used during all sex acts, including anal, vaginal, and oral sex. If you are allergic to latex, use a polyure-thane condom. For oral sex on a woman, she can use a condom split lengthwise to place between her body and her partner's mouth.

If you are thinking about using a spermicide, be aware that re-search has shown that spermicides containing nonoxynol-9 can cause genital irritation and increase your risk of catching an STD. However, using a condom with nonoxynol-9 is better than not using a condom at all.

Use only water-based lubricants (such as K-Y jelly) with condoms. Oil-based lubricants, such as petroleum jelly (such as Vaseline), baby oil, or lotions, cause the rubber in condoms to break.

How to use male condoms: Use a latex or polyurethane condom. Condoms made from natural membranes, such as sheep gut, aren't as good because HIV is small enough to get through the tiny pores in these condoms.

- Put the condom on before any contact is made.

- Unroll the condom over an erect penis. The unrolled ring should be on the outside. Unroll the condom to the base of the penis. Leave about a half-inch of space in the tip so semen can collect there.

- Squeeze the tip of the condom to get the air out.

- Pull out after ejaculating ("coming") and before the penis gets soft. Hold the condom against the base of the penis so it doesn't slip off.

- Throw away the condom. Don't reuse condoms.

What if I share needles?

The best decision for your health is to get help for your drug abuse. If you do share needles and syringes, clean them twice with bleach and water to help kill HIV. Draw bleach into the syringe and needle, then squirt it out. Do the same with water. Do both steps again.

Chapter 24

HIV Prevention through Changing Behavior

Chapter Contents

Section 24.1

Practicing Safer Sex

Definition

Safe sex means taking precautions during sex that can keep you from getting a sexually transmitted disease (STD), or from giving an STD to your partner. These diseases include genital herpes, genital warts, HIV, chlamydia, gonorrhea, syphilis, hepatitis B and C, and others.

Information

A STD is a contagious disease that can be transferred to another person through sexual intercourse or other sexual contact. Many of the organisms that cause sexually-transmitted diseases live on the penis, vagina, anus, mouth, and the skin of surrounding areas.

Most of the diseases are transferred by direct contact with a sore on the genitals or mouth. However, some organisms can be transferred in body fluids without causing a visible sore. They can be transferred to another person during oral, vaginal, or anal intercourse.

Some STDs can also be transferred by nonsexual contact with infected tissues or fluids, such as infected blood. For example, sharing needles when using IV drugs is a major cause of HIV and hepatitis B transmission. An STD can also be transmitted through contaminated blood transfusions and blood products, through the placenta from the mother to the fetus, and sometimes through breastfeeding.

The following factors increase your risk of getting a sexually-transmitted disease (STD):

- not knowing whether a partner has an STD or not
- having a partner with a past history of any STD
- having sex without a male or female condom
- using drugs or alcohol in a situation where sex might occur

- if your partner is an IV drug user
- having anal intercourse

Drinking alcohol or using drugs increase the likelihood that you will participate in high-risk sex. In addition, some diseases can be transferred through the sharing of used needles or other drug paraphernalia.

Abstinence is an absolute answer to preventing STDs. However, abstinence is not always a practical or desirable option.

Next to abstinence, the least risky approach is to have a monogamous sexual relationship with someone that you know is free of any STD. Ideally, before having sex with a new partner, each of you should get screened for STDs, especially HIV and hepatitis B, and share the test results with one another.

Use condoms to avoid contact with semen, vaginal fluids, or blood. Both male and female condoms dramatically reduce the chance you will get or spread an STD. However, condoms must be used properly:

- The condom should be in place from the beginning to end of sexual activity and should be used every time you have sex.

- Lubricants may help reduce the chance a condom will break. Use only water-based lubricants, because oil-based or petroleum-type lubricants can cause latex to weaken and tear. Do NOT use condoms with nonoxynol-9—these help prevent pregnancy, but may increase the chance of HIV transmission.

- Use latex condoms for vaginal, anal, and oral intercourse.

- Keep in mind that STDs can still be spread, even if you use a condom, because a condom does not cover surrounding skin areas. But a condom definitely reduces your risk.

Here are additional safe-sex steps:

- Know your partner. Before having sex, first establish a committed relationship that allows trust and open communication. You should be able to discuss past sexual histories, any previous STDs or IV drug use. You should not feel coerced or forced into having sex.

- Stay sober. Alcohol and drugs impair your judgment, communication abilities, and ability to properly use condoms or lubricants.

- Be responsible. If you have an STD, like HIV or herpes, advise any prospective sexual partner. Allow him or her to decide what

177

to do. If you mutually agree on engaging in sexual activity, use latex condoms and other measures to protect the partner.

- If pregnant, take precautions. If you have an STD, learn about the risk to the infant before becoming pregnant. Ask your provider how to prevent the fetus from becoming infected. HIV-positive women should not breastfeed their infant.

In summary, safe sex requires prior planning and good communication between partners. Given that, couples can enjoy the pleasures of a sexual relationship while reducing the potential risks involved.

References

Polizzotto MJ. "Prevention of sexually transmitted diseases." *Clin Fam Pract.* 2005; 7(1): 1–12.

Cohn SE. "Sexually transmitted diseases, HIV, and AIDS in women." *Med Clin North Am.* 2003; 87(5): 971–995.

Greydanus DE. "Contraception for college students." *Pediatr Clin North Am.* 2005; 52(1): 135–161, ix.

Section 24.2

School Health Education to Prevent the Spread of AIDS

More than half of the 40,000 annual HIV infections in the United States occur in youth ages 13–24. The majority of these 20,000 infections are occurring in two especially at-risk subgroups: young women of color and young gay and bisexual men. School-based HIV prevention education is a critical opportunity to reach all young people with health-promoting HIV prevention messages, and is especially crucial to these subgroups.

The policy arguments regarding school-based sexuality education— including HIV prevention messages—have made for an extremely polarizing debate, in the words of adolescent health expert Dr. Audrey Rogers, "reduc[ing] us all to bumper sticker debates and shouting matches at school boards. Our youth deserve better than this." AIDS Alliance for Children, Youth, and Families offers these recommendations as a statement of principles for the development of HIV prevention education curricula that assure local input and parental choice, while meeting the needs of at-risk youth to not only prevent HIV infection, but also promote their senses of self-worth and self-efficacy so that they may make healthy decisions for a lifetime.

AIDS Alliance recommends: Comprehensive sexuality education for youth with a strong emphasis on all medically accurate HIV prevention strategies, including abstinence-based messages.

Specific Recommendations

1. Schools should provide comprehensive HIV prevention education in grades K–12. HIV prevention education should be age, developmentally, and culturally appropriate. Whenever possible, HIV prevention education should take place within the context

179

of a health education curriculum that addresses STD and teen pregnancy prevention.

2. HIV prevention education should be factual and medically accurate. Programs should provide young people with the knowledge and skills to make lifelong decisions about their health. Programs should be evidence-based, grounded in theories and approaches that have been demonstrated to be effective in reducing HIV, other STDs, and unintended pregnancies.

3. Programs should stress abstinence from sex and drugs as the most effective ways for avoiding HIV infection. However, educational programs should necessarily discuss other strategies for reducing the risk of HIV infection.

4. Age appropriate information about the role of condoms in the prevention of HIV, other STDs, and pregnancies should be a part of education programs. Accurate information about condoms should be a part of HIV prevention programs in every jurisdiction.

5. HIV prevention programs should be locally determined according to the needs of communities and states. School staff, families, students, public health officials, and relevant communities should work together to design and implement HIV prevention programs, closely coordinating prevention priorities with the local HIV community planning groups.

6. Epidemiological data should be used to focus and tailor additional HIV prevention efforts to target those young people most affected by the epidemic.

    • Schools must provide a safe and supporting environment for all students. Stigma and stereotyping of those thought to be at risk for HIV infection are counterproductive to successful prevention efforts, and special attention must be paid to the linkage between stigma and HIV risk-taking behavior.

7. School-based HIV prevention efforts should provide information about the availability of and facilitate access to youth-sensitive confidential or anonymous HIV counseling and testing services.

8. Teachers and staff responsible for sexuality and HIV prevention education should be fully trained for such instruction, and

administrators should provide visible support to these teachers and their efforts.

9. The federal department of education should take a leadership role to encourage the development and prioritization of HIV prevention education in all levels of K–12 instruction, supporting the integration of such programs in both classrooms and throughout all levels of administration.

Section 24.3

Syringe Exchange Programs

"Syringe Exchange Programs," Centers for Disease Control and Prevention (http://www.cdc.gov), December 2005.

In 1997, a report to Congress concluded that needle exchange programs can be an effective component of a comprehensive strategy to prevent HIV and other bloodborne infectious diseases in communities that choose to include them. Federal funding to carry out any program of distributing sterile needles or syringes to injection drug users (IDUs) has been prohibited by Congress since 1988. In addition, several states have restricted the funding or operation of syringe exchange programs (SEPs).

As of 2004, injection drug use accounted for about one-fifth of all HIV infections and most hepatitis C infections in the United States. Injection drug users (IDUs) become infected and transmit the viruses to others through sharing contaminated syringes and other drug injection equipment and through high-risk sexual behaviors. Women who become infected with HIV through sharing needles or having sex with an infected IDU can also transmit the virus to their babies before or during birth or through breastfeeding.

To succeed in effectively reducing the transmission of HIV and other blood-borne infections, programs must consider a comprehensive approach to working with IDUs. Such an approach incorporates a range of pragmatic strategies that address both drug use and sexual risk behaviors. One of the most important of these strategies is ensuring that IDUs who cannot or will not stop injecting drugs have access to sterile syringes. This strategy supports the "one-time-only use of sterile syringes" recommendation of several institutions and governmental bodies, including the U.S. Public Health Service.

What are syringe exchange programs?

It is estimated that an individual IDU injects about 1,000 times a year. This adds up to millions of injections, creating an enormous need for reliable sources of sterile syringes. Syringe exchange programs (SEPs) provide a way for those IDUs who continue to inject to safely dispose of used syringes and to obtain sterile syringes at no cost.

The first organized SEPs in the U.S. were established in the late 1980s in Tacoma, Washington; Portland, Oregon; San Francisco; and New York City. By 2002, there were 184 programs in more than 36 states, Indian lands, and Puerto Rico. These programs exchanged more than 24 million syringes.

In addition to exchanging syringes, many SEPs provide a range of related prevention and care services that are vital to helping IDUs reduce their risks of acquiring and transmitting blood-borne viruses as well as maintain and improve their overall health.

These services may include the following:

- HIV/AIDS education and counseling

- condom distribution to prevent sexual transmission of HIV and other sexually transmitted diseases (STDs)

- referrals to substance abuse treatment and other medical and social services

- distribution of alcohol swabs to help prevent abscesses and other bacterial infections

- on-site HIV testing and counseling and crisis intervention

- screening for tuberculosis (TB), hepatitis B, hepatitis C, and other infections; and

- primary medical services

SEPs operate in a variety of settings, including storefronts, vans, sidewalk tables, health clinics, and places where IDUs gather. They vary in their hours of operation, with some open for two-hour street-based sessions several times a week, and others open continuously.

They also vary in the number of syringes allowed for exchange. Many also conduct outreach efforts in the neighborhoods where IDUs live.

What is the public health impact of SEPs?

SEPs have been shown to be an effective way to link some hard-to-reach IDUs with important public health services, including TB and STD screening and treatment. Through their referrals to substance abuse treatment, SEPs can help IDUs stop using drugs. Studies also show that SEPs do not encourage drug use among SEP participants or the recruitment of first-time drug users. In addition, a number of studies have shown that IDUs will use sterile syringes if they can obtain them. SEPs provide IDUs with an opportunity to use sterile syringes and share less often.

The results of this research, and the clear dangers of syringe sharing, led the National Institutes of Health Consensus Panel on HIV Prevention to state the following:

> "An impressive body of evidence suggests powerful effects from needle exchange programs. ... Studies show reduction in risk behavior as high as 80 percent, with estimates of a 30 percent or greater reduction of HIV in IDUs." (National Institutes of Health, "Consensus Development Statement: Interventions to prevent HIV risk behaviors," February 11–13, 1997:7–8)

Economic studies have concluded that SEPs are also cost effective. At an average cost of $0.97 per syringe distributed, SEPs can save money in all IDU populations where the annual HIV seroincidence exceeds 2.1 per 100 person years. The cost per HIV infection prevented by SEPs has been calculated at $4,000 to $12,000, considerably less than the estimated $190,000 medical costs of treating a person infected with HIV.

What issues do SEPs face?

SEPs face a variety of issues in their operation. One of the most substantial is coverage. For example, Montreal—a city that has active and well-supported SEPs, allows sales of syringes without prescription, and encourages pharmacy sales—was able to meet less than 5 percent of the need for sterile syringes in 1994. Of the 126 SEPs participating in a 2002 survey, the 11 largest exchanged almost half of the 24.8 million syringes exchanged. Most of the remaining SEPs exchanged much smaller numbers (the 22 smallest volume SEPs exchanged fewer than 5,000 syringes each).

SEPs also face significant legal and regulatory restrictions. For example, 47 states have drug paraphernalia laws that establish criminal penalties for the distribution and possession of syringes. Eight states and one territory have laws that prohibit dispensing or possessing syringes without a valid medical prescription. Public health authorities in communities have employed a number of strategies to ensure the legal provision of SEP services, including declaring public health emergencies.

Local community opposition also can be an issue. Residents may be concerned that the programs will encourage drug use and drug traffic and increase the number of used discarded syringes in their neighborhoods. Studies have found no evidence of increases in discarded syringes around SEPs. Finally, some IDUs avoid SEPs because they fear that using a program that serves IDUs will identify them as IDUs. For others, the fear of arrest, fines, and possible incarceration if caught carrying syringes to or from the SEP is a potent deterrent.

What have communities done?

Activities have included the following:

- supporting community-based discussions of the role that SEPs can play in comprehensive HIV and viral hepatitis prevention and care programs, in particular in getting SEP users into substance abuse treatment programs

- educating policy makers about the facts of injection-related transmission of blood-borne pathogens and the public health benefits of providing access to sterile syringes as part of a comprehensive public health approach

- encouraging collaborative review of the public health impact of repealing drug paraphernalia laws that penalize the possession or carrying of syringes

For More Information

Read *A Comprehensive Approach: Preventing Blood-Borne Infections among Injection Drug Users,* available online at http://www.cdc.gov/idu/pubs/ca/toc.htm, which provides extensive background information on HIV and viral hepatitis infection in IDUs and on the legal, social, and policy environment. It also describes strategies and principles for addressing these issues.

Chapter 25

Safety of the Blood Supply

Chapter Contents

Section 25.1

How Safe Is the Blood Supply in the U.S.?

This section contains text from "Blood," Food and Drug Administration (http://www.fda.gov), March 2007, and "How Safe Is the Blood Supply in the United States?" Centers for Disease Control and Prevention (http://www.cdc.gov), October 20, 2006.

Blood

The U.S. Food and Drug Administration (FDA) is responsible for ensuring the safety of our nation's blood supply. The Center for Biologics Evaluation and Research (CBER) regulates the collection of blood and blood components used for transfusion or for the manufacture of pharmaceuticals derived from blood and blood components, such as clotting factors, and establishes standards for the products themselves. CBER also regulates related products such as cell separation devices, blood collection containers, and HIV screening tests that are used to prepare blood products or to ensure the safety of the blood supply. CBER develops and enforces quality standards; inspects blood establishments; and monitors reports of errors, accidents, and adverse clinical events. CBER works closely with other parts of the Public Health Service (PHS) to identify and respond to potential threats to blood safety, to develop safety and technical standards, to monitor blood supplies, and to help industry promote an adequate supply of blood and blood products. While a blood supply with zero risk of transmitting infectious disease may not be possible, the blood supply is safer than it has ever been.

Over a period of years, FDA has progressively strengthened the overlapping safeguards that protect patients from unsuitable blood and blood products. Blood donors are now asked specific and very direct questions about risk factors that could indicate possible infection with a transmissible disease. This "up-front" screening eliminates approximately 90 percent of unsuitable donors. FDA also requires blood centers to maintain lists of unsuitable donors to prevent the use of collections from them. Also, blood donations are now tested for seven different infectious agents. In addition to strengthening these safeguards,

FDA has significantly increased its oversight of the blood industry. The agency inspects all blood facilities at least every two years, and "problem" facilities are inspected more often. Blood establishments are now held to quality standards comparable to those expected of pharmaceutical manufacturers.

In 1997, the FDA initiated the Blood Action Plan to increase the effectiveness of its scientific and regulatory actions, and to ensure greater coordination with our PHS partners. The plan was adopted by the Department of Health and Human Services (DHHS) and is revised as new concerns emerge. As biological products, blood and blood products are likely always to carry an inherent risk of infectious agents. Therefore, zero risk may be unattainable. The role of FDA is to drive that risk to the lowest level reasonably achievable without unduly decreasing the availability of this life saving resource.

How Safe Is the Blood Supply in the United States?

The U.S. blood supply is among the safest in the world. Nearly all people infected with HIV through blood transfusions received those transfusions before 1985, the year HIV testing began for all donated blood.

The Public Health Service has recommended an approach to blood safety in the United States that includes stringent donor selection practices and the use of screening tests. U.S. blood donations have been screened for antibodies to HIV-1 since March 1985 and HIV-2 since

Table 25.1. Tests performed on each unit of donated blood*
(Source: American Red Cross)

Disease	Test	Year Implemented
HIV/AIDS	HIV/AIDS HIV-1 Antibody test	1985
HIV-1/2	Antibody test	1992
HIV-1	p24 Antigen test	1996
HIV/AIDS and Hepatitis C	Nucleic Acid Test (NAT)	1999
Hepatitis C	Hepatitis C Anti-HCV	1990
Hepatitis B	Hepatitis B Surface Antigen test	1971
Hepatitis B	Hepatitis B Core Antibody	1987
Hepatitis	Hepatitis ALT	1986
Syphilis	Syphilis Serologic test	1948
Human T-cell Lymphotropic	HTLV-I Antibody	1989
Virus (HTLV)	HTLV-I/II Antibody	1998

*This list is subject to change as new blood safety opportunities and requirements emerge. Additional tests may be performed to meet special patient needs.

June 1992. The p24 Antigen test was added in 1996. Blood and blood products that test positive for HIV are safely discarded and are not used for transfusions.

The improvement of processing methods for blood products also has reduced the number of infections resulting from the use of these products.

Currently, the risk of infection with HIV in the United States through receiving a blood transfusion or blood products is extremely low and has become progressively lower, even in geographic areas with high HIV prevalence rates.

Section 25.2

Nucleic Acid-Amplification Testing Further Safeguards Blood Supply

"Blood Supply Testing Safeguards: Nucleic Acid-Amplification Testing Further Safeguards Nation's Blood Supply, NHLBI Study Shows," *NIH News,* National Heart, Lung, and Blood Institute (NHLBI), National Institutes of Health (NIH), August 18, 2004.

State-of-the-art testing systems to screen donated blood have improved the safety of the nation's blood supply by preventing the transmission of potentially deadly viruses, according to a study funded by the National Heart, Lung, and Blood Institute (NHLBI), a component of the National Institutes of Health. Nucleic acid-amplification testing (NAT) has helped prevent the transmission of approximately five HIV-1 infections and 56 hepatitis C virus (HCV) infections each year since it began being used in the United States as an investigational screening test in mid-1999. The study is published in the August 19, [2004], issue of the *New England Journal of Medicine.*

"Risks to blood recipients from transfusion-transmitted viruses such as HIV and hepatitis are already extremely low, in part because of increased surveillance and improved testing," said Barbara Alving, MD, NHLBI acting director. "NAT enhances the safety of the nation's blood supply by further reducing these risks."

The study is the first and only one of its scope to show the effectiveness of the NAT assay system nationally. All major blood donation laboratories in the United States participated, accounting for more than 98 percent of tested blood donations. Many organizations collaborated on the research, including the American Red Cross, Blood Systems Research Institute, America's Blood Centers, and the Food and Drug Administration (FDA).

The study investigators analyzed all donations that detected ribonucleic acid (RNA) from HIV-1 and HCV by NAT between 1999 and 2002. The researchers then looked to see which of these infected donations had been missed by tests to detect viral antibodies or antigens (proteins from the virus), the types of screening previously used. They concluded that NAT reduced the risk of HIV-1 and HCV infections associated with blood transfusion to approximately one in 2 million blood units. In comparison, other blood screening tests are associated with rates of one in 1.5 million for HIV-1 and one in 276,000 for HCV.

Blood donors have been tested for evidence of HIV infection since 1985 and for evidence of HCV infection since 1990. Although increasingly sensitive tests to detect HIV and HCV antibodies and HIV antigen were implemented during the past decade, in rare instances infections in donors have been missed. This is due to the "window period" during which a donor can be infected but still test negative on screening tests.

The NAT system, which was approved for use in 2002 by the FDA, can detect HIV and HCV infections in blood donors earlier than other screening tests because it detects viral genes rather than antibodies or antigens. The appearance of antibodies requires time for the donor to develop an immune response, and detection of antigens requires time for a higher level of virus to appear in the bloodstream.

With the use of NAT for HCV, the window period is reduced by approximately 60 days (from an average of 70 days to 10 days). For HIV-1, the average window period with antibody is approximately 22 days. This is reduced to approximately 11 days with the NAT tests used in this study. The use of NAT has allowed blood banks to discontinue two less effective screening tests—HIV-1 antigen testing and a test for a nonspecific marker for HCV. Blood donations continue to be screened with antibody tests for HIV, HCV, and other viruses, which helps ensure the safety of the blood supply.

"NAT not only improves the safety of our already safe blood supply, but the technology can be quickly adapted to screen for emerging viruses," said George Nemo, PhD, project officer of the study and group leader of the Transfusion Medicine and Cell Therapies Scientific Research Group at NHLBI.

For example, screening for West Nile virus was implemented in less than nine months with the collaboration of the Centers for Disease Control and Prevention and FDA and the rapid development of NAT by manufacturers. Nearly 1,000 blood donors with West Nile virus infection were identified by NAT and their donations discarded.

NAT also makes it possible to identify persons in the very early stages of HIV-1 and HCV infection. This information may help the medical community better understand risk factors associated with viral infection and the natural history, disease progression, and treatment for these infections.

One of the NAT systems used in the study was first developed in the mid-1990s by Gen-Probe Incorporated, in collaboration with Chiron Corporation, with support for research and development provided by NHLBI. Results of screening by the NAT system manufactured by Roche Molecular Systems were also included in the study.

Section 25.3

Deferred Blood Donors

Excerpted from "FDA Policy on Blood Donations from Men Who Have Sex with Other Men," Food and Drug Administration (FDA), May 23, 2007. The complete text of this document, including references, is available online at http://www.fda.gov/cber/faq/msmdonor.htm.

What is FDA's policy on blood donations from men who have sex with other men (MSM)?

Men who have had sex with other men, at any time since 1977 (the beginning of the AIDS epidemic in the United States) are currently deferred as blood donors. This is because MSM are, as a group, at increased risk for HIV, hepatitis B, and certain other infections that can be transmitted by transfusion.

Why doesn't FDA allow men who have had sex with men to donate blood?

A history of male-to-male sex is associated with an increased risk for the presence of and transmission of certain infectious diseases, including HIV, the virus that causes AIDS. FDA's policy is intended to protect all people who receive blood transfusions from an increased risk of exposure to potentially infected blood and blood products.

The deferral for men who have had sex with men is based on the following considerations regarding risk of HIV:

- Men who have had sex with men since 1977 have an HIV prevalence (the total number of cases of a disease that are present in a population at a specific point in time) 60 times higher than the general population, 800 times higher than first time blood donors, and 8000 times higher than repeat blood donors (American Red Cross). Even taking into account that 75 percent of HIV infected men who have sex with men already know they are HIV positive and would be unlikely to donate blood, the HIV prevalence in potential donors with history of male sex with males is 200 times higher than first time blood donors and 2000 times higher than repeat blood donors.

- Men who have had sex with men account for the largest single group of blood donors who are found HIV positive by blood donor testing.

- Blood donor testing using current advanced technologies has greatly reduced the risk of HIV transmission but cannot yet detect all infected donors or prevent all transmission by transfusions. While today's highly sensitive tests fail to detect less than one in a million HIV infected donors, it is important to remember that in the U.S. there are over 20 million transfusions of blood, red cell concentrates, plasma or platelets every year. Therefore, even a failure rate of one in a million can be significant if there is an increased risk of undetected HIV in the blood donor population.

- Detection of HIV infection is particularly challenging when very low levels of virus are present in the blood for example during the so-called "window period". The "window period" is the time between being infected with HIV and the ability of an HIV test to detect HIV in an infected person.

- FDA's MSM policy reduces the likelihood that a person would unknowingly donate blood during the "window period" of infection. This is important because the rate of new infections in MSM is higher than in the general population and current blood donors.

- Collection of blood from persons with an increased risk of HIV infection also presents an added risk if blood were to be accidentally given to a patient in error either before testing is completed or following a positive test. Such medical errors occur very rarely, but given that there are over 20 million transfusions every year, in the U.S., they can occur. That is one more reason why FDA and other regulatory authorities work to assure that there are multiple safeguards, not just testing.

- Several scientific models show there would be a small but definite increased risk to people who receive blood transfusions if FDA's MSM policy were changed and that preventable transfusion transmission of HIV could occur as a result.

- No alternate set of donor eligibility criteria (even including practice of safe sex or a low number of lifetime partners) has yet been found to reliably identify MSM who are not at increased risk for HIV or certain other transfusion transmissible infections.

- Today, the risk of getting HIV from a transfusion or a blood product has been nearly eliminated in the United States. Improved procedures, donor screening for risk of infection, and laboratory testing for evidence of HIV infection have made the United States blood supply safer than ever. While appreciative and supportive of the desire of potential blood donors to contribute to the health of others, FDA's first obligation is to assure the safety of the blood supply and protect the health of blood recipients.

- Men who have sex with men also have an increased risk of having other infections that can be transmitted to others by blood transfusion. For example, infection with the hepatitis B virus is about five to six times more common and hepatitis C virus infections are about two times more common in men who have sex with other men than in the general population. Additionally, men who have sex with men have an increased incidence and prevalence of human herpesvirus 8 (HHV-8). HHV-8 causes a cancer called Kaposi sarcoma in immunocompromised individuals.

What is self-deferral?

Self-deferral is a process in which individuals elect not to donate because they identify themselves as having characteristics that place them at potentially higher risk of carrying a transfusion transmissible disease. FDA uses self-deferral as part of a system to protect the blood supply. This system starts by informing donors about the risk of transmitting infectious diseases. Then, potential donors are asked questions about their health and certain behaviors and other factors (like travel and past transfusions) that increase their risk of infection. Screening questions help people, even those who feel well, to identify themselves as potentially at higher risk for transmitting infectious diseases. Screening questions allow individuals to self defer, rather than unknowingly donating blood that may be infected.

Is FDA's policy of excluding MSM blood donors discriminatory?

FDA's deferral policy is based on the documented increased risk of certain transfusion transmissible infections, such as HIV, associated with male-to-male sex and is not based on any judgment concerning the donor's sexual orientation.

Male-to-male sex has been associated with an increased risk of HIV infection at least since 1977. Surveillance data from the Centers for Disease Control and Prevention indicate that men who have sex with men and would be likely to donate have a HIV prevalence that is at present over 15-fold higher than the general population, and over 2000-fold higher than current repeat blood donors (i.e., those who have been negatively screened and tested) in the U.S. MSM continue to account for the largest number of people newly infected with HIV.

Men who have sex with men also have an increased risk of having other infections that can be transmitted to others by blood transfusion.

Are there other donors who have increased risks of HIV or other infections who, as a result, are also excluded from donating blood?

Intravenous drug abusers are excluded from giving blood because they have prevalence rates of HIV, HBV, HCV, and HTLV that are much higher than the general population. People who have received transplants of animal tissue or organs are excluded from giving blood because of the still largely unknown risks of transmitting unknown or emerging pathogens harbored by the animal donors. People who have recently traveled to or lived abroad in certain countries may be excluded because they are at risk for transmitting agents such as malaria or variant Creutzfeldt-Jakob disease (vCJD). People who have engaged in sex in return for money or drugs are also excluded because they are at increased risk for transmitting HIV and other blood-borne infections.

Isn't the HIV test accurate enough to identify all HIV-positive blood donors?

HIV tests currently in use are highly accurate, but still cannot detect HIV 100 percent of the time. It is estimated that the HIV risk from a unit of blood has been reduced to about one per 2 million in the U.S., almost exclusively from so called "window period" donations. The "window period" exists very early after infection, where even current HIV testing methods cannot detect all infections. During this time, a person is infected with HIV, but may not have made enough virus or developed enough antibodies to be detected by available tests. For this reason, a person could test negative, even when they are actually HIV positive and infectious. Therefore, blood donors are not only tested but are also asked questions about behaviors that increase their risk of HIV infection.

Collection of blood from persons with an increased risk of HIV infection also presents an added risk to transfusion recipients due to the possibility that blood may be accidentally given to a patient in error either before testing is completed or following a positive test. Such medical errors occur very rarely, but given that there are over 20 million transfusions every year, in the U.S., they can occur. For these reasons, FDA uses a multi-layered approach to blood safety including pre-donation deferral of potential donors based on risk behaviors and then screening of the donated blood with sensitive tests for infectious agents such as HIV-1, HIV-2, HCV, HBV, and HTLV-I/II.

Chapter 26

Protecting Yourself from Occupational Exposure to HIV: Advice for Health Care Workers

How can HIV be transmitted?

Blood, semen, vaginal secretions, vomitus, breast milk, or pus from a person who is infected with HIV (human immunodeficiency virus) may contain HIV and may cause infection. The risk of acquiring HIV from a needlestick injury is less than 1 percent, and the risk of infection from exposure not involving a puncture or a cut (such as a splash of body fluid onto the skin or the mucous membrane) is less than 0.1 percent. The risk of HIV infection from a human bite is between 0.1 percent and 1 percent.

"Clear" body fluids such as tears, saliva, sweat, and urine contain little or no virus and do not transmit HIV unless they are contaminated with blood.

What should I do if I think I have been exposed?

If a skin puncture has occurred, induce bleeding at the puncture site by applying gentle pressure as you wash the area with soap and water. If skin or mucous membranes have been splashed by body fluid, immediately rinse the area thoroughly with water.

Get the name, address, and phone number of the source person (patient) and the name, address, and phone number of the source person's attending physician. If you do not know the patient's HIV status, ask the attending physician to help. If you are at work, notify your supervisor. Do not spend time now on details of how or why the exposure happened. There will be time for this later.

When do I first need to get medical care?

Seek immediate assessment and treatment from your employee health unit, your private physician, or the emergency department. If anti-HIV medication is indicated, it should be taken as soon as possible. If you have a skin puncture or cut, you might need a tetanus toxoid booster, depending on the nature of the injury. Your physician will need to ask questions about the incident and other details in order to determine what treatment, if any, is necessary.

What details will I need to give my physician?

For a puncture injury: Is it a deep or surface puncture? If the puncture was caused by a needle, what gauge was the needle? Was the needle solid (suturing) or hollow? Could you see blood or bloody material on the surface of the needle or scalpel? Was the device previously in contact with patient's body fluids? If blood was injected into you, how much? Were you wearing protective gloves?

For a skin or mucous membrane splash: Were you exposed to blood or other body fluid? How much? On what part of the body were you exposed? What size was the area of contact? What was the length of contact time? Was there a break in the skin? A rash? A bite? Were you wearing protection (e.g., gloves, eyeglasses)?

What will my physician need to know about the source person?

The HIV status of the source person: If the source person is HIV negative, he or she could be infected but may not yet have positive HIV tests (he or she may be in the "window" period). Will he or she agree to be tested or retested for HIV infection?

If the source person is HIV positive, does he or she have AIDS? Has the source person taken anti-HIV therapy? If so, what medications is he or she taking? Is he or she at the end stage of the disease (with a high quantity of virus in his or her blood and body fluids)?

If the source person will not agree to HIV testing, whether he or she is in a high-risk HIV group: Is the person an intravenous drug user or the sexual partner of an intravenous drug user, a bisexual or homosexual male, and/or a person with multiple partners? Did he or she receive a blood transfusion between 1980 and 1985? Has he or she received a blood transfusion recently?

What will I need to tell my physician about myself?

Information about any medical conditions, medications, and allergies: Have you been exposed to HIV before? If so, when? How? Are you pregnant? Are you breastfeeding? Are you sexually active?

Whether you will agree to testing: Will you agree to confidential testing in order to document seroconversion (in the rare event of HIV transmission by occupational exposure)?

Should I receive post-exposure HIV prophylaxis?

Based on answers to the questions above, your physician may advise you to take medication to reduce your risk of developing HIV. Your doctor may also give medicine to protect you against hepatitis and syphilis. You will need baseline blood work, especially for evaluation of bone marrow, liver, and kidney function. These tests will be repeated during the course of therapy.

Does prophylactic treatment work?

Early post-exposure prophylaxis can reduce the risk of HIV infection ten-fold. Even if infection occurs despite prophylaxis, early suppression of the virus can lower the "set point" for viral load and slow the course of HIV disease substantially.

Does the treatment have side effects?

Some of the medicines used can cause side effects. For example, zidovudine (brand names: AZT; Retrovir) may cause headache, fatigue, insomnia, and gastrointestinal symptoms (nausea, diarrhea, abdominal discomfort). In rare instances, lamivudine (brand name: Epivir) may cause pancreatitis and gastrointestinal symptoms. Indinavir (brand name: Crixivan) and saquinavir (brand name: Invirase) may cause gastrointestinal upset and diarrhea. Indinavir has also been associated with kidney stones. Two quarts of fluid should be taken daily to reduce this risk.

How can I protect others from possible exposure to HIV?

Until HIV infection is ruled out, you should avoid the exchange of body fluids during sex, postpone pregnancy, and refrain from blood or organ donation. If you are breastfeeding, your baby's doctor may ask you to switch to formula feeding.

When should I be retested for HIV?

HIV testing may be repeated at six weeks, three months, and six months. Nearly all people found to be negative at three months are confirmed to be uninfected. However, the Centers for Disease Control and Prevention recommend retesting up to six months following the last possible exposure. If you have not formed antibodies to HIV by six months, then infection did not occur. Until then, you should report and seek medical evaluation if you have any acute illness. An acute illness, especially if accompanied by fever, rash, or swollen lymph nodes, may be a sign of HIV infection or another medical condition.

How can I cope with my feelings?

It is natural to feel anger, self-recrimination, fear, and depression after occupational exposure to HIV. During the difficult time of prevention therapy and waiting, you may want to seek support from employee-assistance programs or local mental health professionals.

Chapter 27

Prevention through Biomedical Advances and Research

Chapter Contents

Section 27.1

Adult Male Circumcision and Risk for HIV Transmission

Excerpted from "CDC HIV/AIDS Science Facts: Male Circumcision and Risk for HIV Transmission: Implications for the United States," Centers for Disease Control and Prevention (CDC), March 2007. The complete text of this document, including references, is available online at http://www.cdc.gov/hiv/resources/factsheets/PDF/circumcision.pdf.

What Is Male Circumcision?

Male circumcision is the surgical removal of some or all of the foreskin (or prepuce) from the penis.

Male Circumcision and Risk for HIV Transmission

Biologic Plausibility

Compared to the dry external skin surface, the inner mucosa of the foreskin has less keratinization (deposition of fibrous protein), a higher density of target cells for HIV infection (Langerhans cells), and is more susceptible to HIV infection in laboratory studies. It has also been argued that the foreskin may have greater susceptibility to traumatic epithelial disruptions (tears) during intercourse, providing a portal of entry for pathogens, including HIV. In addition, the microenvironment in the preputial sac between the unretracted foreskin and the glans penis may be conducive to viral survival. Finally, the higher rates of sexually transmitted genital ulcerative disease, such as syphilis, observed in uncircumcised men may also increase susceptibility to HIV infection.

International Observational Studies

Multiple cross-sectional, prospective, and ecologic (population-level) studies have identified lack of male circumcision as a risk factor for HIV infection.

A systematic review and meta-analysis that focused on hetero-sexual transmission of HIV in Africa was published in 2000. It included 19 cross-sectional studies, five case-control studies, three cohort studies, and one partner study. A substantial protective effect of male circumcision on risk for HIV infection was noted, along with reduced risk for genital ulcer disease. After adjusting for confounding factors in the population-based studies, the relative risk for HIV infection was 44 percent lower in circumcised men. The strongest association was seen in high-risk men, such as patients at sexually transmitted disease (STD) clinics, for whom the adjusted relative risk was 71 percent lower for circumcised men.

A review that included stringent assessment of ten potential confounding factors and was stratified by study type or study population was published in 2004. Most of the studies were from Africa. Of the 35 observational studies included in the review, the 16 in the general population had inconsistent results. The one large prospective cohort study in this group showed a significant protective effect, with the odds of infection being 42 percent lower in circumcised men. The remaining 19 studies were conducted in high-risk populations. These found a consistent, substantial protective effect, which increased with adjustment for confounding. Four of these were cohort studies: all demonstrated a protective effect, with two being statistically significant.

Ecologic studies also indicate a strong association between lack of male circumcision and HIV infection at the population level. Although links between circumcision, culture, religion, and risk behavior may account for some of the differences in HIV infection prevalence, the countries in Africa and Asia with prevalence of male circumcision of less than 20 percent have HIV-infection prevalences several times higher than countries in those regions where more than 80 percent of men are circumcised.

International Clinical Trials

Three randomized, controlled clinical trials have been undertaken in Africa to determine whether circumcision of adult males will reduce their risk for HIV infection. The study conducted in South Africa, was stopped in 2005 and those in Kenya and Uganda were stopped in 2006 after their interim analyses found that medical circumcision reduced male participant's risk of HIV infection.

In these studies, men who had been randomly assigned to the circumcision group had a 60 percent (South Africa), 53 percent (Kenya), and 51 percent (Uganda) lower incidence of HIV infection compared

201

to men assigned to the wait list group to be circumcised at the end of the study. In all three studies, a few men who had been assigned to be circumcised did not undergo the procedure, and vice versa. When the data were reanalyzed to account for these deviations, men who had been circumcised had a 76 percent (South Africa), 60 percent (Kenya), and 55 percent reduction in risk of HIV infection compared to those who were not circumcised. The Uganda study investigators are also examining the following in an ongoing study: 1) safety and acceptability of male circumcision in HIV-infected men and men of unknown HIV-infection status, 2) safety and acceptability of male circumcision in the men's female sex partners, and 3) effect of male circumcision on male-to-female transmission of HIV and other STDs.

Male Circumcision and Male-to-Female Transmission of HIV

In an earlier study of couples in Uganda in which the male partner was HIV infected and the female partner was initially HIV seronegative, the infection rates of the female partners differed by the circumcision status and viral load of the male partners. If the male blood HIV viral load was less than 50,000 copies/ml, there was no HIV transmission if the man was circumcised, compared to a rate of 9.6 per 100 person-years if the man was uncircumcised. If viral load was not controlled for, there was a non-statistically significant trend towards a reduction in the male-to-female transmission rate from circumcised men compared to uncircumcised men. Such an effect may be due to decreased viral shedding from circumcised men or to a reduction in ulcerative sexually transmitted infections acquired by female partners of circumcised men.

HIV Infection and Male Circumcision in the United States

Data on circumcision and risk for HIV infection in the U.S. are limited. In one cross-sectional survey of MSM, lack of circumcision was associated with two-fold increased odds of prevalent HIV infection. In another, prospective study of MSM, lack of circumcision was also associated with a two-fold increased risk for HIV seroconversion. In both studies, the results were statistically significant and controlled statistically for other possible risk factors. In one prospective study of heterosexual men attending an urban STD clinic, when controlling for other risk factors, uncircumcised men had a 3.5-fold higher risk of HIV infection than men who were circumcised. However, this association was not statistically significant.

Status of Male Circumcision in the United States

In a national probability sample of adults in 1992, the National Health and Social Life Survey found that 77 percent of men reported being circumcised including 81 percent of white men, 65 percent of black men, and 54 percent of Hispanic men. It is important to note that reported circumcision status may be subject to misclassification. In a study of adolescents, only 69 percent of circumcised and 65 percent of uncircumcised young men correctly identified their circumcision status as verified by physical exam.

According to the National Hospital Discharge Survey (NHDS), 65 percent of newborns were circumcised in 1999 and the overall proportion of newborns circumcised was stable from 1979 to 1999. Notably, the proportion of black newborns circumcised rose over this reporting period (58 percent to 64 percent), while the proportion of white infants circumcised remained stable (66 percent). In addition, the proportion of newborns who were circumcised in the Midwest increased over the 20-year period from 74 percent in 1979 to 81 percent in 1999, while the proportion of infants born in the West who were circumcised decreased from 64 percent in 1979 to 37 percent in 1999. In another survey, the National Inpatient Sample (NIS), circumcision rates increased from 48 percent during 1988–1991 to 61 percent during 1997–2000. Circumcision was more common among newborns born to families of higher socioeconomic status, in the Northeast or Midwest, and who were black.

In 1999, the American Academy of Pediatrics (AAP) changed from routinely recommending circumcision to a neutral stance on circumcision, noting that: "It is legitimate for the parents to take into account cultural, religious, and ethnic traditions, in addition to medical factors, when making this choice." This position was reaffirmed by the Academy in 2005. This change in policy may influence reimbursement for and practice of neonatal circumcision. In a 1995 review, 61 percent of circumcisions were paid by private insurance, 36 percent were paid for by Medicaid, and 3 percent were self-paid by the parents of the infant. Since 1999, 16 states have eliminated Medicaid payments or circumcisions that were not deemed medically necessary.

Considerations for the United States

There are a number of important differences that must be considered in the possible role of male circumcision in HIV prevention in the U.S. Notably, the overall risk of HIV infection is considerably lower in the United States, changing risk-benefit and cost-effectiveness considerations. Also, studies to date have focused on heterosexual, penile-vaginal sex, the predominant mode of HIV transmission in Africa, while the predominant mode of sexual HIV transmission in the United States is by penile-anal sex among MSM. In addition, while the prevalence of circumcision may be somewhat lower in racial and ethnic groups with higher rates of HIV infection, most Americans are already circumcised, and it is not known if men at higher risk for HIV infection would be willing to be circumcised, nor if parents would be willing to have their infants circumcised to reduce possible future HIV infection risk. Lastly, whether the effect of male circumcision differs by HIV-1 subtype, predominately subtype B in the U.S. and subtypes A, C, and D in Africa, is also unknown.

Summary

Male circumcision has been associated with a lower risk for HIV infection in international observational studies and in three randomized, controlled clinical trials. Male circumcision could also reduce male-to-female transmission of HIV to a lesser extent. It has also been associated with a number of other health benefits. While there are risks to male circumcision, serious complications are rare. Accordingly, male circumcision, together with other prevention interventions, may play an important role in HIV prevention in settings similar to the clinical trials.

Male circumcision may also have a role for the prevention of HIV transmission in the United States. With the results of three clinical trials showing that male circumcision decreases the risk for HIV infection, CDC is undertaking additional research and consultation to evaluate the potential value, risks, and feasibility of circumcision as an HIV prevention intervention in the U.S.

As CDC proceeds with the development of public health recommendations for the U.S., individual men may wish to consider circumcision as an additional HIV prevention measure, but must recognize that circumcision: 1) does carry risks and costs that must be considered in addition to potential benefits; 2) has only proven effective in reducing the risk of infection through insertive vaginal sex; and 3) confers only partial protection and should be considered only in conjunction with other proven prevention measures (abstinence, mutual monogamy, reducing number of sex partners, and correct and consistent condom use).

Section 27.2

Preventive HIV Vaccines

National Institute of Allergies and Infectious Diseases (NIAID), a component of the National Institutes of Health (NIH), May 2006.

What is a vaccine?

A vaccine is a medical product designed to stimulate your body's immune system in order to prevent or control an infection. An effective preventive vaccine trains your immune system to fight off a particular microorganism so that it can't establish a serious infection or make you sick.

What is the difference between a preventive HIV vaccine and a therapeutic HIV vaccine?

Therapeutic HIV vaccines are designed to control HIV infection in people who are already HIV positive. Preventive HIV vaccines are designed to protect HIV negative people from becoming infected or getting sick. This text focuses on preventive HIV vaccines.

Although there is currently no vaccine to prevent HIV, researchers are developing and testing potential HIV vaccines. The goal is to develop a vaccine that can protect people from HIV infection, or at least lessen the chance of getting HIV or AIDS should a person be exposed to the virus.

How does a preventive vaccine work?

When your body encounters a microorganism, your immune system mounts an attack on the invader. After the microorganism is defeated, your immune system continues to "remember" how to quickly beat the invader should it try to infect you again.

A vaccine is designed to resemble a real microorganism. The vaccine trains your immune system to recognize and attack the real microorganism should you ever encounter it. If you've received an effective vaccine, your immune system will "remember" how to quickly attack and defeat a particular microorganism for many years.

Can an HIV vaccine give me HIV or AIDS?

The experimental HIV vaccines currently being studied in clinical trials do not contain any "real" HIV, and therefore cannot cause HIV or AIDS. However, some HIV vaccines in trials could prompt your body to produce antibodies against HIV. These HIV antibodies could cause you to test "positive" on a standard HIV test, even if you don't actually have HIV. New tests are being developed to distinguish between vaccinated and infected people. For more information about this issue, please visit http://www.hvtn.org/science/volunteerfaqs.html (click on "Will I test HIV positive as a result of the vaccine?").

What are the different types of vaccine?

There are three main types of vaccines that are being studied for the prevention of HIV infection and AIDS:

- Subunit vaccines, also known as "component" or "protein" vaccines, contain only individual parts of HIV, rather than the whole virus. Instead of collecting these parts from the virus itself, the HIV subunits are made in the laboratory using genetic engineering techniques. These man-made subunits alone—without the rest of the virus—can prompt the body to produce an anti-HIV immune response, although that response may be too weak to actually protect against future HIV infection.

- Recombinant vector vaccines take advantage of non-HIV viruses that either don't cause disease in humans or have been deliberately weakened so that they can't cause disease. These weakened (attenuated) viruses are used as vectors, or carriers, to deliver copies of HIV genes into the cells of the body. Once inside cells, the body uses the instructions carried in the copies of HIV genes to produce HIV proteins. As with subunit vaccines, these HIV proteins can stimulate an anti-HIV immune response. Most of the recombinant vector vaccines for HIV deliver several HIV genes (but not the complete set) and may therefore create a stronger immune response.

  Some of the virus vectors being studied for HIV vaccines include ALVAC (a canary pox virus), MVA (a type of cowpox virus), VEE (a virus that normally infects horses), and adenovirus 5 (a human virus that doesn't usually cause serious disease) based vectors.

- DNA vaccines also introduce HIV genes into the body. Unlike recombinant vector vaccines, DNA vaccines do not rely on a virus vector. Instead, "naked" DNA containing HIV genes is injected directly into the body. Cells take up this DNA and use it to produce HIV proteins. As with subunit and recombinant vector vaccines, the HIV proteins trigger the body to produce an immune response against HIV.

Again, none of these vaccines contain real HIV or anything else that could cause HIV infection or AIDS.

What is a prime-boost vaccination strategy?

A single type of HIV vaccine may be used alone, or it may be used in combination with another type of HIV vaccine. One approach to combined HIV vaccination is called the prime-boost strategy. In this approach, administration of one type of HIV vaccine (such as a DNA vaccine) is followed by later administration of a second type of HIV vaccine (such as a recombinant vector vaccine). The goal of this approach is to stimulate different parts of the immune system and enhance the body's overall immune response to HIV.

How can I participate in a vaccine clinical trial?

Clinical trial volunteers are tremendously important in the effort to develop a preventive HIV vaccine. To find an HIV vaccine trial near you, contact AIDSinfo toll-free at 800-448-0440 to speak to an Information Specialist, who will help you locate trials in your area. You can also locate research sites using the AIDSinfo Vaccine webpage at http://aidsinfo.nih.gov/Vaccines. On the left side of the screen, under "Preventive HIV Vaccine Trials," click "New and Recruiting Trials" for a complete list of currently recruiting preventive HIV vaccine studies.

Enrolling in a clinical trial isn't the only way to help the HIV vaccine effort—there are other ways to participate. Consider serving on an HIV vaccine Community Advisory Board. Get involved with outreach and community education programs. Lobby your elected officials to support HIV vaccine research and development. Or volunteer in other HIV/AIDS prevention, treatment, and support efforts—all are valuable ways to contribute.

For more information about HIV vaccines, contact your doctor or an AIDSinfo Health Information Specialist at 800-448-0440 or http://aidsinfo.nih.gov.

Section 27.3

Microbicides

"Microbicides," Fact Sheet 157, © 2007 AIDS InfoNet. Reprinted with permission. Fact sheets are regularly updated. Check http://www.aidsinfonet.org for the most recent information.

What Are Microbicides?

Microbicides are anti-HIV substances. They could reduce the risk of HIV infection during vaginal or rectal intercourse. No microbicides are available yet. However, with sufficient funding and demand, microbicides could be available by 2010.

They could be a very important part of global HIV prevention efforts. Currently, male and female condoms are the only tools we have for HIV prevention. However, many men object to wearing condoms. Many women do not feel they can demand, or even ask their male partners to use a condom. Currently, over 50 percent of new HIV infections worldwide occur in women.

The use of microbicides could be controlled by women. They could be applied before sex. They won't require male cooperation to use, the way male and female condoms do. Some might be products women can use without their partners' knowledge.

They will come in gels, foams, and creams. Some may take the form of a sponge or thin film that can be inserted with the fingers. Rings or diaphragms may also be inserted into the vagina to deliver microbicides. Microbicides can also be put in suppositories, small plugs of medication designed to melt at body temperature when placed in the vagina or rectum.

One study estimated that microbicide use could prevent about 2.5 million HIV infections within three years. This is based on a microbicide that only worked 60 percent of the time and was used by only 20 percent of women, in 73 low income countries. Microbicides may also protect women against some other sexually transmitted diseases, in addition to HIV.

Condoms are still the most effective method of preventing infection. Ideally, microbicides would be used along with condoms for added protection. But, for people whose partners won't use condoms, microbicides could offer a way of reducing HIV risk that can be used without a partner's participation.

Microbicides and Vaccines

Vaccines against HIV have gotten much more attention than microbicides in recent years. An effective vaccine would offer important advantages:

- It could be given to a large segment of the population at risk.

- It would be effective for several years.

- It would not depend on people remembering to use it.

Microbicides, on the other hand, depend on people remembering to use them correctly each time they have sex. Once developed, microbicides and vaccines would work together. Microbicides will put the power of prevention directly in women's hands.

After a period of optimism about the development of an HIV vaccine, research has slowed. The virus presents several obstacles to vaccine development. At this point it is not clear when a vaccine might become available. However, it is unlikely to be within the next ten years.

Microbicide research is further along. But microbicide research has also encountered setbacks. Nonoxynol-9 (N-9) is a spermicide that was tested as a microbicide. Research showed that frequent use of N-9 may actually increase the risk of HIV infection. It can damage the lining of the vagina or rectum, making it easier for HIV to get past the body's defenses. N-9 had to be discarded from the list of potential microbicides.

How Do Microbicides Work?

Microbicides could work in various ways:

- They could immobilize the virus.

- They could create a barrier between the virus and the cells of the vagina or rectum to block infection.

- They could prevent HIV from reproducing and establishing an infection after it has entered the body.

Some potential microbicides work in just one of the ways above and some combine two or more methods, to increase effectiveness.

How Many Microbicides Are Near Approval?

No anti-HIV microbicides are currently approved as safe and effective. However, many are being tested. These tests are going on around the world. Large-scale tests are going on mainly in Africa where the HIV rates are highest.

Four microbicides are in Phase III (final) testing. The microbicides closest to approval are Carraguard®, cellulose sulfate gel; PRO 2000 Gel, BufferGel and Savvy. Cellulose sulfate gel is also being studied as a contraceptive.

The Bottom Line

Microbicides are anti-HIV substances designed in various forms to provide additional protection against HIV. They are intended to be used as an additional prevention measure or in cases where a partner is not using condoms.

Dozens of potential microbicides are in various stages of research. Once available, they could help women and men protect themselves. Microbicides may be especially important for women in developing nations who are not always empowered to require partners to wear condoms.

For More Information

The Alliance for Microbicide Development (http://www.microbicide.org) keeps updated listings on microbicides in various stages of development and information on global clinical trials.

The Global Campaign for Microbicides (http://www.global-campaign.org) provides information about global microbicide advocacy efforts. It explains how people can become involved in making microbicides a reality as soon as possible.

Chapter 28

Stigma as a Barrier to HIV Prevention

Stigma Hampers Prevention

Stigma associated with HIV/AIDS continues to profoundly affect prevention efforts, leading people to deny risk, avoid testing, delay treatment, and suffer needlessly. While stigma's pernicious effects are perhaps most obvious in countries other than the U.S., where people may be shunned and physically harmed, stigma negatively affects Americans as well. It is found at the structural level, in the form of laws and regulations, as well as more explicitly at community and individual levels.

Homophobia continues to hamper prevention efforts at all levels: from the individual at risk or infected, who may deny his risk because of internal conflicts, to the broader culture, which delivers anti-gay messages, institutionalizes homophobia through structural mechanisms, such as laws that regulate intimate sexual behavior, and lags in its support of sensitive and honest prevention for gay and bisexual youth, young adults, and older men.

This chapter includes text from "Stigma Hampers Prevention" from *HIV Prevention Strategic Plan through 2005,* Centers for Disease Control and Prevention (http://www.cdc.gov), reviewed/modified April 20, 2007; and, "Stigma as a Barrier to HIV Prevention in the Rural Deep South," reprinted with permission from the Rural Center for AIDS/STD Prevention (RCAP), a joint project of Indiana University, Purdue University, and the University of Colorado, © 2005. The complete text of this document, including list of references, is available online at http://www.indiana.edu/~aids/074077_applied_health_final.pdf.

Stigma associated with addiction and illicit drug use also results in laws and other restrictions on effective prevention. Likewise, persistent social and institutional racism and gender and economic inequities stifle effective HIV prevention. For each of these groups at risk, stigma, stereotyping, and prejudice must be addressed for prevention to be most effective. Political leadership and will are necessary to address these underlying issues, so critical to prevention's success.

Vulnerable Populations Have Multiple Needs

At home and abroad, HIV continues to stalk our most vulnerable populations, people who are marginalized because of race or ethnicity, socioeconomic status, sexual orientation, age, or gender. For HIV/AIDS prevention to succeed, the special needs and life contexts of those populations must be sensitively addressed, by culturally competent programs and staff. Cultural competence must be demonstrated not only by intervention programs and staff, but also by surveillance staff, researchers (and their investigations), as well as by those delivering prevention services, care, and treatment programs to those who are HIV-infected.

Stigma as a Barrier to HIV Prevention in the Rural Deep South

Stigma has been associated with HIV/AIDS since the early 1980s when the U.S. public became aware of a new, fatal sexually-transmitted disease afflicting gay men and other risk groups. The characterization of gay men as vectors of this new disease was a rallying point for HIV prevention in the gay community during the 1980s, but also provided a framework for representing the "AIDS sufferer" in terms of social deviance. This stigma construct has been a potent barrier to HIV/STD prevention, especially in the rural South where conformity to social conservatism is highly valued, and where issues of race, gender, and social class have complicated care-seeking for all sexually transmitted diseases. The stigma context of the Deep South may be fueling the HIV/STD epidemics in the region, since these epidemics are more severe in the Southeast than in any other region of the United States.

How Should HIV-Related Stigma Be Defined?

HIV-positive persons became stigmatized as the result of widespread negative attitudes about people who engage in same-sex activity, injection drug use, or sexual promiscuity. As noted by P. Aggleton

(2002), HIV-related stigmatization is a process that also reinforces existing social inequalities based on race, gender, ethnicity, and sexual orientation. Aggleton's definition of HIV-related stigma distinguishes between the act of stereotyping (e.g., labeling gay men as "disease bearers"), and the act of discrimination (e.g., violence towards HIV-positive persons). There is also a difference between "enacted stigma" which concerns discrimination, prejudice, or blame for violating sexual norms, and "felt stigma" which involves the shame and guilt of being infected. Fear of being blamed for violating sexual norms (i.e., heterosexual monogamy) can lead to non-disclosure to sexual partners if someone is infected. These distinctions play out in culturally specific ways in what Kleinman (1999) describes as "the geography of blame." In the rural Deep South, this moral geography involves notions of sin and sexuality, such as HIV/AIDS being God's punishment for sexual deviance.

HIV/AIDS Is More Stigmatized in the Deep South

Social conservatism is more pronounced in the South compared to the rest of the nation. The measures of social conservatism in Table 28.1 offer a context for understanding stigma as a barrier to HIV prevention in Southern states.

STD-Related Stigma Promotes Feelings of Betrayal or Revenge

STD-related stigma manifests in negative attitudes or actions toward infected persons. In the Deep South, STD-related stigma has had a demonstrable effect on people's willingness to be treated for sexually-transmitted diseases, including HIV/AIDS. In a [2005] telephone survey in Alabama, over 50 percent of the respondents said they would delay seeking medical care for STDs because of stigma, and one-third would not seek treatment at all. Rural residents, especially if they were African American and church-going, were even more likely than others to say that they would avoid screening or treatment for STDs because of stigma. When it came to disclosing the names of sexual partners to health providers (a legal requirement for some infections), almost half of the respondents feared what this disclosure would do to their relationship, and almost one-third said they would refuse because of embarrassment. Almost all of the respondents said they would feel angry, betrayed, and embarrassed if they were infected with a STD. Some respondents would seek revenge against someone who infected them. This revenge typically takes the form of outing infecting partners to family and associates, which can be particularly damaging in small rural communities where people know one another and where stigma can be long-lasting.

Homophobia Is Especially Harmful in Rural Areas

Men in the rural Deep South fear being labeled as homosexual. This fear is more pronounced for African Americans, especially in rural communities where homophobia intersects with religiosity and with cultural constructions of a dominant heterosexual masculinity. Bisexually-active men may deny risky behavior or expect women partners to take responsibility for health checks, including for HIV/AIDS. Bisexually-active men fear being outed in rural communities for another reason—they may be shot and killed. Rural men are sometimes so fearful of being outed that they are publicly homophobic and join in harassing or outing other men. The impact of this stigma for HIV prevention in rural communities often leads bisexually-active men to engage in "sneaky sex" with other men, and to be difficult to reach for safer sex messages. The internet has enhanced the ability of rural, non-identified gay men to avoid being stigmatized in their communities and to seek sexual partners without being detected. However, this trend is not associated with men's greater willingness to use condoms for safer sex, but with desire to "hook up" in ways that avoid local scrutiny.

Table 28.1. Social conservatism and stigma measures for the South compared to all U.S. states

	South	United States
Political Conservatism		
Negative views on homosexuality	55 percent	50 percent
Punitive attitudes towards crime	67 percent	62 percent
Racial prejudice	56 percent	48 percent
Political conservatism	42 percent	35 percent
Religious Conservatism		
Church attendance	49 percent	38 percent
Youth in church weekly	43 percent	35 percent
Religious conservative	21 percent	19 percent
Pro life	10 percent	8 percent

Rural HIV-positive men are unlikely to disclose their diagnosis to women partners. HIV-positive African American men, in particular, are fearful that disclosure might result in being labeled homosexual or in being charged with a crime. This climate of non-disclosure increases the HIV risk of rural African American women whose access to male partners is limited by geography and by the pooling of infection in small or bounded populations. A [2005] study of women and HIV/AIDS in Alabama's Black Belt found that non-disclosing men in rural areas had infected a number of local women, including women who were related to each other. Despite these outbreaks, blame is placed on allegedly "dirty" or "promiscuous" women in relation to heterosexual HIV transmission, and cultural silences over same-sex activity make it almost impossible to counter the blame. This type of gender stigma not only deflects attention from same-sex activity as a likely mode of HIV transmission for African American men in the Deep South, but prevents African American women from knowing why they are being infected at a higher rate than other women.

STD-Related Stigma Is a Heavy Burden for African Americans

African Americans have higher STD/HIV rates than other ethnicities in the United States. This disparity has been reported to occur on a historical basis, with white physicians in the Deep South commonly labeling African Americans as "syphilis soaked" up until the mid-20th century. Several barriers to HIV prevention have occurred as a result of this racist history. The first is African Americans' deep distrust of the "white" health system. The second is the widespread belief among African Americans that official statistics on HIV/AIDS are biased against them. The third is African American men's perceptions that they are being unfairly pursued by the authorities for disease surveillance purposes. The fourth is that African Americans who live in impoverished rural areas lack equitable access to all forms of health care, including for STD/HIV. This barrier particularly occurs in racially segregated areas of the Deep South known as the Black Belt.

Attitudes towards African Americans as disease-ridden were the ideological basis of the Tuskegee Syphilis Study conducted from 1932–1972. In this study, approximately 400 syphilitic African American men in rural Alabama were enrolled without being treated for the disease, with 100 men dying of syphilis-related complications. This public health scandal not only invoked a deep distrust of the medical profession among African Americans, but led to widespread fears of HIV/AIDS being deliberately introduced to reduce the size of the black population. Such fears have been further fueled in recent years by public health warnings of an AIDS crisis in the African American community. In the wake of such warnings, African Americans in the rural Deep South often invoke the specter of a biased public health system, and are sometimes convinced that AIDS is a U.S. government plot to kill blacks. This distrust particularly involves men who are suspicious of the motives of public health workers and who are reluctant parties to partner notification for STDs and testing for HIV/AIDS.

Moral Geography Is a Stumbling Block to HIV Prevention Efforts

Religiosity is highly valued in the Deep South, especially in rural areas. A major stumbling block for HIV prevention, however, is that several church leaders have stated publicly that HIV-positive persons deserve their fate, and some state and local politicians have refused to fund HIV prevention and life-saving medications for infected persons on the basis of their "ungodly lifestyle." There have been numerous reports of church-based responses to HIV/AIDS being absent, inadequate, or condemning. (See reference list online for Fullilove and Fullilove 1999 and Morales and Fullilove 1992 for a discussion of these responses in the black church.)

Frequency of church attendance was positively associated with stigma in Lichtenstein, Hook, and Sharma's (2005) telephone survey. The results of the survey indicated that the most frequent churchgoers, especially in rural areas, were more likely than other respondents to be judgmental, and would be more likely to delay or avoid being treated for STDs. This moral geography also affects HIV prevention when high school students receive abstinence-only sex education and when at-risk persons are denied publicly-funded HIV prevention. The moral geography is further implicated when needle-exchange programs are prohibited, and when condom use is denigrated as a safer sex method.

STD Clinics Can Be Stigmatizing: Enter at Your Own Risk

STD clinics are often avoided because of stigma. Visibility at STD clinics in rural counties may be of such concern that clients travel to other counties for checkups or treatment, or they avoid seeking treatment altogether. A qualitative study found that residents of public housing that was adjacent to a county STD clinic engaged in "patient spotting" and gossiped about their sightings to neighbors. Non-clients have been reported to take snapshots of clients at rural STD clinics with their camera phones. Visibility is particularly damaging at health departments with separate STD clinics or with client sign-up sheets that are visible to the public. In order to avoid this type of stigma, symptomatic persons are sometimes likely to share medications or use herbal remedies, to douche, or to buy non-prescription medicines to treat STDs. None of these informal methods will cure infection, and disease complications or transmission to sexual partners can occur if medical treatment is not sought in a timely manner.

Being the recipient of free public health care is also stigmatizing. "Free care" for STDs was part of an expanded public health policy in the New Deal of the 1930s, when public health clinics were established in low-income, urban neighborhoods and in county health departments. An unintended consequence of this policy in the Deep South is that rural whites have been reluctant to seek treatment at what they consider to be "black" clinics. Clinic employees often mirror the moral attitudes of the community and have been known to discriminate against clients deemed promiscuous or immoral. One multi-site study of health department clinics in Alabama, Mississippi, South Carolina, and Tennessee found that the staff treated African American clients (the large majority) badly, and concluded that they have not learned the lessons of the Tuskegee Syphilis Study. Another study found that clients felt so stigmatized that they feared they would not receive adequate treatment. Other stigmatizing factors in relation to STD clinics in small communities include staff and clients knowing one another, and clients believing that employees divulge confidential personal information to friends and neighbors.

Summary

The topic of HIV prevention in the rural Deep South is so stigmatized that some state and local legislators have refused to fund HIV prevention efforts, many church and other leaders refuse to acknowledge the impact of the epidemic on their communities, and schools are prevented from teaching safer sex methods. As a result, STD services are hampered by pejorative labeling and by lack of funding. Progress towards HIV prevention in the Deep South has stalled, even as the epidemic is having a significant effect on rural communities. The outlook for HIV prevention in the rural Deep South is discouraging. Race, gender, and social inequalities are significant barriers to

HIV prevention, and the moral politics of the region are likely to stymie efforts to protect rural residents from HIV/AIDS in the foreseeable future.

—by Bronwen Lichtenstein, PhD, Department of Criminal Justice, University of Alabama, RCAP Visiting Research Fellow

Part Four

Screening, Diagnosis, and Treatment of HIV/AIDS

Chapter 29

HIV Testing in the United States

HIV testing is integral to HIV prevention, treatment, and care efforts. Knowledge of one's HIV status is important for preventing the spread of disease. Studies show that those who learn they are HIV positive modify their behavior to reduce the risk of HIV transmission.[1,2] Early knowledge of HIV status is also important for linking those with HIV to medical care and services that can reduce morbidity and mortality and improve quality of life.[1,3,4]

Testing Recommendations and Requirements

The U.S. Centers for Disease Control and Prevention (CDC) released revised recommendations for HIV testing in health care settings in 2006,[4] recommending routine HIV screening for all adults aged 13–64, and repeat screening at least annually for those at high risk. Screening should be voluntary, but opt-out—that is, the patient will be notified that the test will be performed and consent is inferred unless the patient declines (as is the case for most laboratory tests in health care settings) versus opt-in, where the test is offered to the patient, who must then explicitly consent to an HIV test, often in

"HIV Testing in the United States—Fact Sheet,"(#6094-05), The Henry J. Kaiser Family Foundation, © September 2006. This information was reprinted with permission from The Henry J. Kaiser Family Foundation. The Kaiser Family Foundation, based in Menlo Park, California, is a nonprofit, private operating foundation focusing on the major health care issues facing the nation and is not associated with Kaiser Permanente or Kaiser Industries.

writing. The CDC is expected to release new testing guidelines for non-clinical settings next year. Currently, the CDC recommends that all persons at high risk for HIV, regardless of setting, be tested routinely for HIV infection.[1] In a recent survey, approximately two-thirds of the U.S. public (65 percent) supported routine HIV testing; 27 percent said that HIV testing should be treated differently, including the need for written consent.[7]

HIV testing is mandatory in the U.S. in certain cases, including for: blood and organ donors;[8] military applicants and active duty personnel;[9] federal and state prison inmates under certain circumstances;[10,11] newborns in some states;[12] and immigrants (waivers for HIV-positive immigrants and visitors may be granted).[13]

Factors considered to increase risk for HIV include ever having:[14,15]

- had unprotected sex with someone who is infected with HIV;

- shared injection drug needles and syringes;

- had a sexually transmitted disease, like chlamydia or gonorrhea;

- received a blood transfusion/blood clotting factor between 1978 and 1985;

- had unprotected sex with anyone who falls into an above category.

Table 29.1. Key dates in history of HIV testing[5]

1981: First AIDS case reported

1984: Human immunodeficiency virus (HIV) identified

1985: First test for HIV licensed (ELISA)

1987: First Western blot blood test kit

1992: First rapid test

1994: First oral fluid test

1996: First home and urine tests

2002: First rapid test using finger prick

2003: Rapid finger prick test granted CLIA [Clinical Laboratory Improvement Amendments][6] waiver

2004: First rapid oral fluid test (also granted CLIA waiver)

2006: CDC releases new U.S. guidelines recommending routine HIV screening of all adults in health care settings[4]

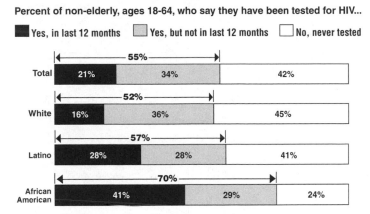

Figure 29.1. Percent non-elderly who report being tested by race/ethnicity, 2006.

Testing Statistics

- More than half (55 percent) of U.S. adults, ages 18–64, report ever having been tested for HIV, including 21 percent who report being tested in the last year. The share of the public saying they have been tested for HIV at some point has increased over time.[7]

- HIV testing rates vary by state, age, and race/ethnicity.[7,16,17,18] For example, African Americans and Latinos are significantly more likely to report having been tested for HIV than whites.[7] (See Figure 29.1.) Forty-one percent of African Americans report being tested in the last year alone.[7]

- Among the more than 1 million[19] people living with HIV/AIDS in the U.S., however, an estimated 25 percent do not know they are infected and knowledge of HIV status is even lower among some populations.[1,20]

- Among those who tested positive at CDC-funded sites in 2000, 31 percent did not return for their test results.[1]

- Many people with HIV are diagnosed late in their illness; in 2004, 39 percent received an AIDS diagnosis within one year of testing HIV positive.[21]

Table 29.2. HIV testing and reporting policies, June 2006[25]

State/Territory	Confidential/Anonymous	HIV Reporting Policy	State/Territory	Confidential/Anonymous	HIV Reporting Policy
Alabama	C	Name	New Hampshire	C, A	Name
Alaska	C, A	Name	New Jersey	C, A	Name
Arizona	C, A	Name	New Mexico	C, A	Name
Arkansas	C, A	Name	New York	C, A	Name
California	C, A	Name	North Carolina	C	Name
Colorado	C, A	Name	North Dakota	C	Name
Connecticut	C, A	Name	Ohio	C, A	Name
Delaware	C, A	Name	Oklahoma	C, A	Name
District of Columbia	C, A	Code	Oregon	C, A	Name
			Pennsylvania	C, A	Name
Florida	C, A	Name	Rhode Island	C, A	Code
Georgia	C, A	Name	South Carolina	C	Name
Hawaii	C, A	Code	South Dakota	C	Name
Idaho	C	Name	Tennessee	C	Name
Illinois	C, A	Name	Texas	C, A	Name
Indiana	C, A	Name	Utah	C, A	Name
Iowa	C	Name	Vermont	C, A	Code
Kansas	C, A	Name	Virginia	C, A	Name
Kentucky	C, A	Name	Washington	C, A	Name
Louisiana	C, A	Name	West Virginia	C, A	Name
Maine	C, A	Name	Wisconsin	C, A	Name
Maryland	C, A	Code	Wyoming	C, A	Name
Massachusetts	C, A	Code	American Samoa	C, A	Name
Michigan	C, A	Name			
Minnesota	C, A	Name	Guam	C, A	Name
Mississippi	C	Name	Northern Mariana Islands	C, A	Name
Missouri	C, A	Name			
Montana	C, A	Name-to-Code			
			Puerto Rico	C, A	Name
Nebraska	C, A	Name	U.S. Virgin Islands	C	Name
Nevada	C	Name			

- The public reports wanting more information about HIV testing including: the different types of HIV tests available (44 percent); how to protect privacy when getting tested (40 percent); and where to get tested (35 percent).[7] African Americans and Latinos are much more likely than whites to say they need these types of information.[7]

Testing Sites and Policies

- HIV testing is offered at CDC-publicly funded testing sites (approximately 11,600 in the U.S.) and in other public and private settings, including free-standing HIV counseling and testing centers, health departments, hospitals, private doctors offices, and STD clinics.[1,22] Most HIV testing is conducted in private doctors' offices.[7]

- Those testing positive for HIV are most likely to have been tested in hospital inpatient settings, followed by private doctors' offices/HMOs, and HIV counseling and testing sites.[23] Those at-risk are most likely to have been tested in private doctors' offices/HMOs or public health clinics.[24]

All states/territories now report HIV cases (in addition to already reporting AIDS cases). HIV reporting is done by name, name-to-code, or code. Most states have already moved to name reporting where a person's name is reported to the state if they are HIV positive (no name or other personally identifying information is reported to CDC; only clinical and basic demographic information are forwarded). As of June 2006, 49 jurisdictions had implemented name reporting; six used codes; and one used name-to-code.[25]

- An HIV test is either confidential or anonymous. With confidential testing, a person's name is recorded with their test result. With anonymous testing, no name is used. All states offer confidential testing but not all offer anonymous testing. As of June 2006, 11 states offered only confidential testing.[25] In those states, a person's name will be reported to the state if they test positive.

Testing Techniques

HIV tests used for screening detect the presence of antibodies produced by the body to fight HIV infection.[26] Detectable antibodies usually develop within three months of infection, but may take longer.[3,15] There are several kinds of HIV tests available in the U.S. They differ based on the type of specimen tested (e.g., whole blood, serum, or plasma; oral fluid; urine); how the specimen is collected (e.g., blood draw/venipuncture, finger prick, oral swab); where the test is done (e.g., laboratory, point-of-care site); and how quickly results are available (conventional or rapid).[1,3,27] The main types of tests are:

- **Conventional blood test:** Blood sample drawn by health care provider; tested at lab. Results: a few days to two weeks.

- **Conventional oral fluid test:** Oral fluid sample collected by health care provider, who swabs inside of mouth; tested at lab. Results: a few days to two weeks. OraSure is the only FDA-approved HIV oral fluid test.

- **Rapid tests:**[27] Sample collected by health care provider at lab or care site, depending on complexity of rapid test. Results: available in as little as ten minutes. If test is negative, no further testing is needed. If positive, test must be confirmed with a more specific test through conventional method. There are four FDA-approved rapid tests: OraQuick Advance Rapid HIV-1/2 Antibody Test (whole blood finger prick or venipuncture, plasma, oral fluid); Reveal Rapid HIV-1 Antibody Test (serum, plasma); Uni-Gold Recombigen HIV Test (whole blood finger prick or venipuncture, serum, plasma); and Multispot HIV-1/HIV-2 Rapid Test (serum, plasma). OraQuick and Uni-Gold have been granted Clinical Laboratory Improvement Amendments (CLIA) waivers for their whole blood rapid tests, which allow them to be performed by persons without formal laboratory training and outside traditional laboratories. OraQuick also has a CLIA-waiver for its oral fluid rapid test. Both OraQuick and UniGold are pursuing over-the-counter (home use) indication for rapid testing with the FDA.[28]

- **Home tests:** Individual performs test by pricking their finger with special device, placing drops of blood on treated card, and mailing to lab for testing. Identification number on card is used when phoning for results; counseling and referral available by phone. Results: in as little as three days. HomeAccess, the only home HIV test currently approved by the FDA, may be purchased from many drug stores and online.

- **Urine test:** Urine sample collected by health care provider; tested at lab. Calypte is the only FDA-approved HIV urine test. Results: a few days to two weeks.

References

1. CDC, *MMWR,* Volume 52, Number 15, 2003.

2. Marks G, et al., "Meta-analysis of High-Risk Sexual Behavior in Persons Aware and Unaware They are Infected with HIV in the United States: Implications for HIV Prevention Programs." *JAIDS*, Volume 39, Number 4, 2005.

3. CDC, *MMWR,* Volume 50, Number RR19, 2001.

4. CDC, *MMWR,* "Revised Recommendations for HIV Testing of Adults, Adolescents, and Pregnant Women in Health Care Settings," September 2006.

5. Kaiser Family Foundation, Global HIV/AIDS Timeline, www.kkff.org/hivaids/timeline.

6. Clinical Laboratory Improvement Amendments (CLIA) waiver.

7. Kaiser Family Foundation, Survey of Americans on HIV/AIDS, 2006.

8. FDA, "Recommendations for the Prevention of Human Immunodeficiency Virus (HIV) Transmission by Blood and Blood Products," 1992.

9. U.S. DOD, May 21, 2004. www.defense.gov/news/May2004/n05212004_200405211.html.

10. U.S. Federal Bureau of Prisons, Legal Resource Guide to the Federal Bureau of Prisons, 2004.

11. DOJ Bureau of Justice Statistics, HIV in Prisons, 2000. Revised 2/24/003.

12. CDC, *MMWR,* Volume 51, Number 45, 2002.

13. U.S. Citizenship and Immigration Services, http://uscis.gov/graphics/Medical_Exam.htm#needed.

14. CDC, HIV and AIDS: Are You at Risk? 2003.

15. www.hivtest.org.

16. CDC, *MMWR,* Volume 52, Number 23, 2003.

17. CDC, Behavioral Risk Factor Surveillance System, www.ccdc.gov/brfss/index.htm.

18. CDC, *MMWR*, Volume 50, Number 47, 2001.

19. Glynn K, Rhodes P, "Estimated HIV Prevalence in the United States at the End of 2003," 2005 National HIV Prevention Conference, June 2005.

20. CDC, *MMWR*, Volume 54, Number 24, 2005.

21. CDC, HIV/AIDS Surveillance Report, Volume 16, 2005.

22. CDC, HIV Counseling and Testing in Publicly Funded Sites, Annual Report, 1997 and 1998, 2001.

23. Kates J, et al., Poster TuPeG 5690, XIV International AIDS Conference, 2002.

24. CDC, "HIV Testing Survey, 2002," HIV/AIDS Special Surveillance Report Number 5, 2004.

25. CDC, Current Status of HIV Infection Surveillance, as of June 2006.

26. There are also HIV tests that can detect HIV before the development of antibodies, but these are not used as general screening tools.

27. Greenwald JL, et al., A Rapid Review of Rapid HIV Antibody Tests, *Current Infectious Disease Reports*, Volume 8, Number 2, 2006.

28. FDA, www.fda.gov/oashi/aids/advisorycom.html#110305.

Chapter 30

Questions and Answers about Voluntary HIV Screening in Health Care Settings

Why should I be tested for HIV?

Centers for Disease Control and Prevention (CDC) believes that everyone should know whether or not they are infected with HIV because there are important health benefits to this knowledge. If you are HIV negative, you can take steps to make sure you stay that way. If you find you are infected with HIV, you can get treatment that can greatly improve your health and extend your life.

If you have HIV, you can also take precautions to protect your partners. Most people who find out they are HIV infected change their behaviors in order to reduce the chance of passing the virus on to others.

Whatever the outcome of your HIV test, knowing your HIV status is valuable information.

How often should I be tested for HIV?

How often you should get an HIV test depends on your circumstances. If you have never been tested for HIV, you should be tested at least once. CDC recommends being tested at least once a year if you do things that can transmit HIV infection. These include the following:

"Questions and Answers for the General Public: Revised Recommendations for HIV Testing of Adults, Adolescents, and Pregnant Women in Healthcare Settings," Centers for Disease Control and Prevention (http://www.cdc.gov), reviewed September 22, 2006.

- injecting drugs or steroids with used injection equipment
- having sex for money or drugs
- having sex with an HIV-infected person
- having more than one sex partner since your last HIV test
- having a sex partner who has had other sex partners since your last HIV test

If you have been tested for HIV and the result is negative and you never do things that might transmit HIV infection, then you and your health care provider can decide whether you need to get tested again. Overall, you should talk to your doctor about how often to get tested for HIV.

Why is the CDC recommending teenagers as young as 13 get an HIV test?

Many teens (even those in high school) are sexually active, which puts them at risk for HIV infection. CDC's surveys of young people have found that almost 47 percent of high-school students reported having sexual intercourse at least once and 37 percent of sexually active students did not use a condom during their last act of sexual intercourse. Because teens may be reluctant to talk about sexual activity with their parents, HIV screening means adolescents can have an HIV test without having to admit whether they have been sexually active. The CDC recommendation for HIV screening does not mean that parents should not talk to their children about HIV. In fact, parents should talk with their children about HIV; parents have a big impact on the health choices their children make.

Starting HIV screening in adolescence offers the best way to raise awareness and develop healthy practices for HIV testing in addition to detecting HIV infection early.

I am over 50 years of age. Why should I be tested for HIV?

People age 50 and older make up 15 percent of new HIV cases. Many older people do not think they are at risk for HIV or other STDs. Doctors do not always address sex with their older patients and their older patients sometimes have limited knowledge about HIV. HIV screening for persons over 50 will not only raise awareness of HIV in older persons, but it will also find new infections in people who thought they were not at risk for HIV.

I have been in a long-term relationship with only one person. Why should I be tested for HIV?

Everyone should know for sure whether or not they have HIV. If you and your partner have been tested and are both HIV negative and you both remain faithful to each other (monogamous) and do not have other risks for HIV infection, then you probably won't need another HIV test unless your situation changes.

Why is CDC recommending HIV screening in medical settings?

CDC believes that voluntary screening for HIV in health care settings can do the following:

- help more people find out if they have HIV
- help those infected with HIV find out earlier, when treatment works best
- further decrease the number of babies born with HIV
- reduce stigma associated with HIV testing
- enable those who are infected to take steps to protect the health of their partners

Experience has shown that HIV screening works. Universal screening of pregnant women for HIV, combined with the right medical care, contributed to the dramatic decrease in the number of babies born with HIV from a high of 1,650 babies in 1991 to fewer than 240 born in 2002.

CDC believes the number of new cases of HIV each year could be decreased up to 30 percent with voluntary HIV screening.

How did CDC develop these recommendations?

These recommendations are the result of a long and careful process that began in 1999 when the Institute of Medicine (IOM) recommended a national policy that all pregnant women should be tested for HIV unless they refuse testing (opt-out). IOM also recommended doing away with pretest counseling and with special written permission for HIV testing.

Between 1999 and 2006, many HIV-infected persons made visits to health care settings but were not tested for HIV. A series of studies

231

has concluded that widespread HIV screening in health care settings was cost effective. CDC proceeded to work with its many partners, such as health care providers, public health officials, persons living with HIV, researchers, community groups, and persons who care for HIV-infected people, to get advice for the recommendations.

Throughout the process, CDC has been committed to involving those most affected by the new recommendations to make sure the recommendations were ethical, fair, and would work.

Do other organizations support these new recommendations?

Yes. In 1999, the Institute of Medicine (IOM) recognized that routine testing and the end of in-depth pretest counseling and separate, written permission, were the best way to increase the number of pregnant women tested for HIV. Other organizations, such as the American Medical Association, the American Academy of HIV Medicine, the National Association of Community Health Centers, and the American Academy of Pediatrics support these new recommendations.

Is the cost of screening all adults, adolescents, and pregnant women for HIV worth the benefits of finding those with HIV (is it cost effective)?

Studies show that HIV screening is cost effective even in areas where there are not that many cases of HIV. For almost all areas, HIV screening is as cost effective as other routine screening programs for diseases such as colon cancer and breast cancer.

Will my test results become part of my medical records?

Yes. Your test results will become part of your medical records. It is important for your doctor or other health care provider to know whether you are infected in order to give you the best care.

How will my privacy be protected?

HIV test results fall under the same strict privacy rules as all of your medical information, including those for other sexually transmitted diseases (STD). Information about your HIV test cannot be released without your permission. If your test shows you are infected with HIV, this information will be reported to the state health department, like other STD results. After all personal information about you (name, address, etc.) is removed, this information, in turn, is forwarded to the CDC. CDC uses this information to keep track of HIV/AIDS in the United States and to direct funding and resources where they are needed the most. CDC does not share this information with anyone else, including insurance companies.

Will my test results be given to my insurance company?

Generally, testing laboratories are not required to share test results with insurance plans and can only share them with the "authorized person" who can be the patient and/or the individual or laboratory (i.e., referral testing) who ordered the test and is responsible for using the results. However, this may vary from state to state and between insurance plans. If you file insurance claims for treatment for HIV or AIDS, your insurance company will know you are infected with HIV.

Will my insurance company drop me if I've been tested for HIV?

An insurance company should not drop you for being tested for HIV. Companies should also not drop you if you are infected with HIV. Certain insurance plans have restrictions on what they will pay for, including pre-existing conditions, but they should not drop you for receiving an HIV test.

Will screening increase fear and anxiety surrounding HIV testing?

By making HIV testing part of routine care, CDC believes that fear and anxiety surrounding HIV testing will decrease. If health care providers test all of their patients, then no one is singled out. A negative HIV test result will not imply that you are at high risk, just that you were tested.

Who will pay for my HIV test?

If you have insurance coverage, your insurer may pay for an HIV test, if it is ordered as part of your routine medical care. Insurance companies usually pay for tests that are ordered as a routine part of medical care, unless they have included a specific provision related to that test. If you have a question about your coverage, please refer to your policy for details.

If your insurance will not pay for an HIV test, there are places where you can get an HIV test at a reduced cost or for free. Visit http://www.hivtest.org or call 800-CDC-INFO to find a testing site in your area. Your public health department or local community-based organizations may also provide that information.

Who will pay for my treatment if the test shows I have HIV?

If you have insurance, your insurer may pay for treatment. If you do not have insurance, or your insurer will not pay for treatment, there are government programs, such as Medicaid, Medicare, Ryan White Care Act treatment centers, and community health centers that may be able to assist if you meet their eligibility criteria (usually income and/or disability). CDC is working with its federal partners that oversee these programs to make sure that all people who need treatment can get it. Your health care provider or local public health department can direct you to HIV treatment programs.

Why should people no longer receive counseling?

CDC strongly believes in prevention counseling, but CDC also believes that such counseling does not have to be linked to HIV testing. For example, if you are visiting your doctor because of a risk related to HIV infection, such as drug abuse or symptoms of an STD, you should receive prevention counseling for HIV. If you are having a detailed physical, reproductive care, or family planning, you should receive HIV counseling as a routine part of care. However, you do not need prevention counseling simply because you are getting an HIV test. One of the purposes of CDC's Revised Recommendations for HIV Testing in Health Care Settings is to reduce or end barriers to testing. Doctors and other health care workers have said that prevention counseling can be a barrier to testing. CDC has seen that when counseling is required with testing in medical care settings, most patients get neither.

Why is CDC recommending the end of a separate, written permission (consent) for an HIV test?

CDC believes HIV testing can be covered under a general permission form (consent form) that is signed for all medical care. CDC's recommendation to end separate, written permission for HIV testing does not mean that CDC encourages testing people without their permission. CDC believes that all HIV testing should be voluntary and only done with the patient's knowledge and agreement.

Is CDC recommending mandatory testing?

No. CDC is recommending voluntary HIV screening. The right to refuse an HIV test is called "opt-out." This means that the patient will be informed that the test will be performed and may choose not to have it.

Will people be tested for HIV without their knowledge or consent?

No one should be tested without their knowledge. Everyone will have the opportunity to refuse HIV testing (opt-out). No one should ever be tested for HIV without their knowledge and permission. The definition of opt-out testing included in the Recommendations clearly states that the HIV test will be given after the patient has been told that the test will be performed and that the patient may decline testing.

Can I choose not to be tested?

Yes. Your health care provider may want to know why you do not want to be tested, but you have the right to refuse any medical screening test, including an HIV test.

Chapter 31

Diagnostic Tests for HIV

Chapter Contents

Section 31.1

ELISA/Western Blot Blood Tests

"HIV ELISA/Western Blot" © 2007 A.D.A.M., Inc.
Reprinted with permission.

Definition

HIV ELISA/Western blot is a set of blood tests used in the diagnosis of chronic infection with human immunodeficiency virus (HIV). The HIV ELISA is a screening test for the diagnosis of HIV infection. If this test is positive, it must be confirmed with a second test called the Western blot, which is more specific and will confirm if someone is truly HIV positive (there are other conditions that may inaccurately produce a positive ELISA test result, including lupus, Lyme disease, and syphilis).

How the Test Is Performed

Blood is drawn from a vein on the inside of the elbow or the back of the hand. The puncture site is cleaned with antiseptic, and an elastic band is placed around the upper arm to apply pressure and restrict blood flow through the vein. This causes veins below the band to fill with blood.

A needle is inserted into the vein, and the blood is collected in an air-tight vial or a syringe. During the procedure, the band is removed to restore circulation. Once the blood has been collected, the needle is removed, and the puncture site is covered to stop any bleeding.

For an infant or young child: The area is cleansed with antiseptic and punctured with a sharp needle or a lancet. The blood may be collected in a pipette (small glass tube), on a slide, onto a test strip, or into a small container. Cotton or a bandage may be applied to the puncture site if there is any continued bleeding.

How to Prepare for the Test

No physical preparation is necessary. HIV testing requires written consent in most U.S. states. For infants and children: The preparation you can provide for this test depends on your child's age and experience.

How the Test Will Feel

When the needle is inserted to draw blood, some people feel moderate pain, while others feel only a prick or stinging sensation. Afterward, there may be some throbbing.

Why the Test Is Performed

Testing for HIV infection is performed and recommended for many reasons. Reasons for testing include screening in high-risk groups (men who have sex with men, injection drug users, commercial sex workers, etc.), screening in pregnant women (proper treatment can often prevent transmission of the virus to the fetus), and screening individuals with certain conditions and infections (such as Kaposi sarcoma, *Pneumocystis carinii* [also called *jiroveci*] pneumonia).

Normal Values

A negative test result is normal. However, early HIV infection (termed acute HIV infection or primary HIV infection) often results in a negative test.

What Abnormal Results Mean

The ELISA is used as a screening test. A positive result does not necessarily mean that the person has HIV infection. There are certain conditions that may lead to a false positive result, such as Lyme disease, syphilis, and lupus. A positive ELISA test is always followed by a confirmatory test termed Western blot. A positive Western blot is generally regarded as conclusive for an HIV infection.

Negative tests do not necessarily rule out HIV infection, because there is an interval (called the "window period") between HIV infection and the appearance of measurable anti-HIV antibodies. If a person is suspected of having acute or primary HIV infection, and of being in the "window period," a negative HIV ELISA and Western blot will not rule out HIV infection. Additional testing for HIV viral load will need to be performed.

What the Risks Are

The risks associated with having blood drawn are:

- excessive bleeding.

- fainting or feeling lightheaded.

- hematoma (blood accumulating under the skin).

- infection (a slight risk any time the skin is broken).

- multiple punctures to locate veins.

Special Considerations

Individuals at high risk (men who have sex with men, injection drug users, commercial sex workers, etc.) should be periodically tested for HIV.

If early (acute or primary HIV infection) is suspected, additional tests (HIV viral load) will be needed to confirm this diagnosis, as the HIV ELISA/Western blot will often be negative during this window period.

Section 31.2

The OraQuick Rapid HIV-1 Antibody Test

"Frequently Asked Questions about the OraQuick Rapid HIV-1 Antibody Test," Centers for Disease Control and Prevention (http://www.cdc.gov), reviewed January 22, 2007.

What is the OraQuick Rapid HIV-1 Antibody Test, and how is it performed?

The OraQuick Rapid HIV-1 Antibody Test checks for HIV-1, the virus that causes AIDS, in a person's blood. The test detects antibodies to HIV-1 found in blood specimens obtained by fingerstick or venipuncture. As is true of all HIV screening tests, a reactive test result needs to be confirmed by an additional, more specific test.

When testing a fingerstick specimen, the fingertip is cleaned with alcohol and pricked with a lancet (needle) to get a small drop of blood. The blood is collected with a specimen loop and transferred to a small plastic vial containing a premeasured volume of developing solution, into which the sample is mixed. The testing process is the same for a whole blood specimen obtained by venipuncture. The specimen loop is inserted into the tube of blood after the tube has been inverted to ensure the blood is well mixed. The loop is then inserted into the test vial. Results of the test can be read in as little as 20 minutes.

How well does the test work?

In the clinical studies by the manufacturer (OraSure Technologies, Inc.), the OraQuick test correctly identified 99.6 percent of people who were infected with HIV-1 (sensitivity) and 100 percent of people who were not infected with HIV-1 (specificity). The Food and Drug Administration expects clinical laboratories to obtain similar results.

What are the limitations of the test? Does this test always give a correct result?

The limitations of this test are similar to the limitations of other HIV antibody tests, including the following:

- **False-positive results:** Although no false-positive results were found in the clinical trial, statistical analysis of the data show that a very small number of people who are not infected with HIV-1 will have reactive test results (that is, tests that show HIV infection). As the test becomes widely used in outreach settings, false-positive results may occur. Reactive results should not be considered definitive until confirmatory testing has been done.

- **False-negative results:** A small number of people who are infected with HIV-1 will have negative test results.

- **Delayed detection of exposure:** OraQuick may not detect HIV-1 infection in people who were exposed within three months before being tested (it can take that long for antibodies to HIV-1 to be detectable in the blood).

- **Follow-up testing:** A reactive result is interpreted as preliminarily positive for HIV-1 infection. Another method should be used to confirm the initial test result.

Because of these limitations, all persons taking this test must receive counseling before being tested and after receiving their test results.

What type of counseling is provided to persons getting a rapid HIV test?

Counseling for rapid HIV tests includes the following:

- information about the importance of HIV testing

- ways to reduce the risk of becoming infected with HIV

- next steps for persons who have a reactive test result

- need for additional testing of persons whose rapid test result is negative but who have had a recent exposure to HIV

The Centers for Disease Control and Prevention (CDC) recently released revised guidelines for HIV counseling and testing. These guidelines include information about post-test counseling for persons tested with rapid HIV tests. The counseling includes information about HIV testing and its importance, as well as specific counseling to help reduce risks for HIV infection. A very important part of counseling persons who have a reactive rapid HIV test result is to make sure they understand that the test result is preliminary and that further testing must be done to confirm the result. Persons who have a negative rapid test result but have had a recent exposure to HIV are counseled to get another test at least three months after the possible exposure to account for the possibility of a false-negative test result. For more information on rapid testing, go to CDC's rapid testing website at: http://www.cdc.gov/hiv/rapid_testing.

Does this test detect antibodies to HIV-2?

The test is approved to detect antibodies to HIV-1. Data on the test's sensitivity to detect antibodies to HIV-2 have not been reviewed, and the Food and Drug Administration has not approved the test for this purpose. Because HIV-2 is very rare in the United States, CDC does not recommend routine screening for HIV-2 at this time.

Are blood donors allowed to be screened by use of the OraQuick test?

No. This test is approved to help diagnose HIV infection, not to screen blood donors.

I heard the rapid test received a CLIA waiver. What does this mean?

CLIA refers to the Clinical Laboratory Improvements Amendments of 1988, which established standards for all laboratory testing to ensure the accuracy, reliability, and timeliness of test results regardless of where a test is performed.

The OraQuick Rapid HIV-1 Antibody Test was categorized as a waived test by the Food and Drug Administration on January 31, 2003. The OraQuick test is simple to use and accurate. Under the waived category, the OraQuick rapid test will face less strict federal controls and can be used at a larger number of clinical and nonclinical testing sites. This categorization will allow nonclinical testing sites to provide the test by applying for a CLIA certificate of waiver or agreeing to work under an organization that has a certificate of waiver. For tests categorized as waived, less stringent guidelines apply. However, before offering testing, an organization that has received a certificate of waiver must have a quality assurance plan and must provide training to ensure that the manufacturer's instructions are followed. For more information on the CLIA waived category and other CLIA categories, go to: http://www.phppo.cdc.gov/clia.

What needs to be done before a site is permitted to purchase and use the test?

Any site offering the rapid HIV test is considered a laboratory under the Clinical Laboratory Improvements Amendments (CLIA) and must meet certain quality assurance requirements before purchasing OraQuick. Under CLIA, a laboratory is defined as any facility that performs examinations, including the OraQuick rapid test, on humans. A facility can be a clinic or hospital with an onsite lab, a voluntary counseling and testing site, or an outreach setting. Only staff of clinical laboratories may use the test. All customers will receive a letter indicating that their purchase of OraQuick means that they agree to meet these requirements.

Any organization or group conducting the OraQuick rapid HIV test must do the following:

- have a CLIA certificate of waiver or be covered under an exception for multiple sites or public health use (The exceptions involve working with a main location that has a CLIA certificate of waiver.)

- ensure that persons administering the test follow the manufacturer's test instructions

- have a quality assurance plan to ensure that certain requirements, such as performing testing correctly and providing staff with appropriate instructional materials, will be met

- agree to allow inspections, announced and unannounced, by the federal Centers for Medicare and Medicaid Services

- follow HIV testing requirements or guidelines from the state health department

How can I obtain a certificate of waiver?

The CLIA program is administered by the federal Centers for Medicare and Medicaid Services. For information on obtaining a certificate of waiver, go to: http://www.cms.gov/clia.

What does it mean to have an "adequate quality assurance system"?

An adequate quality assurance system consists of planned activities to ensure that testing is carried out correctly and that test results are as accurate and reliable as possible for all persons tested. CDC's recommendations for quality assurance systems for rapid HIV testing—*Quality Assurance Guidelines for Testing Using the OraQuick Rapid HIV-1 Antibody Test*—are available at http://www.cdc.gov/hiv/rapid_testing.

Can waived tests be performed at nonclinical sites?

All testing sites, clinical and nonclinical (e.g., mobile vans, health fairs, community clinics, pharmacies) are subject to applicable state requirements. Conducting HIV testing by using the OraQuick Rapid HIV-1 Antibody Test, which is categorized as waived under the Clinical Laboratory Improvements Amendments (CLIA), will allow nonclinical testing sites to participate in HIV screening activities.

How much does the test cost?

The manufacturer and the laboratory performing the test determine the fee for the test.

Reference

Kelen GD, Shahan JB, Quinn TC. Emergency department–based HIV screening and counseling: experience with standard and rapid serologic testing. *Annals of Emergency Medicine* 1999; 33:147-155.

Section 31.3

Home Blood Tests for HIV-1

"Testing Yourself for HIV-1, the Virus that Causes AIDS,"
U.S. Food and Drug Administration (FDA), April 4, 2006.

AIDS is a serious disease that can be fatal. The U.S. Food and Drug Administration (FDA) regulates the tests that detect infection with human immunodeficiency virus-1 (HIV-1), a virus that causes AIDS. A list of FDA approved HIV tests is available on the FDA's Center for Biologics Evaluation and Research (CBER) website at: http://www.fda.gov/cber/products/testkits.htm.

Up until 1996, the only way to get tested for HIV was to be tested under a doctor's supervision. However, in 1996 FDA approved the first home collection HIV testing systems. At this time, only one HIV home collection test system is approved by FDA and legally sold in the United States. This test system, sold as either "The Home Access HIV-1 Test System" or "The Home Access Express HIV-1 Test System" is manufactured by Home Access Health Corporation and allows blood samples to be taken at home, which people then send to a laboratory for testing. This test system may be purchased on the internet.

Consumers should be aware that there are numerous HIV home testing systems that are marketed on the internet, in newspapers, and in magazines that are not FDA approved. These tests claim to detect antibodies to HIV in blood or saliva samples and provide results in the home in 15 minutes or less. The FDA has not approved these rapid HIV-1 home test kits for use and marketing in the United States. Some of these HIV home test kits falsely claim to be approved by the FDA or manufactured in an FDA approved/registered/licensed facility. The only approved HIV test collection system is the "Home Access HIV-1 Test System" manufactured by Home Access Health Corporation. If you are unsure if an HIV test is FDA approved, you can always look for the test on the list of FDA approved HIV tests (http://www.fda.gov/cber/products/testkits.htm).

FDA warned consumers about an unapproved, fraudulently marketed home-use HIV test system labeled "Lei-Home Access HIV test" distributed by Lei-Home Access Care located in Sunnyvale, California, in a press release issued on September 26, 1997. The "Lei-Home Access HIV test" was advertised on the internet as the "Personal HIV Test Kit" and was offered for sale through several Central Valley pharmacies. After an extensive investigation by FDA, the businessman responsible for distributing this fraudulent HIV test kit was sentenced to over five years in prison for selling the unapproved HIV test kits to consumers in the United States.

FDA has also warned consumers about unapproved HIV home test kits marketed by Globus Media (http://www.fda.gov/bbs/topics/ANSWERS/2005/ANS01340.html). These kits were sold over the internet and shipped via overnight delivery services. FDA has not reviewed the tests marketed by Globus Media. Without FDA review and approval, such tests are illegally distributed. Consumers are not assured of getting reliable test results.

CBER will work with FDA's Office of Regulatory Affairs and Office of Criminal Investigations in investigating firms and persons involved in the sale, distribution, and manufacture of unapproved HIV home test kits in the United States.

The following questions and answers may help to explain how HIV-1 home tests differ, and how to select a test that you can trust.

How many different home tests are available in the United States, and how do they work?

Only one HIV home collection test system is approved by FDA and legally sold in the United States. This test, sold as either "The Home Access HIV-1 Test System" or "The Home Access Express HIV-1 Test System" is manufactured by Home Access Health Corporation and allows blood samples to be taken at home, which people then send to a laboratory for testing. However, there are many non-FDA approved tests kits illegally marketed over the internet and in newspaper and magazine advertisements.

What is the difference between a test, a rapid test, test system, and a home-use test kit?

A test is the actual device used to determine whether a sample of blood or other body fluid is HIV positive or not. The sample may be collected in a doctor's office or other clinical setting and sent to a laboratory for analysis. Alternately, a consumer may use a home collection test system to collect a sample, which is then sent anonymously to a laboratory for testing. The consumer, still anonymous, is able to contact the testing facility to obtain their test results.

For a rapid test, a health care worker usually collects the sample. Instead of sending the sample to a laboratory, the test is run at the site where the sample is collected. Rapid tests can produce results within 20 minutes.

With all types of FDA approved testing, the consumer has access to trained health care workers who can help consumers understand their test results.

Home-use test kits are HIV tests kits that require consumers to collect the sample, run the test, and interpret the results. There are currently no FDA approved home-use test kits.

What is an HIV home collection test system and how does it work?

An HIV home collection test system, such as the Home Access test system, consists of multiple components, including materials for specimen collection, a mailing envelope to send the specimen to a laboratory for analysis, and pre- and post-test counseling.

This approved system uses a simple finger prick process for home blood collection which results in dried blood spots on special paper. The dried blood spots are mailed to a laboratory with a confidential and anonymous personal identification number (PIN), and analyzed by trained clinicians in a laboratory using the same tests that are used for samples taken in a doctor's office or clinic. Test results are obtained through a toll free telephone number using the PIN, and post-test counseling is provided by telephone when results are obtained.

How are unapproved test systems different?

The manufacturers of unapproved test systems have not submitted data to FDA to review to determine whether their test systems can reliably detect HIV infection or not. Therefore, FDA cannot give the public any assurance that the results obtained using an unapproved test system are accurate.

How reliable are test kits that are not FDA approved?

FDA cannot ensure the reliability of any test kit that has not undergone FDA review. Diagnostic testing depends on precise science. FDA approved tests have demonstrated that they are reliable. Tests that are not FDA approved have not demonstrated to FDA that they are reliable. Unapproved HIV home test kits do not come with any guarantee of the accuracy of the test. The kits do not train a home user on how to interpret results and they have not demonstrated that home users can use them without that training.

None of the unapproved tests has undergone the review required for FDA marketing approval. Although unapproved tests might be promoted as sensitive and reliable, the consumer has no assurance that test results are accurate.

Simply put, you just can't trust the results of an unapproved test to be correct. Users may get a positive result when they are, in fact, not infected (called a false positive). Or the test may indicate that users are not infected with the virus, when, in fact, they are (called a false negative). Both of these outcomes can have grave consequences in terms of mental anguish, delays in obtaining medical treatment, and transmission of the disease to additional persons.

FDA is unaware of any data to confirm the reliability or accuracy of unapproved HIV home test kits.

How reliable are approved HIV home collection test systems?

Very reliable. Manufacturers of approved test systems have demonstrated that the test system can accurately detect antibodies to the HIV virus that causes AIDS. Approved tests have also demonstrated and that they can detect even low levels of HIV antibodies.

Clinical studies have shown that the FDA approved HIV home collection test system is able to correctly identify 100 percent of known positive blood samples, and 99.5 percent of HIV negative blood samples.

What about counseling?

The approved HIV home collection test system has a built-in mechanism for pre- and post-test counseling provided by the manufacturer. This counseling is anonymous and confidential. Counseling, which uses both printed material and telephone interaction, provides the user with an interpretation of the test result. Counseling also provides information on how to keep from getting infected if you are negative, and how to prevent further transmission of disease if you are infected. Counseling provides you with information about treatment options if you are infected, and can even provide referrals to doctors who treat HIV-infected individuals in your area.

The unapproved HIV home test kits do not provide interactive counseling to help the user understand the test results, answer questions about the test or about HIV infection, or discuss options available to the user, such as medical follow-up.

Are approved HIV collection test systems really confidential?

Yes. The approved HIV home collection test system is confidential. It can be purchased at pharmacies or by mail order from the manufacturer. You mail in your specimen anonymously. Consumers obtain their test results by phone using a confidential code number that is unrelated to the identity of the consumer.

Although some states require testing labs to report new cases of HIV infection to the health department, with the approved test systems the testing lab can report only the number of cases detected with home test systems. The testing lab cannot report the name of the infected person, since the lab does not have that information. The identity of the user remains anonymous.

Is one test better than another?

FDA approved tests have demonstrated their reliability; unapproved tests have not been reviewed by FDA. Therefore, FDA cannot state that unapproved tests are reliable. Since the approved HIV home collection test system has been independently tested, validated, and approved by FDA, the consumer can feel confident that the approved HIV test system will provide accurate results available from an HIV home test. In addition, the user is provided with counseling and referrals if needed.

Are there other ways I can be tested for infection with HIV?

There are several kinds of tests available through your doctor or other trained health care professional to determine if you are infected with HIV, the virus that causes AIDS. In addition to blood tests, there are tests that use oral fluid, collected from between the cheek and gum of the mouth, and a urine test. All of these tests have been reviewed and approved by FDA.

If you are unsure if an HIV test is FDA approved, you can always look for the test on the list of FDA approved HIV tests (http://www.fda.gov/cber/products/testkits.htm). You can also contact the HIV/AIDS Program of FDA, in the Office of Special Health Issues for further information about this topic (http://www.fda.gov/oashi/home.html).

Section 31.4

HIV-1 RNA Qualitative Assay

"FDA News Release: FDA Approves Test to Help Diagnose
Main Virus that Causes AIDS," U.S. Food and Drug Administration
(FDA), October 5, 2006.

The U.S. Food and Drug Administration (FDA) has approved the
APTIMA HIV-1 RNA Qualitative Assay, manufactured by Gen-Probe
Incorporated (San Diego, CA). The APTIMA assay, which detects the
RNA—the nucleic acid or genetic material—of the HIV-1 virus, is the
first test approved for the detection of HIV-1 RNA to help diagnose
HIV-1 infection. HIV-1 is the main virus that causes AIDS.

"This product offers medical diagnostic laboratories the ability to
perform a gene-based test for HIV-1 that, until now, was only available as part of a larger kit used to screen blood and plasma donors,"
said Jay Epstein, MD, director, Office of Blood Research and Review,
Center for Biologics Evaluation and Research (CBER), FDA. "This test
also can detect infection with HIV-1 earlier than HIV antibody tests
when used to detect primary HIV-1 infection."

This test has important implications for medical diagnostic use
because it could be a potential alternative to the traditional Western
blot test now used for confirmation of HIV-1 infection when screening tests for HIV-1 antibodies are positive. In addition, the Western
blot can, in some instances, be difficult to interpret and may not always provide a conclusive result. In such cases, the APTIMA test may
be helpful in HIV-1 diagnosis. The APTIMA test can also be used in
clinical laboratories and public health facilities to detect early HIV-1
infection, before the appearance of antibodies to HIV-1.

The sensitivity of the APTIMA assay is comparable to that of FDA
approved viral load assays that measure the amount of HIV-1 virus
circulating in the blood of patients with established HIV-1 infection
to monitor the treatment and progression of AIDS. Unlike the viral
load tests, the APTIMA test has been approved for the diagnosis of
primary HIV-1 infection, as well as for confirming HIV-1 infection
when tests for antibodies to HIV-1 are positive.

CBER, one of six centers within FDA, is responsible for the regulation of biologically-derived products, including blood intended for transfusion, blood components and derivatives, vaccines and allergenic extracts, and cell, tissue, and gene therapy products. CBER also regulates AIDS-related diagnostic tests.

Section 31.5

P24 Antigen Test

What is being tested?

The p24 test identifies actual HIV viral particles in blood (p24 is a protein found in HIV). However, the p24 test is generally only positive from about one week to three–four weeks after infection with HIV. The p24 protein cannot be detected until about a week after infection with HIV because it generally takes that long for the virus to become established and multiply to sufficient numbers that they can be detected. The p24 proteins then become undetectable again after sufficient antibodies to HIV have been produced because they bind to the p24 protein and eliminate it from the blood. Once antibodies are produced, the p24 test will register negative even in people who are infected with HIV. At that point, the regular HIV antibody test will then be positive. Later in the course of HIV, p24 protein levels again become detectable.

How is the sample collected for testing?

The collection method depends on the type of test kit used. A blood sample can be collected by fingerstick or by drawing blood through a needle placed in a vein in your arm.

How is it used?

P24 testing may be used to detect early HIV infection and to screen donated blood for HIV. Since p24 levels rise and fall with HIV levels, the test may also be used to monitor anti-HIV therapy and to evaluate disease progression. The advantages of the p24 test are that it can detect HIV infection days earlier, before antibodies develop, and that it is a quantitative test that tells the intensity of HIV expression in the body, which is a measure of how fast the disease is progressing.

When is it ordered?

A p24 test may be ordered if you have been recently exposed to HIV and wish to know your HIV status. It may also be ordered if you are donating blood or if you already have HIV and your doctor wants to monitor your response to therapy or to determine if HIV is progressing into AIDS.

What does the test result mean?

A positive result means that you are infected with HIV: the more p24 protein, the higher the amount of HIV in your blood.

Is there anything else I should know?

The p24 test is one of the earlier tests developed to detect HIV infection. Because p24 is only detectable during a short window of time, its utility is limited. However, this test can still be used when other tests are unavailable.

Section 31.6

Viral Load Tests

What is viral load?

The viral load test measures the amount of HIV virus in your blood. There are different techniques for doing this:

- The PCR (polymerase chain reaction) method uses an enzyme to multiply the HIV in the blood sample. Then a chemical reaction marks the virus. The markers are measured and used to calculate the amount of virus. Roche and Abbott produce this type of test.

- The bDNA (branched DNA) method combines a material that gives off light with the sample. This material connects with the HIV particles. The amount of light is measured and converted to a viral count. Bayer produces this test.

- The NASBA (nucleic acid sequence based amplification) method amplifies viral proteins to derive a count. It is manufactured by bioMerieux.

Different test methods often give different results for the same sample. Because the tests are different, you should stick with the same kind of test (PCR or bDNA) to measure your viral load over time.

Viral loads are usually reported as copies of HIV in one milliliter of blood. The tests count up to about one million copies, and are always being improved to be more sensitive. The first bDNA test measured down to 10,000 copies. The second generation could detect as few as 500 copies. Now there are ultra sensitive tests for research that can detect less than five copies.

The best viral load test result is "undetectable." This does not mean that there is no virus in your blood; it just means that there is not enough for the test to find and count. With the first viral load tests, "undetectable" meant up to 9,999 copies! "Undetectable" depends on the sensitivity of the test used on your blood sample.

The first viral load tests all used frozen blood samples. Good results have been obtained using dried samples. This will reduce costs for freezers and shipping.

How is the test used?

The viral load test is helpful in several areas:

- For medical researchers, the test has been used to prove that HIV is never "latent" but is always multiplying. Many people with no symptoms of AIDS and high CD4 cell counts also had high viral loads. If the virus was latent, the test wouldn't have found any HIV in the blood.

- The test can be used for diagnosis, because it can detect a viral load a few days after HIV infection. This is better than the standard HIV (antibody) test, which can be "negative" for two to six months after HIV infection.

- For prognosis, viral load can help predict how long someone will stay healthy. The higher the viral load, the faster HIV disease progresses.

- For prevention, viral load predicts how easy it is to transmit HIV to someone else. The higher the viral load, the higher the risk of transmitting HIV.

- Finally, the viral load test is valuable for managing therapy, to see if antiretroviral drugs are controlling the virus. Current guidelines suggest measuring baseline (pre-treatment) viral load. A drug is "working" if it lowers viral load by at least 90 percent within eight weeks. The viral load should continue to drop to less than 50 copies within six months. The viral load should be measured within two to eight weeks after treatment is started or changed, and every three to four months after that.

How are changes in viral load measured?

Repeat tests of the same blood sample can give results that vary by a factor of three. This means that a meaningful change would be a drop to less than one-third or an increase to more than three times the previous test result. For example, a change from 200,000 to 600,000 is within the normal variability of the test. A drop from 50,000 to 10,000 would be significant. The most important change is to reach an undetectable viral load.

Viral load changes are often described as "log" changes. This refers to scientific notation, which uses powers of ten. For example, a two-log drop is a drop of 10^2 or 100 times. A drop from 60,000 to 600 would be a two-log drop.

Viral load "blips": Recently, researchers have noticed that the viral load of many patients sometimes went from undetectable to a low level (usually less than 500) and then returned to undetectable. Careful study suggests that these "blips" do not indicate that the virus is developing resistance.

What do the numbers mean?

There are no "magic" numbers for viral loads. We don't know how long you'll stay healthy with any particular viral load. All we know so far is that lower is better and seems to mean a longer, healthier life.

U.S. treatment guidelines suggest that anyone with a viral load over 100,000 should be offered treatment.

Some people may think that if their viral load is undetectable, they can't pass the HIV virus to another person. This is not true. There is no "safe" level of viral load. Although the risk is less, you can pass HIV to another person even if your viral load is undetectable.

Are there problems with the viral load test?

There are some concerns with the viral load test:

- Only about 2 percent of the HIV in your body is in the blood. The viral load test does not measure how much HIV is in body tissues like the lymph nodes, spleen, or brain. HIV levels in lymph tissue and semen go down when blood levels go down, but not at the same time or the same rate.

- The viral load test results can be thrown off if your body is fighting an infection, or if you have just received an immunization (like a flu shot). You should not have blood taken for a viral load test within four weeks of any infection or immunization.

Section 31.7

CD4 Cell Tests

"CD4 Cell Tests," Fact Sheet 124, © 2007 AIDS InfoNet. Reprinted with permission. Fact sheets are regularly updated. Check http://www.aidsinfonet.org for the most recent information.

What are CD4 cells?

CD4 cells are a type of lymphocyte (white blood cell). They are an important part of the immune system. CD4 cells are sometimes called T cells. There are two main types of T cells. T-4 cells, also called CD4, are "helper" cells. They lead the attack against infections. T-8 cells, (CD8), are "suppressor" cells that end the immune response. CD8 cells can also be "killer" cells that kill cancer cells and cells infected with a virus.

Researchers can tell these cells apart by specific proteins on the cell surface. A T-4 cell is a T cell with CD4 molecules on its surface. This type of T cell is also called "CD4 positive," or CD4.

Why are CD4 cells important in HIV?

When HIV infects humans, the cells it infects most often are CD4 cells. The virus becomes part of the cells, and when they multiply to fight an infection, they also make more copies of HIV.

When someone is infected with HIV for a long time, the number of CD4 cells they have (their CD4 cell count) goes down. This is a sign that the immune system is being weakened. The lower the CD4 cell count, the more likely the person will get sick.

There are millions of different families of CD4 cells. Each family is designed to fight a specific type of germ. When HIV reduces the number of CD4 cells, some of these families can be totally wiped out. You can lose the ability to fight off the particular germs those families were designed for. If this happens, you might develop an opportunistic infection.

What factors influence a CD4 cell count?

The CD4 cell value bounces around a lot. Time of day, fatigue, and stress can affect the test results. It's best to have blood drawn at the same time of day for each CD4 cell test, and to use the same laboratory.

Infections can have a large impact on CD4 cell counts. When your body fights an infection, the number of white blood cells (lymphocytes) goes up. CD4 and CD8 counts go up, too. Vaccinations can cause the same effects. Don't check your CD4 cells until a couple of weeks after you recover from an infection or get a vaccination.

How are the test results reported?

CD4 cell tests are normally reported as the number of cells in a cubic millimeter of blood, or mm^3. There is some disagreement about the normal range for CD4 cell counts, but normal counts are between 500 and 1600, and CD8 counts are between 375 and 1100. CD4 counts drop dramatically in people with HIV, in some cases down to zero.

The ratio of CD4 cells to CD8 cells is often reported. This is calculated by dividing the CD4 value by the CD8 value. In healthy people, this ratio is between 0.9 and 1.9, meaning that there are about one to two CD4 cells for every CD8 cell. In people with HIV infection, this ratio drops dramatically, meaning that there are many times more CD8 cells than CD4 cells.

Because the CD4 counts are so variable, some health care providers prefer to look at the CD4 cell percentages. These percentages refer to total lymphocytes. If your test reports CD4 percent equals 34 percent, that means that 34 percent of your lymphocytes were CD4 cells. This percentage is more stable than the number of CD4 cells. The normal range is between 20 percent and 40 percent. A CD4 percentage below 14 percent indicates serious immune damage. It is a sign of AIDS in people with HIV infection. A recent study showed that the CD4 percent is a predictor of HIV disease progression.

What do the numbers mean?

The meaning of CD8 cell counts is not clear, but it is being studied.

The CD4 cell count is a key measure of the health of the immune system. The lower the count, the greater damage HIV has done. Anyone who has less than 200 CD4 cells, or a CD4 percentage less than 14 percent, is considered to have AIDS according to the U.S. Centers for Disease Control.

CD4 counts are used together with the viral load to estimate how long someone will stay healthy.

CD4 counts are also used to indicate when to start certain types of drug therapy:

When to start antiretroviral therapy (ART): When the CD4 count goes below 350, most health care providers begin ART. Some health care providers use the CD4 percent going below 15 percent as a sign to start aggressive ART, even if the CD4 count is high. More conservative health care providers might wait until the CD4 count drops to near 200 before starting treatment. A recent study found that starting treatment with a CD4 percent below 5 percent was strongly linked to a poor outcome.

When to start drugs to prevent opportunistic infections: Most health care providers prescribe drugs to prevent opportunistic infections at the following CD4 levels:

- Less than 200: *Pneumocystis* pneumonia (PCP)

- Less than 100: toxoplasmosis and cryptococcosis

- Less than 75: *Mycobacterium avium* complex (MAC)

Because they are such an important indicator of the strength of the immune system, official treatment guidelines in the U.S. suggest that CD4 counts be monitored every three to four months.

Chapter 32

Making Sense of Your Treatment Options If You Have HIV/AIDS

HIV/AIDS Treatment

HIV medicines are giving men and women longer, healthier futures and new strength. While there's no cure for HIV, the treatments today allow men and women to live longer. Making sense of all your treatment options can be hard. By getting the facts, you can decide the best way for you to manage your illness.

You Have Options

If you test positive for HIV, find a doctor you can trust who treats HIV-positive patients. If you need help finding one, call the CDC National AIDS hotline at 800-CDC-INFO (232-4636). This hotline will either point you to a specific doctor or to resources in your area where you can get health care, like a clinic. Your doctor will talk to you about your health. You also will get a physical exam. If you found out about your positive result over the phone from a counselor at a mail-in testing company, follow up with a doctor to talk about your result.

You will have tests to figure out if and when you should start treatment. Some tests may include the following:

This chapter contains text from "Women and HIV/AIDS: Treatment," National Women's Health Information Center (http://www.4women.gov), March 2007; and, "Seeing an HIV Doctor," AIDSInfo, a service of the U.S. Department of Health and Human Services (http://www.aidsinfo.nih.gov), August 2006.

- blood count

- blood chemistry profile (including testing for your kidney and liver)

- hepatitis B test

- hepatitis C test

- viral load test (amount of HIV in your blood)

- CD4 cell count (number of cells in your blood that fight infection, also called "T cells")

- syphilis test

- TB skin test

- toxoplasma antibody test

- gynecologic exam (with Pap test and pregnancy test)—for women

Treatment Will Slow Down the Disease

There is no cure for HIV/AIDS. But there are medicines that slow down the disease. The FDA has approved a number of drugs for treating HIV. Because each HIV drug can't work by itself, patients must take a combination of three or more drugs. When this combination of drugs is taken, it's called "highly active antiretroviral therapy" or HAART. Sometimes, it is also called a "cocktail" or "cocktail therapy." When taken properly, HAART treatment helps people with HIV live longer and have fewer infections or other problems related to their HIV. The drugs work by lowering the amount of HIV in the blood and improving your body's ability to fight infections.

Many medications and other drugs and substances can interact with HIV medicines. These interactions can hurt you or make the HIV medicines weaker. So you should tell your doctor if you are using any other prescribed medications. Also, tell your doctor if you are using any recreational drugs, alcohol, herbal remedies, or over-the-counter medicines.

If you are a woman, make sure to tell your doctor if you are taking birth control pills. Some HIV drugs can make the birth control pill not work as well. Also, tell your doctor if you are pregnant to figure out the best treatment for you and your baby.

There are four classes of drugs used to treat HIV. The names of HIV drugs can be confusing. Many HIV drugs have both a brand name and a generic name. Some also go by a shortened name. For example, Retrovir is the brand name of zidovudine (the generic name), and also goes by "AZT" or "ZDV". Also some drugs now are combined into a single pill. For example, Combivir includes both lamivudine and zidovudine in a single pill. Your doctor will help you decide which medicines should be included in your treatment.

The four classes, along with the drugs that have been FDA approved as of March 2007, are as follows:[1]

Nucleoside/nucleotide reverse transcriptase inhibitors (NRTIs) (also called "nukes") prevent HIV from making copies of itself. Usually, you take two drugs from this class as part of your HAART. These can be combined in one pill or taken separately.

Non-nucleoside reverse transcriptase inhibitors (NNRTIs) (also called "non-nukes") prevent HIV from making copies of itself. You usually take one from this class or one or two from the protease inhibitor class.

Protease inhibitors (PIs) block a protein that HIV makes to stop HIV from making copies of itself and infecting healthy cells. You usually take one or two from this class or one from the NNRTIs class.

Fusion inhibitors work outside of the cell to keep HIV from infecting healthy CD4 cells.

Multi-class combination products combine drugs from more than one class into a single product.

New Information from the Food and Drug Administration (FDA)

- In July 2006, the FDA announced approval of Atripla tablets, the first one-pill, once-a-day product to treat HIV/AIDS. Atripla contains a fixed-dose combination of three widely used antiretroviral drugs in a single tablet. It is taken once a day, either alone or in combination with other antiretroviral products for the treatment of HIV-1 infection in adults. Atripla combines the active ingredients of Sustiva (efavirenz), Emtriva (emtricitabine), and Viread (tenofovir disoproxil fumarate). Atripla was approved in less than three months under the FDA's fast track program.

- In June 2006, the FDA approved Prezista (darunavir), a new drug for adults with HIV who do not respond to other anti-retroviral drugs. Prezista, a protease inhibitor, is approved to be taken with a low dose of ritonavir and other active anti-HIV agents. Ritonavir slows the breakdown of Prezista in the body. Prezista also was approved under the FDA's fast track program.

Table 32.1. Classes of Drugs Used to Treat HIV

Brand Name	Generic Name (pronounciation)	Other Names
Nucleoside/Nucleotide Reverse Transcriptase Inhibitors Class		
Combivir	combination of: lamivudine (la-MY-vyoo-deen) and zidovudine (zye-DOE-vyoo-deen)	ZDV/3TC
Emtriva	emtricitabine (em-trye-SYE-ta-been)	FTC
Epivir	lamivudine (la-MY-vyoo-deen)	3TC
Epzicom	combination of: abacavir (a-BAK-ah-veer) and lamivudine (la-MY-vyoo-deen)	ABC/3TC
HIVID	zalcitabine (zal-SITE-ah-been)	ddC
Retrovir	zidovudine (zye-DOE-vyoo-deen)	AZT, ZDV
Trizivir	combination of: abacavir (a-BAK-ah-veer), lamivudine (la-MY-vyoo-deen), and zidovudine (zye-DOE-vyoo-deen)	ABC/3TC/ZDV
Truvada	combination of: tenofovir (te-NOE-foe-veer) and emtricitabine (em-trye-SYE-ta-been)	TDF/FTC
Videx	didanosine (dye-DAN-oh-seen)	ddl
Videx EC	enteric coated didanosine (dye-DAN-oh-seen)	ddl EC
Viread	tenofovir (te-NOE-foe-veer)	TDF
Zerit	stavudine (STAV-yoo-deen)	d4T
Ziagen	abacavir (a-BAK-ah-veer)	ABC

When to Start Treatment

Talk to your doctor about when to start treatment. The time to start treatment is different for everyone because there are many factors to consider, such as the following:

- **Damage to the immune system:** When to start treatment depends largely on your CD4 cell count, which is a measure of your

Table 32.1. Classes of Drugs Used to Treat HIV (continued)

Brand Name	Generic Name (pronounciation)	Other Names
Non-Nucleoside Reverse Transcriptase Inhibitors Class		
Rescriptor	delavirdine (de-la-VEER-deen)	DLV
Sustiva	efavirenz (eh-FAV-er-enz)	EFV
Viramune	nevirapine (neh-VYE-ra-peen)	NVP
Protease Inhibitors Class		
Agenerase	amprenavir (am-PREN-ah-veer)	APV
Aptivus	tipranavir (tip-RAN-ah-veer)	TPV
Crixivan	indinavir (in-DIN-ah-veer)	IDV
Invirase	saquinavir (sah-KWIN-ah-veer)	SQV
Kaletra	combination of: lopinavir (low-PIN-ah-veer) and ritonavir (ri-TOE-na-veer)	LPV/RTV
Lexiva	fosamprenavir (FOS-am-PREN-ah-veer)	FOS-APV
Norvir	ritonavir (ri-TOE-na-veer)	RTV
Prezista	darunavir (dar-UE-na-veer)	DRV
Reyataz	atazanavir (at-a-ZAN-ah-veer)	ATV
Viracept	nelfinavir (nel-FIN-ah-veer)	NFV
Fusion Inhibitors Class		
Fuzeon	enfuvirtide (en-FYOO-vir-tide)	T-20
Multi-Class Combination Products		
Atripla	combination of: efavirenz (ef-FAH-ver-enz), emtricitabine (em-trye-SYE-tah-been), and tenofovir (te-NOE-foe-veer)	

immune system's strength. CD4 cells are a type of white blood cell that fights infection. With HIV, your CD4 cells are destroyed, causing your immune system to weaken. Treatment should be started before HIV has done too much damage to your immune system.

- **Readiness to stick with treatment:** You will need to take all of the drugs exactly how your doctor tells you to, without missing any doses. Missing doses can result in the virus becoming resistant to the medications. Once this happens, the drugs will not work as well or at all. Since one drug isn't strong enough to fight HIV alone, you will have to take several drugs every day. Whether you must take multiple pills or just one or two pills a day, you must be ready to commit to taking all your medicines as directed and stick with it.

- **Managing side effects:** There is a good chance that you will have some side effects from the drugs. Some of these are tougher to live with than others. And some go away over time, while others will stay. Some side effects are more common and more severe in the first few months of treatment. You must be ready and willing to put up with side effects before you begin treatment. You should make sure to tell your doctor about any side effects you are having so they can help you manage them.

- **Treatment options:** There is more than one way to approach HIV treatment. When you begin treatment and what medicines you will use will depend on the approach you and your doctor agree upon. It is important to start treatment before the HIV has done too much damage to your immune system. But starting very early (based on your CD4 count) if you are not sick is not currently advised. You should talk with your doctor about when is the best time to start. It is important to see your doctor often—even before you start HAART—to keep you as healthy as possible.

There are still a number of things about treatment of HIV that we do not know. This is particularly true for women. Research and clinical trials of what medicines to use and when to start are seeking to answer those questions.

When you begin to discuss treatment options with your doctor, ask about clinical trials. Your doctor can tell you if there are any that would be open to you and how to enroll if you want to participate.

HIV/AIDS Drugs Cause Side Effects

Despite the beneficial effects of HAART, you can get side effects from the drugs. Some are serious. Others are bothersome, but go away with time. These are some side effects:

- nausea
- vomiting
- diarrhea
- weakness
- dizziness
- headache
- rash
- fever
- liver problems
- diabetes
- losing fat in some parts of your body and getting it in other parts (face, legs, arms, buttocks, breasts, neck, stomach)
- high cholesterol
- more bleeding in patients with hemophilia
- decrease in bone density

HIV treatment can be hard because of side effects. Before you start taking HIV drugs, talk to your doctor about side effects you may have, ways to feel better, if/when they will go away, and how long they'll last. Even though you have side effects from the drugs, it's important to take your medicines exactly how and when you're told to and to let your doctor know about your symptoms.

Side Effects Are Different in Women

Women may find that the side effects they're having from the medicines are not the same as other people, especially if the other people are men. Women take the same doses of HIV drugs as men, but have smaller body sizes, higher body fat, and different hormones. Some researchers think these factors affect how women respond to the medicines and believe they cause different side effects in women. For example, Norvir causes more nausea and vomiting in women but less diarrhea than in men. Some studies show that women are more likely to get rashes, fat build-up, and problems with the pancreas and liver. But before treatment doses change, more clinical trials need to be done that include women.

Stick to Your Treatment

HIV drugs can be hard to take. You may need to take a lot of them, and they can cause side effects that are hard to manage. But it's so important that you take all of them as your doctor tells you to. Missing medications can result in the development of drug resistance. This is when the virus is able to "ignore" the medications, and so the medicines do not work as well in fighting the virus or at all. Even people who take their medicines most of the time, but not all of the time, face a high risk of drug resistance. When resistance develops, you will need to change to a new set of medications. The chance of success with your new HAART will not be as high as with the first HAART. You also might get new side effects that you must get used to. Here are some ways to stick to your treatment:

- Know your options and what to expect. Talk to your doctor about all treatment options and drug side effects.

- Think about why you might have a hard time with treatment. For example, it might be hard to take all the drugs when you're supposed to take them or specific times such as the weekend. Talk to your doctor about these problems and how you can make your treatment plan fit your lifestyle. For instance, it is helpful to take them with something you do every day, such as when you get out of bed in the morning.

- Plan your meals. Some drugs have to be taken with food or with no food. If this is true with any of your medicines, plan when you'll eat so you take the right drugs with the right amount and type of food.

- Write down information about the medicines. This includes drug name, when to take it, how much to take, and if you take it when you're eating or on an empty stomach. Use this planner to organize your medicines. Don't leave your doctor's office until you understand how to take your drugs.

- Organize your medicines. Use daily or weekly pill boxes or other organizers (you can even use egg cartons).

- Don't forget! Use timers, alarm clocks, or pagers to remind you to take your medicines. You could even write it in your planner. Some people use family and friends to help them remember.

- Plan ahead. Weekends and holidays make it harder to remember to take your medicines. Come up with a plan ahead of time so you won't forget. If you're traveling, keep medicines with you, just in case your checked luggage is lost. Some people keep an extra dose of medications with them or at work in case they are away from their medications when they are supposed to take them.

- Get refills on time. Don't wait until the last minute. Don't miss a dose.

- Write down the problems you have with the drugs. It will help you remember and track your problems.

- Tell your doctor right away if you have side effects or other problems. Don't wait. Work with your doctor to make your treatment plan work for you—you might be able to change your treatment so it's better for you.

- Talk to people who can help you cope. This process is no easy task. Talk to people who can help you get through this. It is important not to isolate yourself—reach out to those you love. Think about joining a support group to talk to other people with HIV.

How to Know If Treatment Is Working

There are ways to know if your treatment is working. Your doctor will consider these factors:

- viral load (amount of HIV in your blood)—the lower, the better. The goal is for HIV to be "undetectable" in your blood. Undetectable does not mean it is gone, but it is so low that current lab tests cannot find it.

- CD4 cell count (number of cells in your blood that fight infection)—the higher your count, the better able you are to fight your HIV and other infections.

- recent health history (if you are feeling healthy and not getting infections)

- results from physical exams

Even if the treatment is working and the amount of HIV in your blood is so low that that the tests can't find it, you still have HIV or AIDS. You can still give HIV to other people. Keep using condoms, and don't share drug needles. And remember, the HIV will start to increase in your blood again if you stop taking your medicines.

Taking a Drug Holiday

If you take medicines for HIV/AIDS, you may feel like the drugs are running your life. It's tough to take all of the medicines when you're supposed to, some with food, some not. The medicines' side effects can make you long for a break from treatment. Researchers have found that it is not a good idea to stop treatment once started. Stopping can result in you getting sicker and having more side effects from the medications.

The National Institute of Allergy and Infectious Diseases (NIAID) conducted a study of people who had drug-resistant HIV (a type of HIV that does not get better with medicines) and detectable virus in their blood to find out if breaks in their treatments would help them. Unfortunately, it didn't work for this group. Strategy for Management of Antiretroviral Therapy (SMART) is another government-funded study that looked into the possible role of drug holidays in HIV treatment. This study found that even in patients who had not been on HIV medications before, taking planned holidays from drugs was dangerous and resulted in higher risks of getting sick or dying and having more problems with medications. At this time, planned drug holidays are not advised as part of routine care.

Seeing an HIV Doctor

I am HIV positive. What kind of doctor do I need?

Your doctor (or other health care provider) should be experienced in treating HIV and AIDS. You may want to see an infectious disease specialist. You will need to work closely with your doctor to make informed decisions about your treatment, so it is important to find a doctor with whom you are comfortable.

What can I expect at the doctor's office?

Your doctor will ask you questions about your health, do a physical exam, and order blood tests. This is a good time to ask your doctor questions. Write down any questions you have and take them with you to your appointment. Women should have a pregnancy test and a gynecologic examination with Pap smear.

What questions should I ask my doctor?

You should ask your doctor about the following:

- risks and benefits of HIV treatment
- other diseases you may be at risk for
- how your lifestyle will change with HIV infection
- how you can avoid transmitting HIV to others
- how you can achieve and maintain a healthier lifestyle

What tests will my doctor order?

It is very important to have a CD4 count and a viral load test done at your first doctor's visit. You should also have drug resistance testing. The results will provide a baseline measurement for future tests.

- **CD4 count:** CD4 cells, also called CD4+ T cells or CD4 lymphocytes, are a type of white blood cell that fights infection. HIV destroys CD4 cells, weakening your body's immune system. A CD4 count is the number of CD4 cells in a sample of blood.

- **Viral load test:** A viral load test measures the amount of HIV in a sample of blood. This test shows how well your immune system is controlling the virus. The two viral load tests commonly used for HIV are as follows:

  - HIV RNA amplification (RT-PCR) test
  - Branched chain DNA (bDNA) test

- **Drug resistance testing:** Drug resistance testing determines if an individual's HIV strain is resistant to any anti-HIV medications. HIV can mutate (change form), resulting in HIV that cannot be controlled with certain medications.

To ensure accurate results, viral load testing should be done at two different times, by the same laboratory, using the same type of test. The results of different types of tests may differ.

Your doctor may also order the following tests:

- complete blood count

- blood chemistry profile (including liver function tests)

- tests for other sexually transmitted diseases (STDs)

- tests for other infections, such as hepatitis, tuberculosis, or toxoplasmosis

Am I ready to begin HIV treatment?

Once you begin taking anti-HIV medications, you may need to continue taking them for the rest of your life. Deciding when or if to begin treatment depends on your health and your readiness to follow a treatment regimen that may be complicated. You and your doctor should discuss your readiness to begin treatment as well as strategies to make your treatment work for you.

If my doctor and I decide to delay treatment, will I need to have my CD4 count and viral load tested again?

Yes. HIV infected people who have not started drug therapy should have a viral load test every three to four months and a CD4 count every three to six months. You and your doctor will use the test results to monitor your infection and to decide when to start treatment.

For More Information

Contact your doctor or an AIDSinfo Health Information Specialist at 800-448-0440 or http://aidsinfo.nih.gov.

Note

1. In August 2007, the U.S. Food and Drug Administration (FDA) approved maraviroc, for use in combination with other antiretroviral drugs for the treatment of adults with CCR5-tropic HIV-1. Maraviroc, sold under the trade name Selzentry, is the first in a new class of drugs designed to slow the advancement of HIV. Rather than fighting HIV inside white blood cells, maraviroc prevents the virus from entering uninfected cells by blocking the predominant route of entry, the CCR5 co-receptor. (Source: "FDA Approves Novel Antiretroviral Drug," FDA News, FDA, August 6, 2007; http://www.fda.gov/bbs/topics/NEWS/2007/NEW01677.html)

Chapter 33

Anti-HIV Therapy Strategies: Information to Consider When Deciding to Use Therapy

The overall goal of anti-HIV therapy is to slow or stop the ability of HIV to reproduce, and thereby slow or stop the progression of HIV disease and the destruction of the immune system. While other approaches of combating HIV infection have been proposed and tested, thus far only anti-HIV therapy has been proven to slow disease progression and extend life.

While understanding and making decisions about anti-HIV therapy can be an overwhelming process, it isn't insurmountable. With the support of your doctor and reliable information, it's possible to devise a wise anti-HIV strategy. A balanced approach to such a strategy must include knowledge of the benefits, risks, and limitations of existing therapies, and the prospects for improvements offered by combination therapies and newer drugs.

This chapter provides information on these decision points. It is intended to be a tool in making the best possible decision about the use of anti-HIV therapies in adults and adolescents.

The Goals of Anti-HIV Therapy

The goals of anti-HIV therapy should be to:

- **prolong** life and improve quality of life for the long-term;

"Anti-HIV Therapy Strategies: Information to Consider when Deciding to Use Therapy," From Project Inform, © 2007. For more information, contact the National HIV/AIDS Treatment Infoline, 1-800-822-7422, or visit our website at www.projectinform.org.

- **suppress** virus to below the limit of detection on current tests (less than 50 copies HIV RNA), or as low as possible, for as long as possible;

- **optimize** and extend the usefulness of the currently available therapies; and

- **minimize** drug toxicity and manage side effects and drug interactions.

Once HIV was identified as the cause of acquired immunodeficiency syndrome (AIDS), stopping or slowing its replication became a major goal. Significant progress has been made towards reaching this goal, especially with the advent of potent drugs and the use of combination therapy. This has made it possible to develop long-term strategies for managing HIV.

Yet uncertainty remains about when to start and when to switch or how best to combine anti-HIV therapies. Also, the failure of existing drugs to remain completely effective for long periods of time is sometimes misunderstood as meaning that the drugs don't work at all. Making wise decisions about the use of anti-HIV therapies requires understanding the benefits and risks of therapies, good communication with a knowledgeable doctor, and proper use of various lab tests.

It's important to remember that people can live a long time, without symptoms of HIV disease and without using anti-HIV therapy. Thus many, if not most, people don't have to decide about using therapy immediately after learning that they're living with HIV. Assessing your personal risk of HIV disease progression and making decisions that you feel comfortable with and empowered by is part of the key to a successful long-term anti-HIV strategy.

The Challenge of Therapy

Many researchers believe that unless HIV replication can be controlled, other efforts at rebuilding immune health will ultimately fail. Although anti-HIV therapies weaken the virus' ability to replicate, they're not a cure since they have not been shown to totally eradicate HIV from the body. Many scientists fear that it will not be possible to fully eradicate it from the body, no matter how good the drugs become or how early treatment is started.

Over time, the virus mutates or changes itself enough so that it is no longer affected by these drugs. This process is called viral resistance and is likely to happen with almost all anti-HIV drugs to some degree.

It's still clear, however, that suppressing the virus from replicating lengthens a person's survival time and it may be possible, with truly effective therapy, to live out a normal lifespan despite HIV infection.

Even with the limitations of current therapies, however, there's increasing evidence that using potent anti-HIV therapy has had a dramatic impact on decreasing death rates and increasing life and quality of life of people living with HIV. However, the drugs are not without the risk of side effects, and potential short- and long-term side effects must be weighed against their potential short- and long-term benefits when making decisions about using therapies, particularly when considering when to start.

Why Use Anti-HIV Therapy?

When a person is first infected with HIV, high virus levels develop that are often accompanied by flu-like symptoms and a decline in the number of CD4+ cells. These are key cells in maintaining and directing immune responses against disease. They are also a common measure of immune health.

Without using anti-HIV therapy, the immune system produces a dramatic but incomplete suppression of the virus. In most cases, CD4+ cell counts return partially toward normal levels and a person usually regains good health for many years. Studies show that even during this time of seemingly good health, there's an aggressive battle waged daily between HIV and the immune system. Over time the immune system is overwhelmed by HIV's rapid and constant activity.

There's a clear relationship among increased levels of HIV found in blood (viral load), more advanced disease states, and increased risk of disease progression. As a general rule, the more virus being produced in the body, the more rapidly disease progresses. Several studies show that when viral load is reduced and CD4+ cell counts increase for six months or longer, disease progression and death are delayed.

Considering these points, it makes sense to attempt to slow down or stop the replication of HIV as much and for as long as possible. A number of drugs have been shown to significantly reduce HIV levels, and these drugs almost always cause some rise in CD4+ cell counts. The reduction in viral load and increase in CD4+ cell counts indicate some improvement in the immune system. Anti-HIV drugs that fail to reduce HIV levels also generally (but not always) fail to improve measures of immune health such as CD4+ cell counts.

It remains unclear when the best time to start therapy is. The "best" time for one person might not be the "best" time for another. Several factors, including HIV levels, CD4+ cell count as well as how you feel about therapy, are important to consider when determining if and when anti-HIV therapy is right for you. For more information, read Project Inform's publication, *Strategies for When to Start Anti-HIV Therapy* [available online at http://www.projectinform.org].

When Should I Start Treatment?

There's much debate about when to start anti-HIV therapy, which drugs to start with, and in what combinations. Should treatment be used immediately when people first learn they're infected, or should it be saved until there are changes in immune health (noted by a decrease in CD4+ cell counts), increases in HIV levels, or until symptoms of HIV develop? These and other questions need to be considered when deciding when and which combinations to use.

In deciding when to start, switch or change anti-HIV regimens, there are generally three medical factors to consider:

- What's happening with your HIV levels?

- What's happening with measures of your immune health (particularly CD4+ cell counts)?

- What's happening with your general health status (such as symptoms of HIV disease or recurrent health conditions despite treatment)?

The decision to begin treatment is not solely a medical matter. Other factors must be considered, including:

- your feelings about anti-HIV therapy (if you believe a particular drug or treatment regimen will harm you, then you should consider carefully before deciding to take them);

- your readiness and willingness to commit to taking therapy, including your ability to take them as prescribed;

- the impact therapy will have on your quality of life;

- the side effects of the therapies;

- how long therapies can last, and whether or not there will be new and better drugs to replace them if or when they fail; and,

- your risk of disease progression in the short-, middle-, and long-term.

When Is the Right Time to Start?

There's no single, right answer to the question of when to start anti-HIV treatment. Some researchers and doctors believe that nearly everyone who is HIV infected—regardless of viral load, symptoms, or CD4+ cell counts—should be on treatment. Some believe people should begin therapy only when their CD4+ cell count consistently reads below 300 or their viral load consistently exceeds 30,000–55,000. Others believe that only people with symptoms of HIV disease should consider anti-HIV therapy.

One note of agreement is that most researchers and doctors believe that the decision to start therapy should be guided by looking at overall general health and measures of both CD4+ cell counts and viral load. Increasingly information suggests that CD4+ cell counts, coupled with viral load tests, provide the most accurate tool to monitor the risk of HIV disease progression. For more information on these types of tests, read Project Inform's publication, *Blood Work: A Useful Tool for Monitoring HIV,* available at 800-822-7422 and http://www.projectinform.org.

Quality of Life Issues

The ability to tolerate side effects, drug interactions, and the demands of a particular regimen can be as important as the potency of a drug. If you can't take a drug consistently as prescribed, its potency is irrelevant. Not adhering to a drug regimen will quickly contribute to developing drug resistance, which may include concerns about cross-resistance to many or all other drugs in its class. When choosing a combination, consider the daily pill count (anti-HIV drugs, drugs to prevent and treat other infections, and everything else). Also, consider when they have to be taken, whether they can be taken with other medications, and whether they can be taken with food.

It is easiest to combine drugs that require similar conditions for their use (with or without food, etc.). Otherwise, one's life can become dominated by drug schedules. It is also best to avoid mixing drugs with similar side effects, though sometimes this is impossible. And it is critical to learn about the possible side effects of each drug in a regimen as well as possible drug interactions before mixing any of these drugs together. To help with understanding these issues, Project Inform has materials on each anti-HIV drug as well as the publications, *Drug Side Effects Chart* and *Dealing with Drug Side Effects.*

While each drug has potential side effects, not everyone who takes a drug will experience them. Learning about possible side effects before taking a drug will allow you to be aware of what types of side effects to check for and to consider approaches to prevent or manage them, proactively. The more informed you are about the possible side effects and drug interactions of the drugs in a given regimen, the less likely you are to experience severe or life-threatening side effects. Moreover, if someone is prepared for possible side effects, with a plan for managing side effects should they arise, the less likely it is that they'll interfere with adherence.

Information on side effects associated with body composition and the body's ability to process sugars and fats is surfacing. These conditions are generally called lipodystrophy—and include fat accumulation (lipohypertrophy) and/or fat loss (lipoatrophy) and/or changes in lab

Table 33.1. Federal recommendations for when to start therapy.

Advanced stage disease (severe symptoms of AIDS, with any CD4+ cell count or viral load)
All people with severe symptoms of AIDS should be treated with anti-HIV therapy. In this case, anti-HIV therapy is shown to prolong life and is associated with improvements of symptoms. When starting therapy for opportunistic infections at the same time as starting anti-HIV therapy, special care should be taken to avoid drug interactions. A person experiencing an opportunistic infection is generally encouraged to continue anti-HIV therapy.

No symptoms of HIV disease, with CD4+ cell counts below 200 and any viral load
Treatment should be initiated after consideration of the issues affecting treatment decision-making, as the risk for disease progression is very high.

No symptoms of HIV disease, with CD4+ cell counts of 200–350 and any viral load
Treatment should generally be offered, though controversy exists. Some experts believe it's often safe to wait until the CD4+ count falls to 200. Others believe this offers too little room to accommodate individual differences and feel it's safer to start therapy at 350 CD4+ cells.

No symptoms of HIV disease, with CD4+ cell counts above 350 and viral load above 30,000 copies by bDNA or 55,000 by RT-PCR
There are two unproven approaches to treatment in early HIV infection when people do not have symptoms: aggressive and conservative. For people with CD4+ cell counts above 350 and viral load above 30,000 (by bDNA) or 55,000

values of fats (dyslipidemia) or sugars/insulin (diabetes). Another condition, impacting the energy source of cells (mitochondrial toxicity) is particularly associated with using nucleoside reverse transcriptase inhibitors (NRTIs). Reports of some people experiencing bone weakness have also begun to emerge. All of these conditions might result from long-term use of anti-HIV medications. For more information on these conditions, call Project Inform's toll-free hotline at 800-822-7422.

Viral Load and Women: An Additional Consideration?

Several studies have suggested that women have lower HIV levels than men at the same CD4+ cell count. Some suggest that these

Table 33.1. Federal recommendations... *continued*

(by RT-PCR), there are no available data to suggest which approach results in longer survival. Very early, aggressive treatment might lead to longer life. Or it might lead to using up the limited supply of therapies too early in the course of disease. Moreover, it also risks early exposure to possible long-term side effects associated with therapies. As a result many experts would delay starting therapy and continue to check CD4+ cell counts and viral load. On the other hand, the risk of disease progression over the next three years is somewhat high (over 30 percent) in people who meet this definition and other experts prefer to start treatment without further delay.

No symptoms of HIV disease, with CD4+ cell counts above 350 and viral load below 30,000 by bDNA or 55,000 by RT-PCR
Many experts would defer therapy and continue to check CD4+ cell counts and viral load; the risk of disease progression over the next three years in this group is low (below 15 percent).

Acute infection (very early, typically within first weeks after infection)
If infection is suspected, test for HIV using sensitive and sophisticated techniques. (Note: technologies that measure viral load are not approved and are discouraged for use in diagnosing HIV infection.) Experts agree that if treatment is offered in this very early setting, it should only be done in the context of a study. People interested in exploring very early treatment should be made aware of all of its possible risks. The true long-term effect of very early treatment is unclear because current studies are not yet complete, but the hope is that early treatment may alter the course of disease. Whether or not this is the "right" approach remains uncertain.

differences decrease or disappear after the first five years of HIV infection.

Current Public Health Service guidelines acknowledge that viral load may be somewhat lower in women, but these differences don't alter the goals of anti-HIV therapy—to lower HIV levels to as low as possible and impact CD4+ cell count and overall general health. They conclude that these data should not affect the approach to therapy

Table 33.2. Federal recommendations for first line anti-HIV therapy.

	NNRTI-based regimens	**pills/day**
Preferred regimens	efavirenz + 3TC + (AZT or tenofovir or d4T); except for pregnant women or women who wish to become pregnant	3–5
Alternative regimens	efavirenz + (3TC or FTC) + ddl; except for pregnant women or women who wish to become pregnant	3–5
	nevirapine + (3TC or FTC) + (AZT or tenofovir or d4T)	4–6
	PI-based regimens	**pills/day**
Preferred regimens	Kaletra + 3TC + (AZT or d4T)	8–10
Alternative regimens	amprenavir + low dose ritonavir + (3TC or FTC) + (AZT or d4T)	12–14
	atazanavir + (3TC or FTC) + (AZT or d4T)	5–10
	indinavir + (3TC or FTC) + (AZT or d4T)	8–10
	indinavir + low dose ritonavir + (3TC or FTC) + (AZT or d4T)	8–12
	nelfinavir + (3TC or FTC) + (AZT or d4T)	6–14
	saquinavir (soft or hard capsule) + low dose ritonavir + (3TC or FTC) + (AZT or d4T)	14–16
	NRTI regimens **(only when an NNRTI or PI can't be used)**	**pills/day**
Alternative regimens	Trizivir (abacavir + 3TC + AZT)	2
	abacavir + 3TC + stavudine	4–6

for women or for men. More data are needed to confirm the degree and relevance of this noted difference.

The U.S. Department of Health and Human Services released *Guidelines for the Use of Antiretroviral Agents in the Treatment of HIV-Infected Adults and Adolescents*. These are summarized in Table 33.2. The Federal Guidelines describe the recommendations of researchers, and point out that people with HIV and their doctors must take many other factors into consideration, such as the person's readiness to start treatment and concerns about long-term toxicity and drug resistance.

The Risk of Progression to AIDS-Defining Illness

Recent reports show that women progress to HIV disease at a lower viral level than men. While these new data do not currently warrant a new standard of care for women with HIV, women and their doctors should be aware of these reports as they may support starting or switching therapy at lower viral levels than what is currently recommended. CD4+ cell counts, that provide useful measures for the risk of HIV disease progression, are not influenced by sex. For more information on this issue, call Project Inform's toll-free hotline at 800-822-7422.

Points to Think about for People Who Consider Taking Anti-HIV Therapy

There are many issues to consider and discuss with your doctor before taking anti-HIV therapy. (For more information on specific drugs, call Project Inform's Hotline.) The following issues are offered for consideration for people who are starting therapy for the first time (first line therapy) as well as for those who are switching therapies (second or third line therapy).

- **Reducing viral load as low as possible, preferably below the level of detection, should be an important goal of therapy.** Drug regimens that have a larger, more consistent and longer-lasting effect in reducing HIV levels and increasing CD4+ cell counts are more likely to produce longer-lasting health and survival benefits. People with HIV levels below the limit of detection have a much longer lasting anti-HIV response to a given regimen than people with consistently detectable HIV levels. When therapy fails to reduce HIV levels to below the limit of detection, it's usually a sign that it will fail over the next several months.

279

Studies show, however, that occasional "blips" in viral load (a detectable reading every now and again) does not represent a major concern. Trends over time are more important than any single lab report.

Today, viral load tests measure reliably down to 20 copies. Any number below this is considered undetectable. Some researchers believe that people who do not reach undetectable levels after six months on therapy should consider either switching to a new regimen or, if viral levels are detectable but remain very low (like less than 1,000), adding another drug. Others believe it might be okay for a person with few other options to continue using a regimen if it's controlling viral levels at a low (like less than 5,000), yet detectable level. While studies show that reaching "undetectable" viral load is optimal, the cost of side effects or the complexity of a regimen necessary to achieve this goal might not be realistic for everyone.

- **There may be some degree of cross-resistance between the drugs in the same class.** Resistance to a drug occurs when HIV changes or modifies itself such that it's no longer crippled in its replication cycle by the effects of a drug. Cross-resistance is when resistance to one drug also causes resistance to other drugs in the same class. Resistance usually occurs when the drugs being used are not potent enough to completely stop HIV replication or when the drugs are not taken as prescribed.

For instance, someone with resistance to one of the non-nucleoside reverse transcriptase inhibitor (NNRTIs)* is almost certainly going to be cross-resistant with the other approved NNRTIs. What this means is that once resistance to one NNRTI develops, the other drugs in this class are less effective, and possibly wholly ineffective. (*Note: NNRTIs are a class of anti-HIV drugs. See the drug chart, Table 33.3.)

- **Successful long-term use of therapies is more important than short-term gains.** It's possible to get short-term benefits at the cost of wasting potential long-term benefits. An example of this would be starting a two-drug NRTI* regimen in a person with high HIV levels (above 100,000). Studies show that resistance can develop within weeks to months after starting a two-drug NRTI regimen. This may impact the usefulness of other similar drugs as well as eliminating options for future therapies.

(*Note: NRTIs are a class of anti-HIV drugs. See the drug chart, Table 33.3.)

- **Should I get a resistance test?** Several studies show that people who selected therapies based on resistance testing in

Table 33.3. Drug identification chart.

	Generic Name	Trade Name
Protease inhibitor		
	amprenavir	Agenerase
	atazanavir	Reyataz
	fosamprenavir	Lexiva
	indinavir	Crixivan
	lopinavir + ritonavir	Kaletra
	nelfinavir	Viracept
	ritonavir	Norvir
	saquinavir	Invirase
Nucleoside (NRTI) and		
nucleotide (NtRTI) analogue reverse transcriptase inhibitor		
	abacavir	Ziagen
	didanosine (ddI)	Videx
	didanosine enteric-coated (ddI EC)	Videx EC
	emtricitabine (FTC)	Emtriva
	FTC + tenofovir	Truvada
	lamivudine (3TC)	Epivir
	stavudine (d4T)	Zerit
	tenofovir	Viread
	zidovudine (AZT)	Retrovir
	3TC + abacavir	Epzicom
	3TC + AZT	Combivir
	3TC + AZT + abacavir	Trizivir
Non-nucleoside reverse transcriptase inhibitor (NNRTI)		
	delavirdine	Rescriptor
	efavirenz	Sustiva
	nevirapine	Viramune
Entry inhibitor		
	enfuvirtide (T20)	Fuzeon

addition to considering their history of using anti-HIV drug had longer lasting responses to anti-HIV regimens compared to people who didn't get resistance tests before making decisions. Some researchers are proposing that people get a resistance test before they start anti-HIV therapies for the first time as well as before they switch to a new regimen.

Note: In order to run a resistance test, a person must have a viral load above 1,000. Resistance testing cannot be done accurately on people with HIV levels below the limit of detection (50). Also, resistance tests are likely most reliable when conducted while someone is taking anti-HIV therapy.

- **The use of treatment that is only partly effective speeds the development of viral resistance.** If a treatment reduces viral load but still permits a measurable level of viral activity (a measurable viral load), the HIV that's still present is capable of mutating and developing resistance to that treatment. When a three-drug combination doesn't quite succeed in stopping measurable viral activity, many researchers believe it may be wise to either change two of the drugs, or perhaps add a fourth drug.

  It makes sense to try and fully suppress viral replication if this can be done with a reasonable quality of life. When this goal cannot be achieved, people should realize they can still benefit from therapy and that longer-term solutions may become apparent when other therapies are available. Again, using resistance testing may help in guiding which therapies are not working or which ones may be useful to add to a regimen.

- **Learn about drug interactions.** With the number of drugs available to treat HIV and prevent or treat opportunistic infections, as well as other conditions, the potential for drug interactions increases. Not only does each therapy have its own possible side effects, it also may increase or decrease the benefit of other drugs. Drug interactions are not always considered when creating a treatment strategy, but they may play a major role in the success of any treatment plan. Make sure your health care provider knows about all the therapies you take, including experimental and over-the-counter products.

- **Using a drug exactly as prescribed is critical to success.** Using an inadequate dose, reducing the dose below prescribed levels, or failing to take the drug at regularly spaced intervals will increase the risk of developing resistance. If intolerance or side effects develop, it's often better to try to overcome the side effects than to immediately change the regimen. If side effects aren't manageable, it's better to temporarily stop all the drugs in the regimen rather than reduce doses, and try to solve the problem with a doctor's guidance. The fastest way to develop resistance to anti-HIV drugs is to use them at inadequate or inconsistent dose levels.

- **Stopping and starting a regimen frequently (like on a weekly or even bi-weekly basis) will likely lead to an increased risk of drug resistance.** A structured treatment interruption (STI), as discussed later, may include stopping therapy for a two-week period or longer, then restarting it for some period of time. It's important for people considering an STI to be closely checked for viral load and CD4+ cell counts. Many studies show that some people experience a dramatic increase in HIV levels and decrease in CD4+ cells. For more information, read Project Inform's publication, *Structured Treatment Interruptions.*

- **If you need to interrupt therapy, it's best to stop all drugs at the same time (except nevirapine and efavirenz) rather than just stopping one drug.** There are many reasons that people may need to stop taking their meds, including side effects, drug interactions, pregnancy, or their drug supply runs out. Stopping anti-HIV drugs, if they're all stopped at the same time, is unlikely to increase drug resistance. Because nevirapine and efavirenz remain in the body longer than any other anti-HIV therapy, they should be stopped at least two or three days and possibly up to two weeks before stopping the others. Otherwise, there's an increased risk of developing resistance to these drugs.

- **People considering a vacation away from home should wait until they return before starting a new drug regimen.** When side effects occur, they often happen within the first two to four weeks after starting a new regimen. Many resolve after a period of time as the body adjusts to being on new meds. Some, but not all, people experience some mild-to-moderate side effects. Usually, only a small percentage of people experience moderate-to-severe side effects. People should avoid starting a new anti-HIV regimen right before going out of town on vacation. In the unlikely event of serious side effects, it's better to be closer to your doctor who is hopefully experienced with your health and with treating HIV or managing side effects from a specific drug.

Not all people have access to the same treatments, and people respond differently to individual drugs. Treatment options include existing approved drugs and combinations, experimental drugs accessed through studies and access programs, and other unapproved drugs.

How Will I Know If My Treatment Is Working?

The goal of anti-HIV therapy is to reduce HIV levels below the limit of detection (less than 50 copies) with the current viral load tests. However, not everyone can bring their HIV levels to less than 50 copies or to less than 5,000. For these people the minimum change in HIV levels that shows the therapies are active is a three-fold reduction (0.5 logs).

Many doctors believe you need at least ten-fold reduction (1 log) to have a real impact on disease progression. People with lower CD4+ cell counts and high viral load measures may find that HIV levels drop slowly over time, while people who are healthier are likely to see more immediate responses to therapy. Indeed, anecdotal experience suggests that among people in more advanced disease, decreases in HIV levels happen slower (over three to six months).

Considerations for Pregnant Women

In general, the guidelines for treating pregnant women are the same as for treating non-pregnant adults. As in other adults, the decisions to start, change or add anti-HIV therapies should be based on HIV levels, CD4+ cell counts and disease stage. The strategies presented in this section are all valid for pregnant women as well as other adults. The Federal Guidelines recommend that women receive the most effective anti-HIV regimen regardless of pregnancy status.

However, the potential impact of therapy on an infant or unborn child is not wholly known. Therefore, the decision to use anti-HIV therapy during pregnancy should be made by the woman in consideration of the known and unknown benefits and risks to her and her child. Long-term follow-up is recommended for all infants born to women who have taken anti-HIV therapy during pregnancy.

Women in their first trimester (14 weeks) of pregnancy not taking anti-HIV therapy may decide to delay therapy until after 10–12 weeks because of the possible risks to the developing fetus during this time. However, if the woman's own health status warrants starting therapy sooner, most would recommend starting it regardless of how far along a woman is in her pregnancy.

Some women already on therapy may consider temporarily stopping it until after her first trimester. While there are no clear data on the effects of anti-HIV drugs on the developing fetus, most doctors would recommend continuing a highly active anti-HIV regimen regardless of how far along the woman is in her pregnancy. Stopping or delaying therapy may increase HIV levels—possibly increasing her own risk of disease progression as well as the risk of transmitting HIV from her to her child.

Nevertheless, if a woman decides to stop her therapy, all drugs (with the exception of nevirapine) should be stopped at the same time to prevent the development of drug resistance. Similarly, once they're resumed, they should be started at the same time. The use of efavirenz is strongly discouraged in pregnant women due to possible harmful effects on the developing child. For more information, read Project Inform's publication, *Pregnancy and HIV,* available at 800-822-7422 or at http://www.projectinform.org.

When Is It Time to Change Therapies?

The Federal Guidelines recommend that people switch therapies when:

- detectable HIV levels after being undetectable;
- HIV levels remain detectable after four–six months of starting anti-HIV therapy;
- persistent decreases in CD4+ cell counts;
- intolerable side effects occur;
- adherence is poor;
- there is less than a 0.5–0.75 log (three- to six-fold) reduction in HIV levels after four weeks or less than one log after eight weeks of starting anti-HIV therapy (As noted above, however, people who start anti-HIV therapy when CD4+ cell counts are low and HIV levels are high, it may take a longer time to appreciate the capabilities of a regimen.);
- symptoms of HIV disease occur; and/or
- a three-fold or greater increase in HIV levels from their lowest levels.

285

A common infection such as the flu, or even a vaccine shot, can increase HIV levels temporarily. (A flu vaccine can increase HIV levels for up to two months, but they usually fall back to pre-vaccination levels without changes in anti-HIV therapy.) Before making dramatic adjustments in regimens, factor in how other health considerations may be affecting the viral load test results. If necessary, wait and get another test before making decisions. The decision to switch or add therapies should be based on at least two viral load tests and/or two CD4+ cell counts spaced at least two weeks apart, as well as other factors like the readiness to switch and commit to a new regimen.

Write down a list of questions and concerns that you may have for your doctor. It is also helpful to discuss your feelings about taking anti-HIV therapies, especially for the first time. Some of those questions may include:

- How do I know whether I'm ready to start anti-HIV therapy?

- What I think will happen to me after I start therapy is …

- What will happen if I don't start therapy?

- Is it possible for me to wait?

- How I feel about starting therapy is …

It's probably helpful to keep a list of other questions you may have. Some of these may include:

- What is the potency of this regimen?

- What are the side effects of the various drugs and how often do they occur?

- Is there anything I need to do if these side effects occur?

- How do I monitor for these side effects? Are there things I can do to reduce the risk of getting them?

- How often do I need to come in to check and see if the therapies are working?

- How often should I take these drugs?

- What doses should I take?

- Do any of these drugs require a dose change based on my weight or liver or kidney functions?

- Are there any interactions between these drugs and other drugs, herbs, vitamins or supplements that I take?

Other questions for people who may be co-infected with hepatitis B or C may include:

- Will these drugs affect my liver?
- Do any of these drugs have activity against my hepatitis?
- Should I treat the hepatitis as well as the HIV?
- Will these drugs interact with my therapies for hepatitis?

Commentary

In addition to overall general health and quality of life factors, both CD4+ cell counts and viral load must be considered when making decisions about starting anti-HIV therapy or when considering switching therapies. In most studies, as would be expected, there is a direct inverse correlation (when one goes down the other goes up) between viral load and CD4+ cell counts as more virus means more CD4+ cells being infected and destroyed.

There are some people, who despite substantial decreases in HIV levels continue to experience a decline in CD4+ cell counts. In these cases, it is important for doctors to conduct a more extensive diagnosis to see if some other condition is affecting CD4+ cell counts, such as common or even not so common infections.

Ideal combination strategies call for the use of drugs to be started at the same time. This is readily achievable for people beginning therapy for the first time but far more difficult for those who have used many therapies. Existing therapies can sometimes be juggled to achieve the desired effect. At other times, this may be impossible.

For some people, the best choice may sometimes be to delay using protease inhibitors or other new therapies until there are enough new drugs available to start an ideal combination (e.g. at least two drugs never used before by the person). For most people, this will seldom be more than a year away as several new therapies are on the horizon. But getting there will require some people to resist the urge to jump to each new drug as soon as it is available.

This shift toward long-term thinking is the true hallmark of the second decade of anti-HIV therapy. It must become a part of everyone's thinking. The alternative is the perpetuation of the short-term benefits and long-term failures characteristic of the last decade's approach.

All of this emphasizes the importance of a recent study which showed that people who received medical care from doctors with a great deal of experience in treating HIV infection actually lived longer than those with less experienced ones. The complexity of treating HIV has changed dramatically in the last year and the demands on the knowledge of doctors have increased proportionally.

Whatever medical strategy a person chooses, it should begin with finding a doctor who is experienced in treating HIV and who is wise enough to continue studying and learning from new developments in HIV research.

The Basic Message from Project Inform

1. Learn about HIV testing options and choose one that fits your needs. Be sure your privacy is protected.

2. If you're positive, don't panic. If you make your health a priority, chances are you will be reasonably healthy for many years.

3. Learn about your health care options and local support services.

4. Get a complete physical and blood tests for CD4+ cell count and HIV level. Repeat quarterly and watch for trends. Women should get gynecological and Pap tests every six months, more often if abnormal.

5. Work with a doctor to develop a long-term strategy for managing HIV disease.

6. If the CD4+ cell count is below 350 or falling rapidly, consider starting therapy. Test at least twice before taking action.

7. If therapy fails to reduce your HIV level below the "limit of detection" or below 5,000 copies within three to six months, consider a different more aggressive therapy.

8. If the CD4+ count trend stays below 300, consider treatment for preventing *Pneumocystis carinii*[1] pneumonia (PCP). If it stays below 200, start treatment for preventing PCP (if you haven't already done so) and reconsider anti-HIV therapy if not on one. Learn about drug interactions and preventive treatments for opportunistic infections.

9. If you started preventive therapies and your CD4+ cell count rises in response to anti-HIV therapy, ask your doctor whether it might be safe to stop certain preventive therapies.

10. If your CD4+ cell count stays below 75, consider more frequent blood work—perhaps even monthly. Consider therapies for preventing *Mycobacterium avium* complex (MAC)/ *Mycobacterium avium-intracellulare* complex (MAI) and Cytomegalovirus (CMV).

11. Regularly seek support for your personal, spiritual, and emotional needs. It takes more than medicines to keep you well.

Editor's Note

1. *Pneumocystis carinii* is also called *Pneumocystis jiroveci.*

Chapter 34

Once-a-Day Medications for HIV Treatment

Chapter Contents

Section 34.1

More Convenient HIV Treatment as Effective as More Complex Regimens

"New Study Shows More Convenient HIV Treatment as Effective as More Complex Regimens, Press Release," Agency for Healthcare Research and Quality (http://www.ahrq.gov), Rockville, MD, October 27, 2006.

Regimens to treat HIV infection that are based on a non-nucleoside reverse transcriptase inhibitor (NNRTI) are at least as effective as treatment with a protease inhibitor but require patients to take fewer pills each day, according to a new study funded in part by the Department of Health and Human Services (HHS) Agency for Healthcare Research and Quality (AHRQ).

The study, published in the October 28, [2006], online issue of the *Lancet*, found that disease progression was similar for both regimens, but NNRTI-based treatment appeared more effective at decreasing the amount of virus in the blood. The number of patients who stopped treatment because of adverse events was similar for both medications.

The new study is the first to review all published research that directly compares the two classes of antiretroviral drugs used in highly active antiretroviral therapy (HAART). NNRTI-based regimens were found to be up to 60 percent more likely to suppress the amount of virus in patients' blood than protease inhibitor-based regimens. The percentage of patients who died or experienced disease progression were similar between the two treatments, and the number of patients who stopped taking the medications because of side effects or adverse events was also similar.

While some protease inhibitors require four doses each day, one NNRTI, efavirenz, can be taken in one daily dose. This convenience could increase the likelihood that patients will adhere to their HIV regimens.

Publication of the study follows the July 12, [2006], approval by the Food and Drug Administration of the first once-a-day medication to treat HIV. The drug contains emtricitabine and tenofovir, two nucleoside reverse transcriptase inhibitors, plus efavirenz. The components of the drug were previously available, but it is anticipated that the new combined formulation will simplify treatment and improve compliance.

"A simpler regimen offers the potential of improved adherence and better patient outcomes. Combined with the approval of new dosage formulations, this information could improve the management of patients in this country and in regions of the world where access to medical care and treatment compliance can be challenging," said AHRQ Director Carolyn M. Clancy, MD. "These findings highlight the need for additional research that evaluates the extent to which improvements in markers of a disease, such as viral suppression, lead to improved clinical outcomes."

The Centers for Disease Control and Prevention estimates that between 1 million and 1.2 million people in the United States are living with HIV, and at least 40,000 new infections occur each year. Worldwide, approximately 40 million individuals are infected with the virus.

Researchers, led by Roger Chou, MD, at Oregon Health and Science University in Portland, completed an analysis of 26 trials, including 12 head-to-head trials comparing NNRTI-based regimens with protease inhibitor-based regimens. Fourteen other trials compared two-drug regimens with either NNRTI-based or protease inhibitor-based, triple-drug regimens. Among 3,337 patients analyzed in the head-to-head trials, NNRTI-based regimens were better than protease inhibitor-based regimens by 20 percent to 60 percent in their ability to achieve viral suppression.

Dramatic decreases in the rate of HIV-related illnesses and deaths have occurred since the introduction of HAART therapy in which three or more antiretroviral agents are used. However, until now, comparisons of head-to-head trials were not available to support selection of a protease inhibitor or an NNRTI as part of that combination therapy. Researchers concluded that earlier analyses may be unreliable because their results differed dramatically from the analysis of head-to-head trials, even after excluding patients who had previously received HIV therapy and those who had received older NNRTIs, such as delavirdine, that are now used infrequently because they are less effective than newer NNRTIs. Prior antiretroviral treatment can cause drug resistance and treatment failure.

The study was completed as follow-up to an evidence review prepared by Dr. Chou and a team of researchers at AHRQ's Oregon Evidence-based Practice Center (EPC) in Portland. The EPCs were established to synthesize existing scientific literature about important health care topics and promote evidence-based practice and decision-making.

Section 34.2

Once-a-Day Single Tablet Regimens

"Questions and Answers on Atripla (efavirenz, emtricitabine, tenofovir),"
U.S. Food and Drug Administration (http://www.fda.gov), July 12, 2006.

What is Atripla (efavirenz, emtricitabine, tenofovir)?

Atripla (efavirenz, emtricitabine, tenofovir), a fixed dose combination of three widely used antiretroviral drugs, to be taken as one tablet once a day, is indicated for use alone as a complete treatment option or in combination with other antiretroviral agents for the treatment of human immunodeficiency virus-1 (HIV-1) infection in adult patients.

Why is the approval of Atripla (efavirenz, emtricitabine, tenofovir) important?

The approval of Atripla is significant because it markedly simplifies the drug regimen for HIV-1 infected adults. This product offers a one pill, once-a-day treatment option for patients receiving antiretroviral therapy. There has been interest in simplifying treatment options which may potentially improve the patient's ability to adhere to the treatment and result in long-term effective control of HIV-1.

What is meant by a fixed-dose combination?

A fixed-dose combination package has two or three drugs in a single pill. Whereas a co-packaged product refers to two or three pills in a single package, Atripla combines three drugs (efavirenz, emtricitabine, tenofovir) in a single pill.

What were the efficacy results of the main studies that supported the indication?

The evidence of efficacy (viral load reduction and CD4+ cell count increase) of Atripla is based on the analyses of a 48 week-long clinical trial of 244 HIV-1 infected adult patients receiving the drugs contained in Atripla.

What does the FDA know regarding the safety profile of Atripla?

Each component (efavirenz, emtricitabine, and tenofovir) of Atripla is currently approved for use in combination with other antiretroviral agents to treat HIV-1 infected adults. The safety and effectiveness of each component were demonstrated in clinical trials to support their individual approval. FDA approved Sustiva (efavirenz) in 1998, Viread (tenofovir disoproxil fumarate) in 2001, and Emtriva (emtricitabine) in 2003. In addition, the safety and effectiveness of the combination of these three drugs were shown in a 48 week-long clinical study with 244 HIV-1 infected adults receiving the drugs contained in Atripla.

What adverse events are associated with Atripla?

The most common adverse events include headache, dizziness, abdominal pain, nausea, vomiting, and rash.

What other important safety information should I know about Atripla?

The labeling of Atripla includes a boxed warning that the drug's use can cause lactic acidosis (buildup of an acid in the blood). Atripla is not indicated for use in patients with chronic hepatitis B infection. However, discontinuation of the treatment for HIV-1 with Atripla in patients with chronic hepatitis B infection can result in severe flare-ups of hepatitis B infection. Other potential serious adverse events reported for the use of Atripla's ingredients include serious liver toxicity, renal impairment, and severe depression.

Chapter 35

Alternative and Complementary Therapies

Overview

Many people use complementary (sometimes known as alternative) health treatments to go along with the medical care they get from their doctor.

These therapies are called "complementary" therapies because usually they are used alongside the more standard medical care you receive (such as your doctor visits and the anti-HIV drugs you might be taking).

They are sometimes called "alternative" because they don't fit into the more mainstream, Western ways of looking at medicine and health care. These therapies may not fit in with what you usually think of as "health care."

Some common complementary therapies include the following:

- physical (body) therapies, such as yoga, massage, and acupuncture

- relaxation techniques, such as meditation and visualization

- herbal medicine (from plants)

With most complementary therapies, your health is looked at from a holistic (or "whole picture") point of view. Think of your body as working as one big system. From a holistic viewpoint, everything you

---

"Complementary Therapies," U.S. Department of Veterans Affairs, National HIV/AIDS Program (http://www.hiv.va.gov), updated October 16, 2006.

do—from what you eat to what you drink to how stressed you are—affects your health and well-being.

Do These Therapies Work?

Healthy people use these kinds of therapies to try to make their immune systems stronger and to make themselves feel better in general. People who have diseases or illnesses, such as HIV, use these therapies for the same reasons. They also can use these therapies to help deal with symptoms of the disease or side effects from the medicines that treat the disease.

Many people report positive results from using complementary therapies. In most cases, however, there is not enough research to tell if these treatments really help people with HIV.

If you want to try complementary treatments to help you cope with HIV/AIDS, please remember these things:

- Always talk to your health care provider before you start any kind of treatment, even if you think it is safe.

- Just because something is "natural" (an herb, for example) doesn't mean that it is safe to take. Sometimes these products can interact with your HIV medicines or cause side effects on their own. St. John's wort, for example, decreases levels of some HIV medications in your blood.

- The federal government does not require that herbal remedies and dietary supplements be tested in the same way that standard medicines are tested before they are sold. Many of the treatments out there have not been studied as much as the HIV drugs you are taking. It is always a risk to take something or try something that hasn't been fully studied or researched.

- Be careful of treatments that claim to be "miracle cures"—ones that claim to cure HIV/AIDS. There are people out there who may try to trick you into buying an expensive product that doesn't work. Always do your research and ask your doctor for help.

- Complementary therapies are not substitutes for the treatment and drugs you receive from your doctor. Never stop taking your anti-HIV drugs just because you've started another therapy.

- The federal government is funding studies of how well some alternative therapies work to treat disease, so keep your eyes open for news about these studies.

Here you can read about some of the more common complementary therapies that people with HIV use. Sometimes these are used alone, but often they are used in combination with one another. For example, some people combine yoga with meditation.

Physical (Body) Therapies

Physical, or body, therapies include such activities as yoga, massage, and aromatherapy. These types of therapies focus on using a person's body and senses to promote healing and well-being. Here you can learn about examples of these types of therapies.

Yoga

Yoga is a set of exercises that people use to improve their fitness, reduce stress, and increase flexibility.

Yoga can involve breathing exercises, certain stretches and poses, and meditation.

Many people, including people with HIV, use yoga to reduce stress and to become more relaxed and calm. Some people think that yoga helps make them healthier in general, because it can make a person's body stronger.

If you would like to try yoga, talk to your health care provider. There are many different types of yoga and various classes you can take. You can also try out yoga by following a program on videotape.

Before you begin any kind of exercise program, always talk with your doctor.

Massage

Many people believe that massage therapy is an excellent way to deal with the stress and side effects that go along with having an illness, including HIV.

During massage therapy, a trained therapist moves and rubs your body tissues (such as your muscles). There are many kinds of massage therapy.

You can try massage therapy for reducing muscle and back pain, headaches, and soreness. Massages also can improve your blood flow (your circulation) and reduce tension. Some people think that massages might even make your immune system stronger.

If you are interested in learning more about massage, you should ask your doctor to recommend a trained therapist. Your doctor may have a list of trained massage therapists, so if you want to learn more about massage, ask.

Acupuncture

Acupuncture is part of a whole healing system known as traditional Chinese medicine. During acupuncture treatment, tiny needles (about as wide as a hair) are inserted into certain areas of a person's body. Most people say that they don't feel any pain at all from the needles.

Many people with HIV use acupuncture. Some people think that acupuncture can help treat symptoms of HIV and side effects from the medicine, like fatigue and stomach aches.

Some people say that acupuncture can be used to help with neuropathy (body pain caused by nerve damage from HIV or the medicines used to treat HIV). Others report that acupuncture gives them more energy.

If you are interested in trying it out, ask your doctor to recommend an expert.

Aromatherapy

Aromatherapy is based on the idea that certain smells can change the way you feel. The smells used in aromatherapy come from plant oils, and they can be inhaled (breathed in) or used in baths or massages.

People use aromatherapy to help them deal with stress or to help with fatigue. For example, some people report that lavender oil calms them down and helps them sleep better.

You can also ask friends or family if they've tried aromatherapy or know someone who has.

Please remember: The oils used in aromatherapy can be very strong and even harmful. Always talk with an expert before buying and using these oils yourself.

Relaxation Techniques

Relaxation therapies, such as meditation and visualization, focus on how a person's mind and imagination can promote overall health and well-being. In this section, you can read about some examples of how you can use relaxation therapies to reduce stress and relax.

Meditation

Meditation is a certain way of concentrating that allows your mind and body to become very relaxed. Meditation helps people to focus and be quiet.

There are many different forms of meditation. Most involve deep breathing and paying attention to your body and mind.

Sometimes people sit still and close their eyes to meditate. Meditation also can be casual. For instance, you can meditate when you are taking a walk or watching a sunrise.

People with HIV can use meditation to relax. It can help them deal with the stress that comes with any illness. Meditation can help you to calm down and focus if you are feeling overwhelmed.

If you are interested in learning more about meditation, you should ask your health care provider for more information. There may be meditation classes you can take.

Visualization

Visualization is another method people use to feel more relaxed and less anxious. People who use visualization imagine that they are in a safe, relaxing place (such as the beach). Most of us use visualization without realizing it—for example, when we daydream or remember a fun, happy time in our lives.

Focusing on a safe, comfortable place can help you to feel less stress, and sometimes it can lessen the pain or side effects from HIV or the medicines you are taking.

You can ask your doctor where you can learn more about visualization. There are classes you can take, and there are self-help tapes that you can listen to that lead you through the process.

Herbal Medicine

Many people, including people with HIV, use herbal medicines to improve their health. Herbal medicines are substances that come from plants, and they work like standard medicine. They can be taken from all parts of a plant, including the roots, leaves, berries, and flowers.

People with HIV sometimes take these medicines to help deal with side effects from anti-HIV medicines or with symptoms from the illness.

An important note about St. John's wort: St. John's wort has become a popular herbal medicine for treating depression. It interacts with the liver and can change how some drugs work in your body, including some anti-HIV drugs (protease inhibitors and NNRTIs). If you are taking antiviral drugs for your HIV, you should not take St. John's wort. Be sure you tell you doctor if you are using St. John's wort. You should also not take St. John's wort if you are taking other antidepressants.

- It is important to remember to always use herbs carefully. Learn the proper dosage and use. Don't take too much of anything.

- Always ask your doctor before taking anything new. Just because something is "natural" or "non-drug" doesn't mean that it is safe.

- Finally, learn about the possible side effects of an herbal therapy. Remember: Some herbs can interfere with your HIV medications.

Points to Remember

- In addition to getting mainstream medical care, more and more people are turning to complementary treatments to improve their overall health or to help with specific health problems.

- Complementary therapies can include physical therapies (such as yoga and acupuncture), relaxation techniques (such as meditation), and herbal medicines.

- Many people report that these therapies make them feel better and help with symptoms and side effects.

- It is important to remember that not all complementary therapies are safe for you. In fact, some therapies (including certain herbs) can be very dangerous because they can interact with your HIV drugs or cause severe side effects.

- Always be sure to let your doctor know what medicines you are taking—whether they are prescription or not.

Chapter 36

Resistance Testing

What is HIV drug resistance?

HIV drug resistance means that the virus can adapt, grow, and multiply in the presence of drugs. HIV is considered to be drug resistant when a drug or class of drugs is no longer effective against it.

What causes drug resistance?

HIV replicates very rapidly and makes many mistakes (mutations) in the process. However, HIV doesn't have the ability to correct these mistakes. This results in mutant viruses that can be resistant to one or more of the drugs used in HIV therapy. These mutant viruses continue to make copies of themselves, further reducing the effectiveness of an individual's HIV therapy.

How common is drug resistance?

According to recent data, in three out of four people currently taking HIV drugs, treatment failure is linked to drug resistance. Additionally, one in four newly infected individuals is already resistant to at least one HIV drug.

Excerpted from "Resistance Basics," reprinted with permission from www.hivdrugresistance.com. © 2007 Monogram Biosciences, Inc. You can view the complete text of this document online at http://www.hivdrugresistance.com/210ResistanceBasics.asp.

Why is drug resistance testing important?

When used in combination with treatment history, viral load, and CD4 cell count information, drug resistance testing gives health care providers a more complete picture of an individual's therapy options. This allows providers to develop a treatment plan that is more likely to be effective. In addition, resistance testing may help avoid unnecessary drug side effects and medical costs associated with taking drugs that are not likely to work.

How is drug resistance tested?

A blood sample is taken and sent to a laboratory where one or both types of resistance testing—phenotypic and genotypic—are performed.

- **Phenotypic testing** is performed by testing a sample of a person's HIV against all of the available antiretroviral drugs. By directly measuring the ability of HIV to grow in the presence of these drugs, the laboratory can determine which drugs will work and which are no longer good options. The activity of a person's HIV in the presence of the antiretroviral drugs is compared to the activity of a control strain of HIV that is known to be susceptible to all drugs. This comparison determines how well a drug is likely to work.

- **Genotypic testing** is performed by identifying genetic mutations, or changes in genes, in an individual's HIV that are known to be associated with drug-resistant HIV. Once the mutations have been identified, a computer is usually used to interpret the results for the health care provider.

Can phenotypic and genotypic tests be used together?

Yes. PhenoSense GT is a test from Monogram that combines both types of tests to make up one convenient evaluation of drug resistance that is measured from the same blood sample and is reported on the same report form. The PhenoSense GT report displays phenotypic and genotypic results side by side so that health care providers can select the best possible therapy for a person living with HIV. PhenoSense GT is direct, uses proven technology, and offers consistency because both phenotypic and genotypic results come from the same blood sample.

What do drug resistance test results look like?

The report forms used for Monogram's resistance tests include genotypic and/or phenotypic drug resistance information for all of the approved nucleoside reverse transcriptase inhibitors (NRTIs), non-nucleoside reverse transcriptase inhibitors (NNRTIs), and protease inhibitors (PIs). [Sample report forms for each of the following tests are available online at http://www.hivdrugresistance.com/210ResistanceBasics.asp]:

- GeneSeq™ HIV
- PhenoSense™ HIV
- PhenoSense GT™

When should drug resistance testing be used?

Before therapy begins: Because drug-resistant strains of HIV can be passed from one person to another, resistance testing can be used to evaluate drug resistance in recently infected or newly diagnosed people. The results can help a health care provider work with an individual to design a targeted treatment plan that is more likely to be effective for a longer period of time. By using information about how resistance develops when certain drugs are used, health care providers can design combinations of drugs that will preserve more treatment options if therapy failure occurs later on down the road.

Following treatment failure: When a person no longer benefits from his or her HIV therapy (treatment failure) and viral load is increasing, drug resistance testing can help determine which drug or combination of drugs is no longer effective. A treatment plan can then be developed that is more likely to slow HIV replication.

Throughout therapy: Drug resistance testing can also be used during the course of an individual's therapy. Periodic testing when HIV is detected in plasma can help gauge therapy effectiveness and drug resistance, so that treatments can be altered as needed.

How can HIV-positive people prevent drug resistance?

In addition to working with their health care providers and using drug resistance tests as appropriate, people living with HIV can fight drug resistance by:

- taking HIV drugs on time, every time. If people under HIV treatment skip their medications, stop taking them or don't stick to their schedules, it becomes easier for the virus to develop resistance.

- not sharing needles or having sex without a condom with someone else who has HIV. This way, HIV-positive people avoid exposure to additional, drug-resistant strains of the virus.

Chapter 37

Salvage Therapy

What Is Salvage Therapy?

Antiretroviral therapy (ART) sometimes needs to be changed. This usually happens when the viral load increases instead of staying very low. This treatment failure almost always means that HIV has developed resistance to the antiretroviral drugs (ARVs) someone is taking. Then HIV can multiply even when someone is taking ART.

Before the use of triple combinations of antiretroviral drugs (ARVs) many health care providers changed ART at the first sign of an increase in viral load. Patients were given just one new ARV at a time. This approach is called "sequential monotherapy" or "virtual monotherapy." The goal was just to keep the patient alive for a few more months.

We now know that this is not the best way to control viral load. If the virus is only exposed to one new drug, it's much easier for the virus to develop resistance. Also, as we learn more about salvage therapy, the goal has shifted to be the same as for anyone else: to control viral load and maintain CD4 count.

As a patient's virus accumulates more and more resistance mutations, it becomes harder to choose ARVs that can control it. When there are no good treatment options, ART for these patients is referred to as "salvage therapy." The number of people with HIV in the U.S. who need salvage therapy is unknown, but is estimated to be between 20,000 and 40,000.

How Can You Avoid Salvage Therapy?

The best way to avoid salvage therapy is to make each regimen of ART last as long as you can. Be sure to miss as few doses as possible. Learn about the pattern of resistance of your virus. Ask your health care provider about any changes in your ART.

If possible, you should always have two or more "active drugs" in your ART regimen. An active drug is one that is expected to work against HIV based on the mutations in your virus. Your health care provider will need to review the results of a resistance test. This can be a genotypic test or a phenotypic test.

Remember, the best way to get into trouble is to just add one new drug at a time to failing ART. That will set you up for resistance to the new drug in a very short time.

When Does Someone Need Salvage Therapy?

Once HIV has acquired several resistance mutations, the chances of serious HIV disease are higher. This is especially true for patients with low CD4 counts. You may need to make immediate changes if:

- you are losing weight;
- your CD4 count is dropping;
- you have serious side effects;
- you have increasing symptoms.

However, if your health and CD4 count are stable, you can go onto a "holding regimen" while you wait for new drugs to be developed. Do not stop taking medications to prevent opportunistic infections (OIs). The drugs you need to take to prevent OIs are based on your CD4 count.

What Is a "Holding Regimen"?

If you don't have at least two active ARVs to use, you need to pre-serve your CD4 count and keep your viral load as low as possible. You also want to preserve your treatment options. This normally means stopping any ARVs that are only partly effective so that your virus doesn't develop more resistance to them. This would make them totally ineffective. However, stopping all ARVs can be harmful.

An important concept is viral fitness, how well the virus can multiply. The more mutations HIV has, the slower it multiplies. If you can keep the virus "handicapped" with key mutations, you may be able to stop taking some ARVs. For example, the M184V mutation gives HIV resistance to Epivir (lamivudine, 3TC) and reduces viral fitness. It is helpful to keep Epivir in a holding regimen.

On the other hand, stopping NNRTIs (delavirdine, nevirapine, or efavirenz) does not lead to increases in viral load or drops in CD4 cells. There's no benefit to keeping an NNRTI in a holding regimen. It appears that stopping protease inhibitors is less risky than stopping nukes (reverse transcriptase inhibitors.)

It can be scary to wait until you have two active ARVs available. The alternative is to "use up" a new ARV and lose its benefits quickly due to viral resistance.

Getting Access to New Drugs

You may not have to wait until new drugs are approved before you can use them. You may have access to a clinical trial of a drug in development. Some ARVs become available through an expanded access program long before they are approved. Currently Prezista (darunavir or TMC114) is available in expanded access. Sometimes these programs continue after approval for patients with special needs. You may be able to get Aptivus this way.

Remember that you want to be able to combine a new drug with at least one other active drug. You should review clinical trials carefully with your health care provider to make sure you're not exposed to sequential monotherapy. This is most likely if you get assigned to a "placebo" arm and don't receive the new drug being studied. More information on clinical trials is available at the following websites:

- http://www.salvagetherapies.org/clinical.html,

- http://www.acria.org/clinical_trials/index.html, and

- http://www.clinicaltrials.gov.

The best option is being able to use a drug in a new class. Your virus will almost certainly not have any resistance mutations to a fusion or attachment inhibitor, or an integrase inhibitor. Right now, you might have access to T-20 (Fuzeon, enfuvirtide) which is a fusion inhibitor.

There are also clinical trials of attachment inhibitors and integrase inhibitors and other ARVs.

The Bottom Line

There are more options today for people with advanced HIV disease than at any time in the past. Treatment can have excellent results, even for people whose virus is resistant to most existing ARVs. An experienced health care provider is very important in helping you decide when to change treatment and when to wait.

Part Five

Complications Associated with HIV/AIDS

Chapter 38

Infections Associated with HIV/AIDS

Chapter Contents

Section 38.1

HIV and Hepatitis C Virus (HCV) Co-Infection

"Frequently Asked Questions and Answers about Co-Infection
with Hepatitis C Virus," Centers for Disease Control and Prevention
(http://www.cdc.gov), reviewed January 23, 2007.

Why should HIV-infected persons be concerned about co-infection with HCV?

About one-quarter of HIV-infected persons in the United States are also infected with hepatitis C virus (HCV). HCV is one of the most important causes of chronic liver disease in the United States and HCV infection progresses more rapidly to liver damage in HIV-infected persons. HCV infection may also impact the course and management of HIV infection.

The latest U.S. Public Health Service/Infectious Diseases Society of America (USPHS/IDSA) guidelines recommend that all HIV-infected persons should be screened for HCV infection. Prevention of HCV infection for those not already infected and reducing chronic liver disease in those who are infected are important concerns for HIV-infected individuals and their health care providers.

Who is likely to have HIV-HCV co-infection?

The hepatitis C virus (HCV) is transmitted primarily by large or repeated direct percutaneous (i.e., passage through the skin by puncture) exposures to contaminated blood. Therefore, co-infection with HIV and HCV is common (50 percent–90 percent) among HIV-infected injection drug users (IDUs). Co-infection is also common among persons with hemophilia who received clotting factor concentrates before concentrates were effectively treated to inactivate both viruses (i.e., products made before 1987). The risk for acquiring infection through perinatal or sexual exposures is much lower for HCV than for HIV. For persons infected with HIV through sexual exposure (e.g., male-to-male sexual activity), co-infection with HCV is no more common than among similarly aged adults in the general population (3 percent–5 percent).

What are the effects of co-infection on disease progression of HCV and HIV?

Chronic HCV infection develops in 75 percent–85 percent of infected persons and leads to chronic liver disease in 70 percent of these chronically infected persons. HIV-HCV co-infection has been associated with higher titers of HCV, more rapid progression to HCV-related liver disease, and an increased risk for HCV-related cirrhosis (scarring) of the liver. Because of this, HCV infection has been viewed as an opportunistic infection in HIV-infected persons and was included in the 1999 USPHS/IDSA *Guidelines for the Prevention of Opportunistic Infections in Persons Infected with Human Immunodeficiency Virus.* It is not, however, considered an AIDS-defining illness. As highly active antiretroviral therapy (HAART) and prophylaxis of opportunistic infections increase the life span of persons living with HIV, HCV-related liver disease has become a major cause of hospital admissions and deaths among HIV-infected persons.

The effects of HCV co-infection on HIV disease progression are less certain. Some studies have suggested that infection with certain HCV genotypes is associated with more rapid progression to AIDS or death. However, the subject remains controversial. Since co-infected patients are living longer on HAART, more data are needed to determine if HCV infection influences the long-term natural history of HIV infection.

How can co-infection with HCV be prevented?

Persons living with HIV who are not already co-infected with HCV can adopt measures to prevent acquiring HCV. Such measures will also reduce the chance of transmitting their HIV infection to others.

Not injecting or stopping injection drug use would eliminate the chief route of HCV transmission; substance-abuse treatment and relapse-prevention programs should be recommended. If patients continue to inject, they should be counseled about safer injection practices; that is, to use new, sterile syringes every time they inject drugs and never reuse or share syringes, needles, water, or drug preparation equipment.

Toothbrushes, razors, and other personal care items that might be contaminated with blood should not be shared. Although there are no data from the United States indicating that tattooing and body piercing place persons at increased risk for HCV infection, these procedures may be a source for infection with any bloodborne pathogen if proper infection control practices are not followed.

Although consistent data are lacking regarding the extent to which sexual activity contributes to HCV transmission, persons having multiple sex partners are at risk for other sexually transmitted diseases (STDs) as well as for transmitting HIV to others. They should be counseled accordingly.

How should patients co-infected with HIV and HCV be managed?

General guidelines: Patients co-infected with HIV and HCV should be encouraged to adopt safe behaviors (as described in the previous section) to prevent transmission of HIV and HCV to others.

Individuals with evidence of HCV infection should be given information about prevention of liver damage, undergo evaluation for chronic liver disease and, if indicated, be considered for treatment. Persons co-infected with HIV and HCV should be advised not to drink excessive amounts of alcohol. Avoiding alcohol altogether might be wise because the effects of even moderate or low amounts of alcohol (e.g., 12 ounces of beer, 5 ounces of wine, or 1.5 ounces of hard liquor per day) on disease progression are unknown. When appropriate, referral should be made to alcohol treatment and relapse-prevention programs. Because of possible effects on the liver, HCV-infected patients should consult with their health care professional before taking any new medicines, including over-the-counter, alternative or herbal medicines.

Susceptible co-infected patients should receive hepatitis A vaccine because the risk for fulminant hepatitis associated with hepatitis A is increased in persons with chronic liver disease. Susceptible patients should receive hepatitis B vaccine because most HIV-infected persons are at risk for HBV infection. The vaccines appear safe for these patients and more than two-thirds of those vaccinated develop antibody responses. Prevaccination screening for antibodies against hepatitis A and hepatitis B in this high-prevalence population is generally cost-effective. Postvaccination testing for hepatitis A is not recommended, but testing for antibody to hepatitis B surface antigen (anti-HBs) should be performed one to two months after completion of the primary series of hepatitis B vaccine. Persons who fail to respond should be revaccinated with up to three additional doses.

HAART has no significant effect on HCV. However, co-infected persons may be at increased risk for HAART-associated liver toxicity and should be closely monitored during antiretroviral therapy. Data suggest that the majority of these persons do not appear to develop significant and/or symptomatic hepatitis after initiation of antiretroviral therapy.

Treatment for HCV infection: A Consensus Development Conference Panel convened by The National Institutes of Health in 1997 recommended antiviral therapy for patients with chronic hepatitis C who are at the greatest risk for progression to cirrhosis. These persons include anti-HCV positive patients with persistently elevated liver enzymes, detectable HCV RNA, and a liver biopsy that indicates either portal or bridging fibrosis or at least moderate degrees of inflammation and necrosis. Patients with less severe histological disease should be managed on an individual basis.

In the United States, two different regimens have been approved as therapy for chronic hepatitis C: monotherapy with alpha interferon and combination therapy with alpha interferon and ribavirin. Among HIV-negative persons with chronic hepatitis C, combination therapy consistently yields higher rates (30 percent–40 percent) of sustained response than monotherapy (10 percent–20 percent). Combination therapy is more effective against viral genotypes 2 and 3, and requires a shorter course of treatment; however, viral genotype 1 is the most common among U.S. patients. Combination therapy is associated with more side effects than monotherapy, but, in most situations, it is preferable. At present, interferon monotherapy is reserved for patients who have contraindications to the use of ribavirin.

Studies thus far, although not extensive, have indicated that response rates in HIV-infected patients to alpha interferon monotherapy for HCV were lower than in non-HIV-infected patients, but the differences were not statistically significant. Monotherapy appears to be reasonably well tolerated in co-infected patients, but studies currently underway suggest it is superior to monotherapy. However, the side effects of combination therapy are greater in co-infected patients. Thus, combination therapy should be used with caution until more data are available.

The decision to treat people co-infected with HIV and HCV must also take into consideration their concurrent medications and medical conditions. If CD4 counts are normal or minimally abnormal (greater than 400/ul), there is little difference in treatment success rates between those who are co-infected and those who are infected with HCV alone.

Other treatment considerations: Persons with chronic hepatitis C who continue to abuse alcohol are at risk for ongoing liver injury, and antiviral therapy may be ineffective. Therefore, strict abstinence from alcohol is recommended during antiviral therapy, and interferon should be given with caution to a patient who has only recently stopped alcohol abuse. Typically, a six-month abstinence is recommended for alcohol abusers before starting therapy; such patients should be treated with the support and collaboration of alcohol abuse treatment programs.

Although there is limited experience with antiviral treatment for chronic hepatitis C of persons who are recovering from long-term injection drug use, there are concerns that interferon therapy could be associated with relapse into drug use, both because of its side effects and because it is administered by injection. There is even less experience with treatment of persons who are active injection drug users, and an additional concern for this group is the risk for reinfection with HCV. Although a six-month abstinence before starting therapy also has been recommended for injection drug users, additional research is needed on the benefits and drawbacks of treating these patients. Regardless, when patients with past or continuing problems of substance abuse are being considered for treatment, such patients should be treated only in collaboration with substance abuse specialists or counselors. Patients can be successfully treated while on methadone maintenance treatment of addiction.

Because many co-infected patients have conditions or factors (such as major depression or active illicit drug or alcohol use) that may prevent or complicate antiviral therapy, treatment for chronic hepatitis C in HIV-infected patients should be coordinated by health care providers with experience in treating co-infected patients or in clinical trials. It is not known if maintenance therapy is needed after successful therapy, but patients should be counseled to avoid injection drug use and other behaviors that could lead to reinfection with HCV and should continue to abstain from alcohol.

Infections in infants and children: The average rate of HCV infection among infants born to women co-infected with HCV and HIV is 14 percent to 17 percent, higher than among infants born to women infected with HCV alone. Data are limited on the natural history of HCV infection in children, and antiviral drugs for chronic hepatitis C are not FDA-approved for use in children under age 18 years. Therefore, children should be referred to a pediatric hepatologist or similar specialist for management and for determination for eligibility in clinical trials.

What research is needed on HIV-HCV co-infection?

Many important questions remain about HIV-HCV co-infection:

- By what mechanism does HIV infection affect the natural history of hepatitis C?

- Does HAART affect the impact of HIV on the natural history of HCV infection?

- Does HCV affect the natural history of HIV and, if so, by what mechanism?

- How can we effectively and safely treat chronic hepatitis C in HIV-infected patients?

- How can we distinguish between liver toxicity caused by anti-retrovirals and that caused by HCV infection?

- What is the best protocol for treating both HIV and chronic hepatitis C in the co-infected patient?

Section 38.2

Herpes Simplex Virus (HSV) and HIV-1

"Herpes Simplex (Cold Sores and Genital Herpes)," Fact Sheet 508, © 2007 AIDS InfoNet. Reprinted with permission. Fact sheets are regularly updated. Check http://www.aidsinfonet.org for the most recent information.

What Is Herpes?

Herpes simplex refers to a group of viruses that infect humans. Like herpes zoster (shingles), herpes simplex causes very painful skin eruptions. Itching and tingling are usually the first signs, followed by a bump that breaks open and becomes very painful. The infection goes dormant for periods of time. It can become active again with no warning.

Herpes simplex virus 1 (HSV-1) is the common cause of cold sores (oral herpes) around the mouth. HSV-2 normally causes genital herpes. However, through sexual activity, HSV-1 can cause infections in the genital area, and HSV-2 can infect the mouth area.

HSV is a very common disease. Approximately 45 million people in the U.S. have HSV infection—about one in five people over the age of 12. The U.S. Centers for Disease Control estimates that there are 1 million new genital herpes infections each year. The rates of HSV infection have increased significantly in the past ten years or so. About 80 percent of people with HIV are also infected with genital herpes.

HSV-2 infection is more common in women. It infects about one out of four women and about one out of five men. Genital HSV can cause potentially fatal infections in babies. If a woman has active genital herpes at delivery, a cesarean delivery is usually performed.

Repeat outbreaks of HSV are most likely to occur in people with a weakened immune system. This includes people with HIV disease, and anyone over 50 years old. Some people also believe that repeat outbreaks are more common when someone is very tired or experiencing a lot of stress.

HSV and HIV

HSV is not one of the infections that are part of the official diagnosis of AIDS. However, people infected with both HIV and HSV are likely to have more frequent outbreaks of herpes. These outbreaks can be more serious, and last longer than for people without HIV.

Herpes sores provide a way for HIV to get past the body's immune defenses and make it easier to get HIV infection. A recent study found that people with HSV had three times the risk of becoming infected with HIV as people without HSV. People with active herpes should be very careful during sexual activity to avoid becoming infected with HIV.

People with both HIV and HSV also need to be very careful during outbreaks of HSV. Their HIV viral load usually goes up, which can make it easier to transmit HIV to others.

How Is HSV Transmitted?

HSV infections are passed from person to person by direct contact with an infected area. You don't have to have an open HSV sore to spread the infection!

Also, most people with HSV don't know that they are infected and aren't aware that they could be spreading it. In fact, in the U.S. only about 9 percent of people with HSV-2 infection knew that they had it.

How Is Herpes Treated?

The standard treatment for HSV is the drug acyclovir, given orally (in pill form) up to five times a day. Another form of acyclovir is valacyclovir. It can be taken just twice a day, but it is much more expensive than acyclovir. Famciclovir is another drug used to treat HSV. New drugs are being tested. ME-609 (by Medivir) for oral herpes is finishing Phase II trials. PCL-016 (by Novactyl) for oral or genital herpes is in Phase II trials.

These drugs do not cure HSV infections. However, they can make the outbreaks shorter and less severe. Doctors may prescribe "maintenance" therapy—daily anti-herpes medications—for people with HIV who have had repeated outbreaks. Maintenance therapy will prevent most future outbreaks.

Can Herpes Be Prevented?

It is difficult to prevent the spread of HSV. Partly this is because many infected people don't know that they carry HSV and can spread it. Even people who know they are infected with HSV may not realize they can transmit the infection even without an open herpes sore.

Condoms can reduce the rate of HSV transmission. However, they cannot prevent it. HSV infections can be transmitted to and from a larger genital area, such as that area covered by "boxer shorts"—and also around the mouth. If people with herpes take valacyclovir every day, they can reduce the risk of transmitting herpes to others.

Drug companies are working on vaccines to prevent HSV. One vaccine showed good results against HSV-2 in women, but not in men. No vaccines have been approved yet to prevent HSV infection, but research is ongoing in this area.

The Bottom Line

Herpes simplex is a viral infection that can cause genital herpes or "cold sores" around the mouth. Most people infected with HSV don't know it. HSV is transmitted easily from person to person during sexual activity or other direct contact with a herpes infection site. Herpes can be transmitted even when there is no visible open sore.

There is no cure for herpes. It is a permanent infection. People with herpes have occasional outbreaks of painful blisters. When each outbreak ends, the infection becomes latent for a while. People with HIV have more frequent and more serious outbreaks of HSV.

Section 38.3

Cryptosporidiosis

- Cryptosporidiosis [krip-toe-spo-rid-ee-OH-sis] is a parasitic illness that causes diarrhea. It is an important emerging infection in the United States.

- Cryptosporidiosis parasites are passed in the stool of infected persons and animals. People get cryptosporidiosis when they swallow the parasites. Sources of disease include parasite-containing stool, food, and water.

- Anyone can get cryptosporidiosis, but persons with weakened immune systems can develop serious, life-threatening illness.

- There is no specific treatment for cryptosporidiosis.

- Cryptosporidiosis can be prevented by washing hands, drinking safe water, eating safe food, and avoiding all contact with the stool of infected persons or animals.

What is cryptosporidiosis?

Cryptosporidiosis is a parasitic illness that causes diarrhea.

What is the infectious agent that causes cryptosporidiosis?

Cryptosporidiosis is caused by *Cryptosporidium parvum*, a microscopic one-celled parasite that can live in the intestines of humans, farm animals, wild animals, and pets.

The parasite is protected by an outer shell called an oocyst [oh-oh-cist]. This protective shell allows it to survive outside the body for a long time. When a person or animal swallows a *Cryptosporidium* oocyst, the parasite comes out of its shell and can cause infection.

Then, more oocysts are produced and passed in the stool of the infected person or animal.

Where is cryptosporidiosis found?

Cryptosporidium parasites can be found anywhere in the environment that is contaminated by animal droppings or human waste. *Cryptosporidium* oocysts can contaminate soil and the food grown in it. They can get onto objects and surfaces that people touch. They can get into lakes, rivers, streams, and pools where people swim. They are also in many of the reservoirs that provide drinking water in the United States.

How do people get cryptosporidiosis?

People get cryptosporidiosis by swallowing *Cryptosporidium* oocysts. Even a few can cause infection. Some sources of cryptosporidiosis are as follows:

Human and Animal Waste

- Diapers, clothing, bedding, or other items can be soiled with stool from an infected person or animal.

- Infected persons might have small amounts of *Cryptosporidium*-containing stool on their skin in the genital area. Sexual activities that might involve contact with stool can lead to infection with *Cryptosporidium*.

- The feces of animals, especially young animals and animals with diarrhea, can contain *Cryptosporidium*. People can be exposed to the parasite when touching animals, cleaning up their droppings, cleaning cages or stalls, or visiting barns and other places where animals live.

Food

- Food can be grown in or can fall on soil contaminated with human or animal waste.

- Unpasteurized milk and dairy products can be contaminated after contact with stool from an infected animal.

- Food can be contaminated when it is handled by someone who is infected or when it is washed with *Cryptosporidium*-contaminated water.

Water

- Water in lakes, rivers, streams, ocean bays, swimming pools, hot tubs, and recreational water parks can be contaminated with *Cryptosporidium*. People can get cryptosporidiosis if they drink this water or accidentally swallow it when swimming. Neither the chlorine used to disinfect swimming pools nor the types of filters used in most pools can be depended on to kill or remove *Cryptosporidium*.

- Contaminated drinking water or ice can be a source of *Cryptosporidium* infection. Unlike most disease-causing organisms, *Cryptosporidium* is not completely removed or killed by the treatment methods most commonly used for drinking water.

What are the signs and symptoms of cryptosporidiosis?

- watery diarrhea
- stomach cramps
- upset stomach
- slight fever

People with healthy immune systems will usually have symptoms for two weeks or less, although during that time symptoms might improve and then worsen. People who recover from their initial illness can continue to pass *Cryptosporidium* in their stool for up to two months. During this two-month period they can spread the disease to others. Although some people who swallow *Cryptosporidium* oocysts will not get sick, they can still pass the organism in their stool.

People with severely weakened immune systems often cannot clear the parasite. They can suffer more severe diarrhea that can last long enough to be life threatening. People with HIV infection, cancer, and transplant patients taking certain immune-suppressing drugs, and persons with inherited diseases that affect the immune system should talk to their health care providers about how to avoid cryptosporidiosis.

How soon after exposure do symptoms appear?

Symptoms appear two to ten days after swallowing *Cryptosporidium* oocysts.

How is cryptosporidiosis diagnosed?

Cryptosporidiosis is diagnosed in a laboratory by examining a stool sample for oocysts. A health care worker who suspects cryptosporidiosis must specifically order testing for *Cryptosporidium*, since routine tests do not test for this parasite.

Who is at risk for cryptosporidiosis?

Anyone can get cryptosporidiosis, but some persons are at increased risk:

- child-care workers and diaper-aged children who attend day-care centers

- persons who take care of infected persons at home or in a group setting

- persons exposed to human stool during sexual contact

- persons with weakened immune systems, such as cancer patients, organ transplant recipients, and persons with HIV infection

What is the treatment for cryptosporidiosis?

There is no specific treatment for cryptosporidiosis. Healthy persons with normal immune systems usually get better on their own. The recommended treatment is to drink plenty of fluids and to get extra rest. Doctors may prescribe medicine to slow the diarrhea. Young children and persons with weakened immune systems might need special treatment from a health care provider to replace fluids lost during the illness.

How common is cryptosporidiosis?

Cases of cryptosporidiosis occur singly and in outbreaks. Individual cases have been reported most often in persons with weakened immune systems, and infection with *Cryptosporidium* is among the most common causes of diarrhea in persons with AIDS in the United States. With the help of new techniques to diagnose the infection, however, cases in persons with healthy immune systems are being reported more often.

Six well-documented outbreaks of cryptosporidiosis attributed to municipal drinking water have been recognized in the United States, including an outbreak in Milwaukee, Wisconsin, that affected more than 400,000 persons. The sources of drinking water linked to these outbreaks included surface water (lakes, rivers, streams), well water, and spring water. Studies show that *Cryptosporidium* oocysts are in 65 percent to 97 percent of surface water tested around the country. Outbreaks have also been associated with swimming pools and amusement park wave pools and water slides.

Is cryptosporidiosis an emerging infectious disease?

Yes. Cryptosporidiosis is an important emerging infection in the United States and a cause of severe, life-threatening disease in persons with weakened immune systems. *Cryptosporidium* was recognized as a cause of human disease in 1976, but was rarely reported until 1982, when cases increased dramatically as part of the HIV/AIDS epidemic. Still, few people had heard of cryptosporidiosis until the 1993 outbreak in Milwaukee. Since then, concern about the safety of drinking water in the United States has increased, and attention has been focused on determining and reducing the risk for cryptosporidiosis from water supplies and other sources.

How can cryptosporidiosis be prevented?

The risk of infection associated with each of the sources of *Cryptosporidium* parasites is still unknown. Until more is learned about this organism, it is important to follow these basic prevention steps:

- Keep hands clean. Wash hands thoroughly with soap and warm water after using the toilet, after changing diapers, and before handling or eating food. Wash hands well after touching faucet handles, clothing, bedding, toilets, or bed pans soiled by someone with diarrhea. Wash hands after gardening, after cleaning up after pets or other animals, and after touching anything that might have had contact with even small amounts of human or animal stool. Supervise children to make sure they wash their hands well.

- Avoid sexual activity that might involve contact with stool.

- Drink safe water. Know the source of your drinking water. Avoid swallowing water when swimming in lakes, rivers, the ocean, or pools, and when using hot tubs. When camping or traveling in a less developed region, avoid drinking water that has not been boiled or filtered to remove *Cryptosporidium*.

- Eat safe food. Prepare food carefully. Wash all vegetables or fruits that you eat raw, even those that you peel before eating. Wash foods with purified (boiled or filtered) water. Use only pasteurized milk, dairy products, juices, and ciders.

- Comply with any water advisories issued by local and state authorities.

What extra precautions should persons with weakened immune systems take to reduce the risk?

Cryptosporidiosis can be a severe, life-threatening disease in persons with weakened immune systems. If you have a weakened immune system, talk to your health care provider about the need for extra precautions to minimize the risk of infection. These might include the following steps:

- Boil all drinking water, or use filters or bottled water for all drinking water, including water for tooth brushing.

- Wash hands thoroughly after any contact with stool.

- Avoid sexual practices that can result in hand or mouth exposure to stool.

- Avoid direct exposure to cattle and other farm animals. If exposure cannot be avoided, wash hands well immediately after contact.

This section is for information only and is not meant to be used for self-diagnosis or as a substitute for consultation with a health care provider. If you have any questions about the disease described above or think that you might have a parasitic infection, consult a health care provider.

Section 38.4

Mycobacterium Avium *Complex*

"Mycobacterium Avium Complex," From Project Inform, © 2004. For more information, contact the National HIV/AIDS Treatment Infoline, 1-800-822-7422, or visit our website at www.projectinform.org.

Mycobacterium avium complex (my-koe-back-teer-ee-um ay-vee-um com-plecks) disease is among the most common bacterial infections in people living with HIV. In one study, MAC bacteria were found in the blood of 43 percent of people within two years of diagnosis with AIDS. MAC is most likely to occur in people with CD4+ cell counts below 50 and at least one other opportunistic infection (OI).

Routine blood tests from people with low CD4+ cell counts can detect MAC at an early stage when it can be treated fairly easily. Drugs can also be used to prevent MAC disease in people with low CD4+ cell counts.

If you develop MAC disease, treatment can ease symptoms and improve your quality of life. And, if you have had MAC disease, then you will need to continue taking drugs to stop the disease from returning. Drug resistance is a serious issue in treating MAC, but potent treatments can slow the development of drug-resistant MAC bacteria.

Cause

MAC is the term for two related bacteria: *Mycobacterium avium* and *Mycobacterium intracellulare* (MAI). These bacteria are found in water, dust, soil, and bird droppings. They enter the body in food and water or sometimes through the lungs.

Most people usually have small numbers of these bacteria growing in their gut or lungs, but do not have any symptoms. This is because a weakened immune system allows the bacteria to attack the lining of the gut and multiply. From there, they can enter the blood and spread through the body, which is called disseminated infection.

Diagnosis

MAC is diagnosed by culture from blood, tissue or bone marrow. If MAC bacteria are found in stool and sputum samples, this could mean the infection has spread. Doctors may have to use special methods to get cells or tissue for MAC diagnosis. These include taking bone marrow from the hip using a needle, or inserting a flexible tube into the stomach or bowels (endoscopy) or the lungs (bronchoscopy).

Some doctors choose to treat MAC infection while waiting for the test results, which can take several weeks. New tests are being developed to give a faster diagnosis. These include polymerase chain reaction (PCR) and branched DNA (bDNA) tests for MAC (the same methods used for HIV viral load tests). Severe anemia and liver problems can occur in MAC, so doctors may take blood samples to look for a low red blood cell count or raised alkaline phosphatase levels.

Symptoms

The most common symptoms of MAC are persistent fevers plus night sweats, loss of appetite, weight loss, tiredness or worsening diarrhea. Symptoms of early disease often involve the gut: stomach cramps, nausea, and vomiting. Disseminated disease can lead to bone, brain or skin infections, or cause painful joints.

Signs of MAC include swollen abdominal lymph nodes, usually on only one side of the body, and an enlarged liver and spleen. Coughing and wheezing are less common. Since many of these symptoms are similar to symptoms of other OIs, it's important to get a correct diagnosis before you start treatment. If you have symptoms like these, talk to your doctor.

A recent study showed that people who already have MAC when they start potent anti-HIV therapy sometimes have an unusual response. It has been called MAC reversal syndrome and results from improved immune function (increases in CD4+ cell counts). It involves fevers and the growth of lumps usually around the neck or spine. The drug prednisone can reduce these symptoms.

Over time, these people still benefit from anti-HIV therapy and their MAC infection stabilizes. So anti-HIV therapy does not always stop MAC in people with early MAC infection, but overall it seems to be beneficial whether or not MAC occurs. However, it may be useful to screen for MAC in people with symptoms like fevers before they start anti-HIV therapy.

Treating Mycobacterium Avium Complex

Treatment reduces the symptoms of MAC disease and improves your quality of life. However, treating MAC is difficult for several reasons:

- **MAC can easily become drug-resistant.** MAC strains found in people with HIV are naturally more drug-resistant than those found in most HIV-negative people. Treatment usually involves taking several drugs for a long time. Combining several drugs increases the chance of side effects and drug interactions and can be expensive. This may mean that people do not finish the full treatment, which can lead to drug resistance.

- **The needed dose of drug may cause serious side effects.** Some drugs used to treat MAC are destroyed by stomach juices or cannot be dissolved in body fluids. It is particularly difficult for drugs to get into cells called macrophages, where MAC bacteria are found. In order to have high enough levels of the drug at the site of infection, higher doses may be needed. This may then lead to side effects.

- **The effect of a drug on MAC bacteria in a lab test is not a reliable guide to treating someone with MAC.** Resistance patterns of MAC bacteria vary a lot. It may be difficult to work out the best MAC treatment for an individual.

Treating MAC infection requires several drugs because no one drug by itself is effective. MAC bacteria can quickly become resistant to a drug and to other drugs in the same family. Combination therapy is more effective and may slow the development of drug resistance.

The Public Health Service Task Force recommends that MAC treatment includes: clarithromycin (Biaxin) 500 mg twice a day, or azithromycin (Zithromax) 500–600 mg/day PLUS ethambutol (Myambutol) 15 mg/kg/day PLUS one or more of rifabutin (Mycobutin), rifampin (Rifadin, Rimactane), ciprofloxacin (Cipro) or amikacin (Amikin).

Use of clofazimine (Lamprene) has been shown to increase the risk of death during MAC treatment in several studies, so it should not be used.

Azithromycin and clarithromycin are related antibiotics. They are approved for treating serious bacterial infections including MAC in combination with at least one other drug. Resistance to clarithromycin develops quickly when used alone. The higher the level of bacteria in the blood before starting therapy, the more rapid resistance develops.

Clarithromycin has been studied together with various anti-MAC therapies. Studies show that a combination of clarithromycin, ethambutol, and rifabutin may prevent developing resistance to clarithromycin, which is common with two-drug combinations. One study also showed that people using the three drugs had fewer symptoms and lower levels of MAC bacteria in their blood. Survival was also longer on three-drug regimens.

This suggests that using clarithromycin or azithromycin together with ethambutol and rifabutin should now be the standard treatment for people with MAC disease. However, several studies have shown that people taking 1,000 mg of clarithromycin twice a day had a higher death rate than those taking 500 mg twice a day. The higher dose should not be used.

Doctors have had less experience with azithromycin for treating MAC compared to clarithromycin. Studies are underway to find the best treatment combination using azithromycin.

Several pharmaceutical companies have payment assistance programs for their anti-MAC drugs. Doctors should call the toll-free number:

- Azithromycin: Pfizer, Inc., 800-869-9979

- Ethambutol: Dura Pharmaceuticals, 800-859-8586

Side Effects

The most common side effects with azithromycin and clarithromycin are nausea, vomiting, diarrhea, and abdominal pain. A rare side effect is hearing loss. Azithromycin may also cause swelling of the blood vessels and liver damage.

Ethambutol can cause nausea and vomiting. It may lead to impaired vision, so people taking this drug should have regular eye checkups.

Common side effects of rifabutin include orange urine, stomach upsets, and rashes. In some studies, up to a quarter of people taking rifabutin developed uveitis, a painful inflammation in the eye. This occurred more often among people who also took clarithromycin.

Drug Interactions

Interactions may occur between clarithromycin and rifabutin. Rifabutin can decrease clarithromycin levels in the blood by 50 percent, while clarithromycin can increase rifabutin levels by as much as 80 percent. Fluconazole, an antifungal drug, can also increase rifabutin levels by up to 80 percent. Increased levels of rifabutin could cause more severe side effects like uveitis. It's important to talk to your doctor about potential drug interactions.

Rifabutin and clarithromycin may interact with protease inhibitors (PIs). Azithromycin is not thought to interact with PIs so it may be the best choice for people taking a protease inhibitor.

In general, people taking PIs should avoid rifabutin. If a person has to take rifabutin, indinavir is the PI of choice, and the dose of rifabutin should be cut in half. Rifabutin may also interact with some non-nucleoside reverse transcriptase inhibitors.

Although PIs might also raise clarithromycin levels, there are not enough data on this to say whether the dose of either drug should be changed. Clarithromycin may also decrease blood levels of zidovudine. For more details about interactions of anti-MAC treatments with other drugs, read Project Inform's publication, *Drug Interactions*, available at 800-822-7422 or http://www.projectinform.org.

Cytokines

Because MAC bacteria often live in cells called macrophages, new treatments for MAC may target these cells. Macrophages are scavenger cells that eat up and kill bacteria and viruses. They circulate in the blood or live in organs like the liver, spleen, or lungs. In people with HIV, macrophages can eat but not kill MAC bacteria. The bacteria grow inside the macrophages and can be spread through the body.

Cells of the immune system release chemicals, called cytokines, that enable them to signal and work with each other to fight infections. In the future, cytokines may be given to enhance the effect of anti-MAC drugs by helping macrophages kill MAC bacteria. A study combining azithromycin with granulocyte macrophage-colony stimulating factor (GM-CSF) is looking at this. Interleukin-12 (IL-12) is in early studies as well.

Preventing the Infection

It is difficult to avoid contact with MAC bacteria, but there are some ways to reduce the risk.

- Boil drinking water. MAC bacteria are found in most water systems, hospital water supplies, and bottled water.

- Do not eat raw foods, especially salads, root vegetables, and unpasteurized milk and cheese.

- MAC bacteria are killed at 176° F, so they are destroyed during normal cooking.

- Rinse and peel fruit and vegetables thoroughly.

- Avoid contact with animals, especially birds and bird droppings. Pigeons—common in most cities—can also transmit cryptococcosis, an OI affecting people with HIV.

- Avoid or reduce alcohol intake. Drinking alcohol regularly can help MAC infection to spread more quickly in people with HIV.

Drugs can be used to prevent or delay the onset of MAC in people with HIV. Three drugs are approved by the Food and Drug Administration (FDA) for MAC prevention: azithromycin, clarithromycin, and rifabutin. The decision to start MAC prevention should take into account possible drug side effects and interactions with other drugs. In addition, MAC bacteria may become resistant to a drug when it is used alone for preventing the disease.

The Public Health Service recommends that people with CD4+ cell counts below 50 should take either clarithromycin (500 mg twice a day) or azithromycin (1,200 mg once a week) for preventing MAC disease. Rifabutin (300 mg/day) should only be used if clarithromycin or azithromycin cannot be taken. There is a risk of developing resistance to clarithromycin, so azithromycin might be the best first choice.

Studies have shown that clarithromycin can reduce the chance of developing MAC by 70 percent. Another study showed that outbreaks of MAC disease were reduced by 65 percent in people who took azithromycin. Both drugs also protect against bacterial infections in the lungs and airways. Rifabutin can reduce the risk of developing MAC by 30–50 percent. Combinations of these drugs have been tested for MAC prevention, but in all cases increased side effects and cost outweigh any added protection from disease.

One worrying outcome of these studies was that some people develop resistant MAC. MAC bacteria were three times as likely to become resistant to clarithromycin taken alone than to azithromycin. Taking clarithromycin with rifabutin did not decrease the risk of resistance to clarithromycin.

As clarithromycin is often the drug of choice to treat MAC, some doctors choose not to use it for MAC prevention. That way, it is still an option for treating the disease later if necessary. However, the chance of having an outbreak of MAC disease is very low when on preventive therapy with clarithromycin or azithromycin, so resistant bacteria are quite rare.

No studies have yet compared clarithromycin and azithromycin for MAC prevention. The two drugs are very similar, so developing resistance to one is likely to result in some level of resistance to the other (cross-resistance). Rifabutin belongs to a different class of drugs, so there should be no cross-resistance between rifabutin and either azithromycin or clarithromycin.

It's important to make sure that you do not have disseminated MAC disease before you start preventive therapy, as this may lead to drug-resistant bacteria. It is also essential to have a chest x-ray and tuberculosis (TB) skin test. The bacteria that cause MAC and TB are related. Some drugs used to treat MAC are also used for TB. If you have active TB, using a single anti-MAC drug may lead to resistant TB. This is most important before starting MAC prevention with rifabutin. Rifabutin is closely related to rifampin, a drug used to treat TB, and cross-resistance can develop.

Stopping Preventive Therapy

Many studies have shown that OIs and deaths have been reduced since protease inhibitors were first used. Now several studies show that it may be safe for people on potent anti-HIV therapy to stop OI prevention if there is evidence of immune reconstitution.

One study looked at 643 people whose CD4+ cell counts had risen from below 50 to over 100 following potent anti-HIV therapy. About 60 percent of people in the study had viral loads below 500 copies HIV RNA. They were given either azithromycin (1,200 mg once a week) or placebo (sugar pill).

After one year there were only two cases of MAC, and both cases were in the placebo group. So, people who have had a CD4+ cell count over 100 and a low viral load for at least three to six months may be able to stop taking MAC prevention. You should think about restarting MAC prevention if your CD4+ cell count falls back below 50.

Maintenance Therapy

People who have been treated for MAC disease have to take anti-MAC drugs for life as symptoms will often return if therapy is stopped. This is called maintenance therapy. The best maintenance therapy should lower the risk of drug resistance and should have few side effects. The current recommendation is to use clarithromycin or azithromycin plus ethambutol with or without rifabutin.

Successful treatment with potent anti-HIV therapy for several months may reduce the risk of relapse for people on maintenance therapy for MAC. However, it is not recommended that people stop their maintenance therapy as this has not been studied in enough people.

When Making a Decision about OI Prevention, Consider These Guidelines

- Potent anti-HIV therapy restores the immune response slowly over time. It may be wise to wait until you establish a good response to anti-HIV therapy (HIV levels decrease and CD4+ cell counts increase) for at least a few months before changing prevention strategies.

- The risk of stopping prevention is likely to be lowest in people who have never had an OI before they started anti-HIV therapy.

- People who have the strongest and longest lasting improvement in CD4+ cell count due to anti-HIV therapy probably stand the best chance of success when stopping OI prevention.

- A person's tolerance for the risk of getting an OI must be weighed against their willingness to take extra drugs and risk side effects.

Children

Children with advanced HIV have a high risk of developing disseminated MAC. It is recommended that preventive MAC therapy with azithromycin (20 mg/kg once a week, max. 1,200 mg/day) or clarithromycin (7.5 mg/kg twice a day, max. 1,000 mg/ day) be started in children in the following categories:

- older than six years, CD4+ cells below 50

- two to six years old, CD4+ cells below 75

- one to two years old, CD4+ cells below 500

- less than twelve months old, CD4+ cells below 750

Azithromycin and clarithromycin are both available as a liquid for children. A solution of rifabutin can be made by a pharmacist using the powder from capsules. There have not been any studies on the safety of stopping MAC prevention in children whose CD4+ cell counts have increased due to potent anti-HIV therapy.

The guidelines for treating children with MAC are the same as those for adults. To stop MAC returning in children, they should take the following maintenance therapy: clarithromycin (30 mg/kg per day in two doses) plus at least one of ethambutol (15 mg/kg once a day), and rifabutin (5 mg/kg once a day).

Pregnancy

Pregnant women should take the same MAC preventive therapy as other adults. Animal studies suggest that clarithromycin, ethambutol or rifabutin may cause some harm to the developing child during the first three months of pregnancy. Doctors may prefer to wait until the second trimester to begin or continue preventive therapy.

Azithromycin should be the drug of choice in pregnant women. Clarithromycin should only be used if no other therapy can be taken. For maintenance therapy, azithromycin plus ethambutol are the preferred drugs.

Commentary

Researchers are developing and testing new drugs and drug combinations that are more effective and have fewer side effects. More novel treatment ideas and better methods of drug testing are needed.

A better understanding of how MAC bacteria function will help pave the way to finding more effective drugs to kill them. There are many questions that still need to be answered:

- What makes one strain of MAC bacteria more harmful than another?

- How does the immune response affect how the bacteria behave?

- What factors influence the bacteria becoming drug-resistant?

- What are the differences between HIV-infected and normal macrophages?

- How does HIV change the complex system of cytokines that cells of the immune system use to signal to each other?

The Bottom Line on MAC

Mycobacterium avium complex is a bacterial infection found in water, dust, soil, and bird droppings.

Symptoms: Persistent fever, night sweats, fatigue, weight loss, anemia, abdominal pain, dizziness, diarrhea, and weakness.

Diagnosis: Culture from a sterile site such as blood, bone marrow or cerebral spinal fluid.

Preventive therapy (prophylaxis): People whose CD4+ cell counts stay consistently below 50 should start preventive therapy.

- Preferred: Clarithromycin (500 mg twice a day); or azithromycin (1,200 mg once a week)

- Alternative: Rifabutin (300 mg once a day)

Stopping preventive therapy: People with sustained CD4+ cells above 100 for three–six months and sustained viral load suppression may consider stopping preventive therapy.

Treatment—Preferred: Azithromycin (500–600 mg once a day); or clarithromycin (500 mg twice a day) plus ethambutol (15 mg/kg/day) plus rifabutin (300 mg once a day).

Alternative: Azithromycin or clarithromycin plus ethambutol plus rifabutin plus/minus ciprofloxacin (500–750 mg twice a day) plus/minus IV amikacin (10–15 mg/kg/day). IV amikacin can be added for severe disease.

Higher doses of clarithromycin (1,000 mg twice a day) may be linked with increased risk of death. Clofazimine may be associated with increased side effects and risk of death and it should not be used.

Maintenance therapy: Everyone who has had MAC should be on maintenance therapy with either clarithromycin (500 mg twice a day) or azithromycin (500 mg once a day) if it has been proven there is no resistance to either drug plus ethambutol (15 mg/kg once a day) plus/minus rifabutin (300 mg once a day).

Stopping maintenance therapy: People with sustained CD4+ cells above 100 for six to twelve months as a result of potent anti-HIV therapy may consider stopping maintenance therapy.

1999 Public Health Service Prevention Guidelines on MAC

Prevention

- Preventive MAC therapy is needed for adults with CD4+ cell counts below 50.
- First choice: clarithromycin or azithromycin; second choice: rifabutin.
- Before starting preventive therapy, rule out active MAC or TB infection.
- Check for potential drug interactions.

Maintenance

- Clarithromycin or azithromycin plus ethambutol and with or without rifabutin.

Prevention in Children

- Clarithromycin or azithromycin are the drugs of choice for children:
  - over six years, CD4+ cells below 50.
  - two to six years, CD4+ cells below 75.
  - one to two years, CD4+ cells below 500.
  - less than 12 months, CD4+ cells below 750.

Prevention during Pregnancy

- MAC preventive therapy is needed for pregnant women with CD4+ cell counts below 50.
- Azithromycin is the drug of choice.

Section 38.5

Histoplasmosis Fungal Infection

"Histoplasmosis," *Healthbeat*, Illinois Department of Public Health
(http://www.idph.state.il.us), updated August 8, 2006.

What is histoplasmosis?

Histoplasmosis is an infection caused by a fungus, *Histoplasma capsulatum*. The principal habitat for this fungus is soil enriched by bird droppings and in bat droppings. In the United States, the fungus is found most often along the Mississippi and Ohio River valleys, but also is present in other central, southeastern, and mid-Atlantic states. In people, this uncommon disease affects the lungs and may occasionally invade other parts of the body. Dogs, cats, rats, skunks, opossum, foxes, and other animals also can get histoplasmosis.

Who gets histoplasmosis?

Anyone can get histoplasmosis. In some areas where the fungus is prevalent, 80 percent or more of the population has been exposed to infection through breathing in airborne spores. The initial infection often occurs without causing symptoms, and most persons usually will not develop subsequent disease, unless the exposure was heavy.

Long-term smokers and those with preexisting lung disease may be at higher risk for developing the disease.

People with severely damaged immune systems—such as those with AIDS or leukemia, those who are on corticosteroid therapy, and recent transplant recipients—are vulnerable to a very serious disease known as progressive, disseminated histoplasmosis. Nationwide, about 5 percent of people with AIDS will develop histoplasmosis. In geographic areas where the fungus is common, people with AIDS are at higher risk for disseminated histoplasmosis.

How is the fungus spread?

The organism is found throughout the world and grows in soil that has been enriched with bat or bird droppings or in bat droppings themselves, for example, around old chicken houses, in caves and other areas harboring bats, and around starling and blackbird roosts. The fungus produces spores that can become airborne if the soil is disturbed. Inhalation of these spores may cause infection. The disease is not acquired through person-to-person transmission, nor is it acquired from animals that have the disease.

What are the symptoms of histoplasmosis?

The majority of infected persons have no symptoms. When symptoms occur, they vary widely, depending on the form of disease. The acute pulmonary form of the disease is a "flu"-like illness characterized by respiratory symptoms, general malaise, fever, chest pains, and a dry or nonproductive cough. Distinct patterns are seen on chest x-rays. Chronic pulmonary disease resembles chronic tuberculosis and progresses over months or years. The disseminated form of histoplasmosis is usually fatal unless treated.

How soon after exposure do symptoms appear?

If symptoms occur, they will usually appear within three to seventeen days after exposure; the average is ten days. However, disease onset could occur sooner if exposure is heavy. Most people do not experience symptoms.

Does past infection with histoplasmosis make a person immune?

Infection usually results in increased resistance to infection, but the immunity may not be complete.

How is histoplasmosis treated?

Specific antifungal medications are used to treat severe cases of acute histoplasmosis and all cases of chronic and disseminated disease. Mild disease usually resolves without treatment.

What can be done to prevent the spread of histoplasmosis?

The following steps can be taken to minimize exposure to *Histoplasma capsulatum:*

- Avoid areas that may harbor the fungus, particularly those areas with accumulations of bird or bat droppings.

- Minimize exposure to dust by spraying with a mist of water before working in potentially contaminated sites.

- When working in high-risk areas, all persons should wear disposable clothing and a face mask capable of filtering out particulate matter above 1 millimicron in diameter.

Section 38.6

Bacillary Angiomatosis

"Bacillary Angiomatosis (Bartonella Infection)," this information is reprinted with the permission from DermNet, the website of the New Zealand Dermatological Society. Visit www.dermnet.org.nz for patient information on numerous skin conditions and their treatment. © 2006 New Zealand Dermatological Society.

Bacillary angiomatosis is a systemic illness characterized by lesions similar to those of Kaposi sarcoma in the skin, mucosal surfaces, liver, spleen, and other organs. It is caused by bacterial infection with *Bartonella quintana* and *Bartonella henselae* (cause of catscratch disease). The disease is only rarely seen in healthy immunocompetent people. It mostly affects immunocompromised patients, particularly those with AIDS or HIV.

How do you get bacillary angiomatosis?

Bacillary angiomatosis is caused equally by *Bartonella quintana* and *Bartonella henselae*. It is usually a result of exposure to flea-infested cats with *Bartonella henselae* and the human body louse for *Bartonella quintana* (cause of trench fever in soldiers during World War I). Nowadays, the disease occurs mainly in AIDS patients. It may also be a complication of catscratch disease in immunocompetent patients.

What are the signs and symptoms of bacillary angiomatosis?

The first sign is usually the appearance of numerous pinpoint purplish to bright red raised spots and nodules up to 10 cm on or just

341

under the skin. These lesions resemble Kaposi sarcoma and often the disease is mistaken for this. There can be anywhere between one to 100 lesions occurring on any part of the body, although they are rarely found on the palms, soles, or in the mouth. Lesions may be pinhead sized spots or nodules up to 10 cm in diameter. Nodules are firm lumps and do not turn white with firm pressure. If injured, the lesions bleed profusely.

As the number of lesions increase, the patient may develop high fever, tender and swollen lymph nodes, nausea, vomiting, sweats, chills, and poor appetite.

The infection can also causes blood vessels to grow out of control and form tumor-like masses in other organs including the bone, liver, spleen, lymph nodes, heart, gastrointestinal tract and respiratory tract where airway obstruction may occur. The condition can become life threatening if not diagnosed and treated promptly.

What is the treatment of bacillary angiomatosis?

Bacillary angiomatosis is effectively treated with antibiotics. Erythromycin appears to be the antibiotic of choice and is given until lesions resolve, usually within three to four weeks of starting therapy. Other antibiotics used include doxycycline, co-trimoxazole, tetracycline, and rifampicin.

Large pus-filled lymph nodes or blisters may need to be drained. Supportive therapy includes hydration and analgesics for pain and fever. Warm moist compresses to affected nodes may decrease swelling and tenderness.

Chapter 39

Opportunistic Lung Diseases

Chapter Contents

Section 39.1

HIV/AIDS and Lung Disease

The lung is a major target of attack in HIV-positive and AIDS patients because the human immunodeficiency virus inhibits the body's ability to defend itself against infections and some kinds of cancer. People with HIV or AIDS in the U.S. are at a greater risk for contracting "opportunistic" lung diseases because these diseases take advantage of the body's lowered defenses. Some of these are described below. In addition the virus itself may cause lung damage.

***Pneumocystis jiroveci* pneumonia (PCP),** formerly known as *Pneumocystis carinii* pneumonia, is the most common opportunistic respiratory infection in patients infected with HIV:

- Symptoms include shortness of breath, fever, and cough without sputum. The shortness of breath worsens over a period of days to weeks. PCP is not contagious.

- With the advent of preventive therapy and effective antiretroviral therapy the incidence of PCP has declined substantially in the U.S. Without preventive medicine over 80 percent of Americans with HIV will likely get PCP.[1]

- The most common form of preventive treatment is an antibiotic combination of trimethoprim and sulfamethoxazole (TMP-SMX) or co-trimoxazole (Bactrim, Cotrim, Septra), given intravenously or orally. Another frequently used drug is pentamidine, which is given intravenously for treatment. For prevention, it is given in the form of aerosol mist, in order to deliver the major portion directly to the lungs, avoiding adverse side effects on other organs.[2]

Tuberculosis (TB) is an airborne infection caused by the bacillus *Mycobacterium tuberculosis* that primarily affects the lungs:

- Symptoms of pulmonary TB include a productive cough, fever, weight loss, coughing up blood, chest pain, loss of appetite, fatigue, and/or night sweats.

- HIV's suppression of the immune system allows new active TB infection and permits activation of latent TB disease. An individual who is infected with both HIV and TB has a 7 to 10 percent chance per year of developing active TB compared to a 10 percent lifetime chance in people without HIV.[3]

- The percentage of patients with both TB and HIV is declining in the U.S. because of improved infection control practices and better diagnosis and treatment of both HIV infection and TB.

- Treatment of HIV-related TB usually consists of four drugs— isoniazid, rifampin, pyrazinamide, and ethambutol. Duration of treatment varies but on average it lasts from six to twelve months. Directly observed therapy is strongly recommended for all patients with TB especially those with HIV infection.[4]

Mycobacterium avium **complex (MAC)** is caused by an organism closely related to *tuberculosis bacillus* that causes lung disease, anemia, and swollen lymph nodes, and infects the blood and entire body in HIV-positive persons:

- In the absence of effective combination antiretrovirals or preventative medications, the incidence of MAC disease is up to 30 to 50 percent of HIV-infected persons that are severely immunosuppressed (CD4 counts of less than 50 cells/µl).[5]

- Antimycobacterial drugs, such as clarithromycin, are available to treat MAC.[6] Treatment regimens should be made by a doctor experienced in dealing with MAC HIV-positive patients.

Bacterial pneumonia is a common cause of HIV-positive related morbidity:

- Approximately 100 cases per 1,000 HIV-positive persons occur each year. This rate is much higher than in the noninfected population.[7]

345

- Bacterial pneumonia can be an early sign of HIV disease. Patients with relatively preserved CD4 counts can develop serious pneumococcal infections.

- Symptoms are similar to bacterial pneumonia in noninfected persons, i.e., chills, fever, chest pain, and thick sputum.

- Well-established antibiotic treatments are used for bacterial pneumonia. Treatment is also similar to noninfected persons, with therapy targeting the most commonly identified causative agent, particularly *S. pneumoniae* and *H. influenzae.*[8]

Viral pneumonia is also easily contracted by persons with HIV and AIDS:

- The prominent causes of viral pneumonia in persons with HIV are members of the virus group herpesvirus, which have shown to be stubbornly resistant to treatment.

Candidiasis is a common fungal infection that causes illness in both the AIDS and the non-AIDS population. Other fungal infections may also occur:

- Fungal infections are often more common, more severe, and more difficult to treat in AIDS patients.

- A number of antifungal drugs are in established use; among those currently employed are amphotericin B, miconazole, and flucytosine. Fungal infections of the lung are not transmissible to healthy people.

There are other less common types of lung disease that also afflict persons with AIDS. Kaposi sarcoma, a cancer which also affects other parts of the body, can cause damage to the lungs. Nonspecific interstitial pneumonitis, small airways disease, and pulmonary hypertension are other forms of lung disease that affect people with HIV infection.

A person who has AIDS or is HIV-positive can take precautions to help prevent lung disease, although it is impossible to guarantee that these steps will enable the person to avoid these diseases. The patient should be inoculated against pneumococcal pneumonia and influenza, and receive PCP prophylaxis.

It is essential that persons with AIDS or HIV avoid smoking and secondhand smoke since they will further weaken the body's defenses against infection.

For more information call the American Lung Association at 800-LUNG-USA (800-586-4872), or visit their website at http://www.lung usa.org.

Sources

1. Wilken A, Feinberg J. Pneumocystis carinii Pneumonia: a clinical review. *American Family Physician,* October 15, 1999.

2. Centers for Disease Control. Treating Opportunistic Infections among HIV-Infected Adults and Adolescents. *Morbidity and Mortality Weekly Report.* Volume 53(RR15), December 2004.

3. Girardi E, Raviglione MC, Antonucci G, et al. Impact of the HIV epidemic on the spread of other diseases: the case of tuberculosis. *AIDS 2000;* Volume 14 (Suppl 3): 47-56.

4. Centers for Disease Control. Treating Opportunistic Infections among HIV-Infected Adults and Adolescents. *Morbidity and Mortality Weekly Report.* Volume 53(RR15), December 2004.

5. Jacobson MA, Aberg JA. Mycobacterium avium complex and atypical mycobacterial infections in the setting of HIV infection. HIV InSite Knowledge Base Chapter. May 2002.

6. Centers for Disease Control. Treating Opportunistic Infections among HIV-Infected Adults and Adolescents. *Morbidity and Mortality Weekly Report.* Volume 53(RR15), December 2004.

7. Ibid.

8. Ibid.

Section 39.2

AIDS, HIV, and Tuberculosis (TB)

What Is TB?

Tuberculosis (TB) is a contagious disease that kills around 1.6 million people each year. One-third of the world's population is currently infected with TB and someone is newly infected every few seconds.

What Is the Relationship between TB and HIV?

TB is the leading cause of death among HIV-infected people; the World Health Organization (WHO) estimates that TB accounts for up to a third of AIDS deaths worldwide.[1] When someone is infected with TB, the likelihood of them becoming sick with the disease is increased many times if they are also HIV positive.

What Causes TB?

TB is caused by an organism called *Mycobacterium tuberculosis*. These bacteria can attack any part of the body, but they most commonly attack the lungs. TB bacteria are very common in many resource-poor countries and in poor urban "pockets" of industrialized countries.

The Spread of TB

A person can have active or inactive TB. Active TB or TB disease means the bacteria are active in the body and the immune system is unable to stop them from causing illness. People with active TB in their lungs can pass the bacteria on to anyone they come into close contact with. When a person with active TB coughs, sneezes, or spits, people nearby may breathe in the TB bacteria and become infected. Left untreated, each person with active TB will infect on average between 10 and 15 people every year.

People can also be infected with TB that is not active in the body. Inactive TB infection is also called latent TB. If a person has latent TB, it means their body has been able to successfully fight the bacteria and stop them from causing illness. People who have latent TB do not feel sick, do not have symptoms, and cannot spread TB. In some people TB bacteria remain inactive for a lifetime without becoming active. But in some other people the inactive TB may become active TB if their immune system becomes weakened—for example, by HIV. People with inactive TB are also called TB carriers.

TB and HIV-Positive People

Because TB can spread through the air, the increase in active TB among people infected with both TB and HIV results in the following:

- more transmission of the TB bacteria

- more people with latent TB

- more TB disease in the whole population

People with latent TB are increasingly becoming infected with HIV, and many more are developing active TB because HIV is weakening their immune system. People who are co-infected with both HIV and latent TB have an up to 800 times greater risk of developing active TB disease and becoming infectious compared to people not infected with HIV.[2]

People with advanced HIV infection are vulnerable to a wide range of infections and malignancies that are called "opportunistic infections" because they take advantage of the opportunity offered by a weakened immune system. TB is an HIV-related opportunistic infection. A person that has both HIV and active TB has an AIDS-defining illness.

The HIV/AIDS epidemic is reviving an old problem in well-resourced countries and greatly worsening an existing problem in resource-poor countries. The are several important associations between epidemics of HIV and TB:

- TB is harder to diagnose in HIV-positive people.

- TB progresses faster in HIV-infected people.

- TB in HIV-positive people is more likely to be fatal if undiagnosed or left untreated.

- TB occurs earlier in the course of HIV infection than other opportunistic infections.

- TB is the only major AIDS-related opportunistic infection that poses a risk to HIV-negative people.

What Are the Symptoms of TB?

Symptoms of TB depend on where in the body the TB bacteria are growing. TB bacteria often grow in the lungs, causing pulmonary tuberculosis. Pulmonary TB may cause a bad cough that lasts longer than two weeks, pain in the chest, and coughing up of blood or sputum. Other symptoms of TB disease include weakness or fatigue, weight loss, lack of appetite, chills, fever, and night sweats.

Inactive TB has no symptoms.

How Is TB Diagnosed?

TB can be diagnosed by injecting a protein found in TB bacteria into the skin of an arm. If the skin reacts by swelling then the person is probably infected with TB. However, this method is not wholly reliable at detecting TB infections among HIV-infected people because their weakened immune systems often cannot mount a strong enough defense against the injected proteins to cause swelling. It also detects both active and latent TB, meaning the test is not very accurate at diagnosing active TB disease in people who live in areas where TB (and, thus, latent TB infection) is very common.

Diagnosis of TB in the lungs may be made using an x-ray or sputum test, but again, these may not give a clear indication of active TB infection in HIV-positive people, because their immune systems are not strong enough to mount an inflammatory reaction against the bacteria. In cases of extra-pulmonary TB (where the disease is affecting organs other than the lungs), fluid or tissue samples may be tested.

If there is doubt about the diagnosis of TB, a culture of TB bacteria can also be grown in a laboratory. However, this requires specialized and costly equipment and can take six to eight weeks to produce a result.

If the necessary facilities are not available then the TB diagnosis is often based on symptoms.

How Is TB Treated?

Active TB disease can almost always be cured with a combination of antibiotics. The variety of treatments and drug options depend on the country you are in. A proper combination of anti-TB drugs provides both prevention and cure. Effective treatment quickly makes the person with TB non-contagious and, therefore, prevents further spread of TB. Achieving a cure takes about six to eight months of daily treatment.

Several drugs are needed to treat active TB. Taking several drugs does a better job of killing all of the bacteria and is more likely to prevent them from becoming resistant to the drugs. To ensure thorough treatment, it is often recommended that the patient take his or her pills in the presence of someone who can supervise the therapy. This approach is called DOTS (directly observed treatment, short course). DOTS cures TB in 95 percent of cases, and a six-month supply of DOTS costs as little as $10 per person in some parts of the world.

Can TB Be Prevented?

There is a vaccine against TB called bacille Calmette-Guérin (BCG),[3] but the vaccine is now very old (it was first used in the 1920s), and tests have found it to be very variable in its ability to protect people from infection in modern settings. When it does provide protection, this generally only lasts for around 15 years. The BCG can also cause false-positive readings on the tuberculin skin test, and if given to HIV-positive adults or children with very weak immune systems, it can occasionally cause disseminated BCG disease. This is often fatal.

A drug called isoniazid (INH) can be used as a preventative therapy for those who are at high risk of becoming infected with TB or for those who have inactive TB. People who have inactive TB but are not yet sick can take a course of isoniazid for several months to stop them developing active TB.

The WHO recommends that HIV-positive people who have latent TB (but definitely not active TB) should be offered isoniazid preventive therapy as needed.

TB Treatment and HIV

It is vitally important for people with HIV to have treatment if they have active TB. This will cure them and prevent transmission to others.

351

Even in settings where antiretroviral drugs are unavailable or inaccessible, it is crucial that the health system is able to offer HIV-positive people the simple antibiotics needed for DOTS.

For some people it can be difficult to take drugs for both TB and HIV at the same time. Some anti-HIV drugs can also interact with some TB drugs making the treatment more difficult. It is important that the TB treatment is taken regularly and exactly as the health care provider has advised. If the drugs are not taken regularly, the bacteria can become resistant to the drugs and this can be dangerous.

As one of the first opportunistic infections to appear in HIV-infected people, TB may be one of the earlier signs of HIV infection. Addressing TB offers the opportunity for early HIV intervention. Although treatment of TB can improve the quality of life of HIV-positive people and prolong their life, it cannot stop them from dying of AIDS. This is why access to antiretroviral treatment is also vitally important.

Around the world, attempts are being made to improve collaboration between TB and HIV programs. It is being proposed that everyone diagnosed with TB should be tested for HIV and vice-versa, and that treatment programs should share facilities and expertise. However, achieving such collaboration is not straightforward:

"The different cultures of the TB and HIV communities raise many challenges in achieving an effective and productive partnership.... TB services are geared towards chronic-care services with simple and standardized technical procedures, while HIV/AIDS services are clinically oriented and tend to be more individual-patient-oriented."[4]

What Are Multi-Drug Resistant TB (MDR-TB) and Extreme Drug Resistant TB (XDR-TB)?

When a strain of TB is resistant to two or more "first-line" antibiotic drugs, it is called multi-drug resistant TB or MDR-TB. When it is resistant to three or more "second-line" antibiotics as well, it is classed as extreme drug resistant TB, or XDR-TB. Drug resistance usually arises when TB patients do not or cannot take their medicine as prescribed and drug-resistant mutations of the TB bacteria are allowed to replicate. People can also catch MDR and XDR-TB from others.

MDR-TB is a serious problem and is very difficult to treat. In normal first-line treatment, patients take the drugs isoniazid and rifampicin (the most effective TB drug available) plus two or three other first-line drugs for around six to eight months. If a person is resistant to isoniazid and rifampicin however, they are said to have MDR-TB, and will need to change to a regime containing newer and often less widely-available "second-line" drugs. Treatment with second-line drugs can take a very long time, and is usually far more expensive than standard DOTS therapy because most of the drugs are still under patent.

XDR-TB is even more serious. If someone has XDR-TB, it means they are not only resistant to isoniazid and rifampicin, but to three or more of the six available second-line drugs too. This can make it virtually impossible to formulate an effective treatment regime for them. Many people with XDR-TB will die before it is even realized that they have the extreme resistant strain.

In 2006, 53 people in the province of KwaZulu Natal in South Africa were identified as having XDR-TB. Fifty-two of these people died within 25 days of TB being diagnosed. The majority were HIV positive.

Being HIV positive does not of itself increase the chance of drug resistance, but both MDR-TB, and XDR-TB are a serious problem for HIV-positive people, whose weakened immune systems mean they are unlikely to fight off TB naturally (often the only hope for those with a resistant strain).

TB and HIV around the World

The importance of TB to the global HIV epidemic is enormous. Tuberculosis is a serious health problem in its own right, but it is also the most likely cause of death for HIV-positive people. Like HIV, TB has had an uneven impact around the world. In some parts of the world, TB is increasing after almost 40 years of decline. Escalating TB rates over the past decade in many countries in sub-Saharan Africa and in parts of Southeast Asia are mainly due to the HIV epidemic.

Between 1990 and 2005, TB incidence rates tripled in African countries with high HIV prevalence. In 2005, Africa accounted for an estimated 80 percent of TB among HIV-positive people worldwide.

The largest number of TB cases occurs in the Southeast Asia region, which in 2005 accounted for an estimated 3 million new cases (one-third of the global total). However, the estimated incidence per capita in sub-Saharan Africa is nearly twice that of the Southeast Asia, at 356 cases per 100,000 population in 2005. The countries of Eastern Europe are facing a serious epidemic; there were an estimated 170,000 new cases in Russia alone in 2005.

TB is not only a problem in low- and middle-income countries. For example, there were 14,097 new cases reported in the U.S. in 2005.[5] In the United Kingdom (UK), TB has been dubbed "the disease that has never went away," with 8,113 new cases reported in England,

Wales, and Northern Ireland in 2005.[6] Although the UK's national rate is very low in comparison with most of the world, London has become one of the world's TB hotspots. In parts of London, TB rates are ten times the national rate—higher than in some countries of the former Soviet Union. About 10 percent of people with TB in London are likely to be co-infected with HIV.[7]

Worldwide TB Control

The discovery of antibiotic drugs that kill bacteria, was a turning point in TB control. In well-resourced countries, TB was previously treated with a special diet and bed rest, usually in a sanatorium. In the late 1950s, it was found that this was unnecessary and TB could be cured with well-supervised antibiotic treatment at home.

Since DOTS was introduced on a global scale in 1991, more than 26 million people have received the treatment. By the end of 2000, all 22 of the countries with the highest number of TB infections, which together have 80 percent of the world's estimated incident cases, had adopted the DOTS strategy. In total, 187 countries were implementing the DOTS strategy by the end of 2005, and 89 percent of the global population was living in parts of countries where the DOTS strategy was in place. Around 46 percent of new smear-positive (active) TB cases were detected and then treated successfully with DOTS in 2005.

However, improved diagnostic methods for detecting the infection are desperately required, as is a more effective vaccine against the disease. New and more potent drugs are also needed to help simplify and shorten treatment, and fight multi-drug resistant TB. The emergence of MDR, and especially XDR-TB, threatens TB control efforts across the globe, including those in well-resourced countries. Due to antibiotic supply problems in the late 1970s and early 1980s, MDR-TB is now particularly common in former Soviet Union countries. It has also been found in a large number of cases in China, Ecuador, and Israel. Central Europe and Africa, in contrast, have reported the lowest median levels of drug resistance, but the numbers are rising rapidly.

The WHO's leading infectious disease experts estimate there are more than 400,000 new cases of MDR-TB worldwide each year. About half of these are among new TB patients, and the other half are among patients who have previously received treatment. There is also new evidence that drug resistant strains are becoming more resistant and unresponsive to current treatments. More than three-quarters of MDR-TB cases are now "super strains," resistant to at least three of the four main drugs used to cure TB in first-line treatment. The number of these that could also be classed as extreme drug resistant strains is, however, unknown.

For many years, TB remained relatively overlooked on the global scale, but MDR and XDR-TB, and other problematic issues are now being recognized internationally. In 2006, the Stop TB Partnership launched "The Global Plan to Stop TB,"[8] an initiative that aims to halve the death rates and prevalence of tuberculosis worldwide by 2015. If successful, the plan will save over 14 million lives, and will pave the way for the ultimate goal of eradicating tuberculosis by 2050. However, much more still needs to be done to achieve this aim, both by directly combating TB, and by addressing the HIV epidemic that is fueling its spread.

References

1. World Health Organization, *Joint HIV/Tuberculosis (TB) Interventions.*

2. CDC NCHSTP Division of Tuberculosis Elimination, *TB and HIV Coinfection.*

3. Davies PDO, Tuberculosis Research Unit, *Frequently Asked Questions about BCG,* Liverpool, UK.

4. WHO and Stop TB Partnership, *Scaling up prevention and treatment for TB and HIV-Report of the Fourth Global TB/ HIV Working Group Meeting,* September 2004.

5. CDC, *Reported Tuberculosis in the United States, 2005,* September 2006.

6. Health Protection Agency (HPA), *Case Reports (Enhanced TB Surveillance),* March 2007.

7. HPA, *Annual Report and Accounts 2004.*

8. Stop TB Partnership, *Actions for Life: The Global Plan to Stop TB 2006–2015,* 2006.

Sources

WHO Report 2007, *Global Tuberculosis Control—Surveillance, Planning, Financing*

WHO, *Fact Sheet No. 104*

WHO/IUATLD Global Project on Anti-Tuberculosis Drug Resistance Surveillance 1999–2002

TB-Alert website (http://www.tbalert.org)

Section 39.3

Multi-Drug Resistant TB

Drug Resistant TB by the Numbers

- Many TB patients do not complete their full six- to nine-month drug regimen. The TB bacillus develops resistance through incomplete, erratic, or inadequate treatment.

- Four percent or more of new TB cases may be multi-drug resistant. Ten percent of those may be extremely drug resistant.

- In some TB hot-spots, up to 15 percent of patients are infected with drug resistant strains.

- 450,000 new MDR-TB cases are estimated to occur each year.

Drug resistant strains of tuberculosis are complicating efforts to control the global TB pandemic and putting thousands of lives at risk.

Drug resistant TB is the man-made result of interrupted, erratic, or inadequate TB therapy; it develops when the long, complex, decades-old TB drug regimen is poorly administered, or when patients stop taking their medicines before the disease has been fully eradicated. Once a drug resistant strain has developed, it may also be transmitted directly to others.

Multi-Drug Resistant TB (MDR-TB)

Multi-Drug Resistant TB (MDR-TB) is defined by resistance to the two most commonly used drugs in the current four-drug (or first-line) regimen, isoniazid and rifampin. World Health Organization (WHO) treatment standards require that at least four drugs be used to treat TB, to avoid the development of further resistance.

MDR-TB is not limited to the developing world. During the late 1980s and early 1990s, outbreaks of MDR-TB in North America and Europe killed over 80 percent of those who contracted the disease.

During a major TB outbreak in New York City in the early 1990s, one in ten cases proved to be drug-resistant.

450,000 new MDR-TB cases are estimated to occur every year. The WHO estimates that MDR-TB makes up greater than 4 percent of all new TB cases in those regions most affected by the disease: Eastern Europe, Latin America, Africa, and Asia. Rates of up to 6 percent have been reported in many countries, while in some parts of the former Soviet Union, up to 15 percent of all patients with TB have resistant strains.

MDR-TB cannot be cured using two of the four recommended first-line drugs. When those drugs fail, second-line drugs are used. But some second-line drugs are toxic and fraught with side-effects. They must be taken for up to two years in order to eradicate the infection. The costs of curing MDR-TB can be staggering—as much as 1400 times that of regular treatment. Patients can ill-afford the time and money required. At the same time, MDR-TB poses a significant challenge to national health care systems. In 1998, the WHO introduced DOTS-Plus, an enhanced program that targets MDR-TB with second-line treatments. But DOTS-Plus is still in development, and its reach remains limited.

Extremely Drug Resistant TB (XDR-TB)

Extremely Drug Resistant TB (XDR-TB), also known as Extensively Drug Resistant TB, is emerging as an even more ominous threat. XDR-TB is defined as MDR-TB, with additional resistance to two classes of antibiotics used as second-line drugs: the fluoroquinolones and the aminoglycosides. This makes XDR-TB treatment extremely complicated, and some strains are virtually untreatable.

In March 2006, the Centers for Disease Control (CDC) released the first known data on XDR-TB. The CDC and the WHO surveyed TB strains from a global network of TB laboratories, and identified XDR-TB cases in all regions of the world. In the worst-affected areas, 10 percent of MDR-TB cases were XDR-TB.

In August 2006, at the International AIDS Conference, researchers announced initial findings from an outbreak of particularly virulent XDR-TB in KwaZulu Natal, South Africa. Fifty-two of 53 patients died, on average within 25 days of diagnosis. Most of the patients were co-infected with HIV/AIDS. However, the deaths included those who were taking antiretroviral drugs. These numbers have since risen. The WHO and others are now mounting an intensified global response to escalating global resistance.

So long as TB is treated with a long, complex, decades-old drug regimen, drug resistance will continue to develop. Yet novel TB drugs, working through new biological mechanisms of action, are designed to be effective against drug-susceptible and drug-resistant strains alike, saving lives. A shorter regimen, reliably administered, would also minimize the potential for further resistance.

Chapter 40

HIV/AIDS and Cancer

Why do people with HIV seem to get cancer more often than people without HIV?

HIV itself plays a role in how cancer grows in people who are HIV-positive. HIV attacks the immune system, which protects the body from infections and disease. A weaker immune system is less able to fight off diseases, like cancer. People with HIV often have weakened immune systems, which means they will have a greater chance of getting cancer.

Here are some reasons why cancer seems to be more common among people with HIV:

People with HIV and AIDS are living longer. HIV medications are helping people with HIV live longer, healthier lives. But their immune systems do not get fully healthy. As people with HIV live longer, their chances of having other health problems, like cancer, increase.

HIV and other viruses work together. Having HIV and a weakened immune system makes it easier for other viruses to stay alive in your body. HIV and these other viruses work together to help cancer cells start growing. Once cancer starts in people with weakened

"HIV and Cancer: What Is the Link?" March 2006, reprinted with permission from the AIDS Institute of the New York State Department of Health (http://www.health.state.ny.us).

immune systems, it grows faster than in healthy people. Some of these viruses are as follows:

- hepatitis B and hepatitis C
- herpes
- human papillomavirus (HPV)
- Epstein-Barr virus (EBV)

Most people with HIV smoke cigarettes. About 60 percent to 70 percent of people with HIV smoke. Smoking is a risk factor for many different types of cancer. As people with HIV live longer and continue to smoke, they increase their risk of developing smoking-related cancers.

Is it true that HIV medications cause cancer?

No. There is no proof that HIV medications increase the risk of getting any type of cancer.

What is a "risk factor"?

A "risk factor" means anything that increases your chances of getting cancer. For example, smoking is a major risk factor for lung cancer. You can protect yourself from a lot of that risk by not smoking or by quitting smoking. Other risk factors are out of your control, like having a family history or genetic history of cancer. For example, if a parent or grandparent had cancer, your risk of getting that type of cancer will be greater.

Take action on the risk factors that you have some control over. If you have a family history of cancer, ask your doctor or health care worker about ways to prevent that cancer and test for it.

What kinds of cancer do people with HIV usually get?

AIDS-related cancers: In the past, people with HIV often got three types of cancer: Kaposi sarcoma, non-Hodgkin lymphoma, and cervical cancer (in women).These are called AIDS-related cancers because they occur more often in people whose immune systems have been weakened by HIV/AIDS. Here are some facts about these cancers:

- *Kaposi sarcoma:* This cancer grows into reddish-purple patches on your skin that cannot kill you. It can be deadly if it gets in your throat or lungs. A herpesvirus causes Kaposi sarcoma.

- *Non-Hodgkin lymphoma:* This cancer usually starts in the lymph glands, which are part of your immune system and help fight off disease. Lymph glands are mainly in the neck, under the arms, in the groin, and inside the belly. Epstein-Barr virus is a risk factor for this cancer.

- *Invasive cervical cancer* affects the cervix, the entrance from the vagina to the uterus. Almost all women who get cervical cancer also have HPV. Having HIV and HPV makes cervical cancer grow faster.

Non-AIDS-related cancers: People with HIV are getting more non-AIDS-related cancers. This happens even if they take HIV medications and have healthier immune systems. These cancers affect many different parts of the body. Smoking is a risk factor for many of these cancers. Here are some facts about non-AIDS-related cancers:

- *Lung cancer:* Smoking is the main risk factor. Lung cancer among people with HIV has become more common since people began taking HIV medications and living longer. Quitting smoking, exercising, and keeping your immune system strong greatly lowers your lung cancer risk.

- *Hodgkin lymphoma* is another cancer that occurs mainly in the lymph glands. It grows quickly in people who have weak immune systems.

- *Anal cancer:* Men who have sex with men have a greater risk of anal cancer. Anal sex does not directly cause anal cancer. But it can lead to getting HPV, which makes your risk for anal cancer much higher.

- *Liver cancer:* Having hepatitis B or hepatitis C and HIV makes your risk of liver cancer very high. Smoking, drinking alcohol, using street drugs, and sharing needles or other equipment to shoot drugs are also risk factors.

- *Other skin cancers:* Skin cancers other than Kaposi sarcoma are becoming more common.

What can you do to lower your chances of getting cancer?

You can lower your cancer risk a lot, and manage your HIV at the same time, by making healthy choices. Finding cancer in its early stages (early detection) and treating it right away can raise your chances of living longer with HIV. Cancer treatments can also be very hard on the immune systems of people with HIV. So it is also important for people with HIV to not let cancer start growing (prevention) and find cancer in its early stages.

Healthy Living to Prevent Cancer

Quitting smoking is the biggest step to protecting yourself from cancer. If you quit smoking, you can greatly lower your risk of cancer of the mouth, throat, lungs, stomach, kidneys, liver, pancreas, and bladder. As soon as you stop smoking, your body starts to heal and your cancer risk drops. Ask your doctor about treatment and counseling to help you quit.

Take all your HIV medications on schedule. A stronger immune system is your best protection against many types of cancer. Take all your medications on schedule and try not to skip doses. HIV medications have helped to greatly reduce Kaposi sarcoma.

Protect yourself and others from HIV and other viruses. HIV, HPV, hepatitis, and herpes are passed through sex or sharing needles or other equipment used to inject drugs. Use a condom the right way every time you have sex. Never share needles or drug works.

Eat healthy foods. You can lower your risk of cancers of the breast, prostate, stomach, colon, and rectum with a healthy diet.

- Fruits and vegetables have lots of minerals, vitamins, and fiber. Try to eat them five times a day—as part of every meal and as snacks.

- Eat whole wheat bread, pasta, rice, and beans.

- Eat lean meats (lower fat) like chicken and fish and low-fat dairy products, such as skim milk and cottage cheese.

- Cook with canola oil or olive oil instead of butter.

- Try to get your vitamins and minerals from healthy foods—not from pills, drinks, and powders.

- Talk with your doctor or a nutritionist about what foods are right for you.

Get plenty of exercise; stay at a healthy weight. Regular exercise can lower your risk of getting some types of cancer.

- Try walking, jogging, or riding a bike four or five days a week. A lot of things can count as exercise—as long as you move your body on a regular basis.

- Do something that you enjoy. That will make it easier to stick with it.

- People with HIV or AIDS sometimes have trouble keeping enough weight on. Ask your doctor about how to exercise enough and eat enough to stay at a healthy weight.

Avoid drugs and alcohol. Drugs are not a direct cancer risk, but they can hurt your immune system and make it harder to stay healthy with HIV. You can lower your risk of mouth, throat, liver, and breast cancer (in women) by not drinking alcohol. If you have chronic hepatitis C and liver disease, don't drink at all.

Protect yourself from the sun. Wear sunscreen that is rated SPF [sun protection factor] 15 or higher. Wear a hat, sunglasses, and clothing to protect you from the sun.

Finding Cancer in Its Early Stages (Early Detection)

Have regular medical checkups. Talk with your doctor or health care provider about your cancer risk and problems to watch for. Ask about tests you can get even if you have no signs of cancer:

- Pap smear for cervical cancer or anal Pap smear for anal cancer

- mammogram for female breast cancer

- colon/rectal exam

- prostate exam for men over age 50

- oral exam by a dentist every six months

Know the warning signs of cancer and do self-exams. If you notice any of these warning signs, tell your doctor or dentist right away:

- a sore that does not heal (Look for new growths on your skin or any changes in the size, color, or shape of moles or warts.)

- a lump or hardness in the skin, especially in female breasts and in the male testicles and groin area

- oral exam (Check the inside of your mouth, lips, gums, and tongue for sores, swelling or bleeding, white patches, scabs, or cracks.)

- bleeding or loss of body fluids that is not normal

- changes in your bowel or bladder habits

- a cough or a sore throat that lasts for a long time

- heartburn or trouble swallowing that does not go away

Staying Healthy and Preventing Cancer

HIV weakens the immune system and allows the growth of other viruses that can cause cancer. Scientists are working hard to figure out the links between HIV, other viruses, and cancer and to make medications that prevent and treat these diseases. In the meantime, do what you can to stay healthy and prevent cancer.

Chapter 41

Bone and Joint Problems with AIDS

You might think that your bones stay pretty much the same once you become an adult, but that isn't the case. In fact, each one of your bones is in a constant state of change and renewal; experts say that your entire skeleton gets replaced every 10 to 20 years.

Some of your bone cells make the materials that will become bone, while other bone cells eat up and remodel those materials.

Occasionally, though, something goes wrong with this process of bone creation and renewal. This is when bone problems occur.

What Causes Bone Problems?

Some experts believe that HIV itself may affect bones in ways that we don't yet understand. In addition, you may be more likely to develop bone problems if you are:

- a woman (especially if you've gone through menopause or have low levels of estrogen).

- older (bone mass peaks at around age 25, after which bones become less dense).

- white.

- underweight.

- not getting much exercise.
- a smoker.
- a heavy alcohol drinker.
- someone who has used corticosteroids (such as Prednisone or Cortisone), either as pills or through injections.
- extremely fond of caffeine (too much coffee, tea, cola, chocolate, etc.).
- part of a family with a history of bone problems.

Types of Bone Problems

Osteonecrosis (also called avascular necrosis) is a condition in which bone tissue dies because not enough blood is being supplied to the bone, usually because of damage to blood vessels in the area. It usually happens to bone tissue about the hip joints, although it can occur in bone tissue near other joints.

Osteoporosis is a condition in which your bones become smaller and less dense, which may make them more likely to break.

Osteopenia is like osteoporosis, only less severe.

Are HIV Meds to Blame?

Researchers are still trying to figure out how much of a role HIV meds play in bone problems. Most of what we know suggests that, even if HIV meds do play a role, the factors listed previously are more important.

We know that some bone problems, like osteonecrosis and osteopenia, have occurred more often in HIV-positive people over the last ten years, especially in people taking protease inhibitors. However, it's not clear whether there's a direct cause-and-effect relationship. Since people with HIV are now living longer, it's possible that the long-term effects of HIV, rather than HIV meds, are to blame. Some research has shown that HIV-positive people are at a higher risk for bone problems than HIV-negative people, even if they've never taken HIV meds.

Still, there are early signs that some HIV meds, including Viread and Zerit, may at least have some effect on people's bones. Hopefully, researchers will take a closer look at these possible links in the future.

366

What Can You Do?

The best weapon against bone problems is to keep them from happening in the first place. There are a few commonsense things you can do if you and your doctor think you may be at risk for bone problems:

Calcium: Calcium is one of the key ingredients in bones, so it should not come as a surprise that calcium-rich foods—like milk, cheese, yogurt, and other dairy products—are an essential part of a bone-healthy diet. Besides dairy, a growing number of foods are "calcium-fortified," including some breads and orange juice.

Calcium supplements can also help. The daily recommended intake of calcium is 1,000 mg, but you should talk to your doctor or a nutritionist to find the dosage that is right for you before you start taking a supplement. Some calcium supplements can reduce the strength of HIV meds. (Tums, for example, can weaken Reyataz.)

Vitamin D: This vitamin helps your body absorb calcium. Experts recommend you take between 400 and 800 IU (international units) per day. Many over-the-counter supplements contain both calcium and vitamin D.

Phosphorous: Phosphorous is also essential in bones, so make sure you get enough. Dairy products often have phosphorous in them, as do beans and peanuts. You can also find supplements that contain phosphorous.

Exercise: Regular exercise—especially the kind that involves weights or resistance—can help prevent a bone fracture by strengthening the muscles that support the bones. Walking, jogging, stair-climbing, and weight-lifting can all be helpful. And we're not talking about once in a while, either; consistent exercise is the key to healthy bones.

Prescription medications: Several medications have been found to make bones denser. These include Fosamax and Actonel; both are approved for use in women and men with certain types of osteopenia. Fosamax, in particular, has been found to be effective in studies of HIV-positive people who have reduced bone density. If Fosamax or Actonel don't work, your doctor can recommend other prescription medications.

Hormone replacement: Estrogen and testosterone, the main female and male hormones, appear to help keep bones healthy. But as we get older, production of these hormones begins to drop. This is especially a concern for women who have been through menopause. If your doctor finds that your hormone levels are low, the two of you should discuss the risks and benefits of hormone replacement therapy.

Conclusion

Metabolic complications may not be the most dangerous, or even the most common, type of side effect that HIV-positive people experience. But they are among the most frightening for many people. In the case of body shape changes, they can affect how you look and feel about yourself and, in the case of high cholesterol/triglycerides, they can affect your heart.

Although much is still unknown about metabolic complications, there are clearly ways to avoid at least some of them. We hope this chapter has helped you better understand how metabolic complications happen and what you can do about them if they happen to you.

Of course, don't let that be the end of the story. There are a million people in the United States living with HIV—many of whom, whether on meds or not, are worried about metabolic complications. You and your doctor should work together, as a team, to figure out how to balance your concerns about metabolic complications with your other health needs.

One thing to always keep in mind: You are not alone. There are a million people in the United States living with HIV—many of whom, whether on meds or not, are worried about metabolic complications. Connect with others who are dealing with metabolic complications by signing up for e-mail lists and browsing reputable websites. AIDS organizations across the country also provide educational workshops on HIV medications and dealing with side effects. How you do it isn't important; what matters is that you stay informed and connect with others.

Chapter 42

Neurological Complications of AIDS

What is AIDS?

AIDS (acquired immunodeficiency syndrome) is a condition that occurs in the most advanced stages of human immunodeficiency virus (HIV) infection. It may take many years for AIDS to develop following the initial HIV infection.

Although AIDS is primarily an immune system disorder, it also affects the nervous system and can lead to a wide range of severe neurological disorders.

How does AIDS affect the nervous system?

The virus does not appear to directly invade nerve cells, but it jeopardizes their health and function. The resulting inflammation may damage the brain and spinal cord and cause symptoms such as confusion and forgetfulness, behavioral changes, severe headaches, progressive weakness, loss of sensation in the arms and legs, and stroke. Cognitive motor impairment or damage to the peripheral nerves is also common. Research has shown that the HIV infection can significantly alter the size of certain brain structures involved in learning and information processing.

Other nervous system complications that occur as a result of the disease or the drugs used to treat it include pain, seizures, shingles,

---

"Neurological Complications of AIDS Fact Sheet," National Institute of Neurological Disorders and Stroke (http://www.ninds.nih.gov), National Institutes of Health (NIH), updated February 14, 2007.

spinal cord problems, lack of coordination, difficult or painful swallowing, anxiety disorder, depression, fever, vision loss, gait disorders, destruction of brain tissue, and coma. These symptoms may be mild in the early stages of AIDS, but can become progressively severe.

In the United States, neurological complications are seen in more than 40 percent of adult patients with AIDS. They can occur at any age, but tend to progress more rapidly in children. Nervous system complications in children may include developmental delays, loss of previously achieved milestones, brain lesions, nerve pain, smaller than normal skull size, slow growth, eye problems, and recurring bacterial infections.

What are some of the neurological complications that are associated with AIDS?

AIDS-related disorders of the nervous system may be caused directly by the HIV virus, by certain cancers and opportunistic infections (illnesses caused by bacteria, fungi, and other viruses that would not otherwise affect people with healthy immune systems), or by toxic effects of the drugs used to treat symptoms. Other neuro-AIDS disorders of unknown origin may be influenced by but are not caused directly by the virus.

AIDS dementia complex (ADC), or HIV-associated encephalopathy, occurs primarily in persons with more advanced HIV infection. Symptoms include encephalitis (inflammation of the brain), behavioral changes, and a gradual decline in cognitive function, including trouble with concentration, memory, and attention. Persons with ADC also show progressive slowing of motor function and loss of dexterity and coordination. When left untreated, ADC can be fatal.

Central nervous system (CNS) lymphomas are cancerous tumors that either begin in the brain or result from a cancer that has spread from another site in the body. CNS lymphomas are almost always associated with the Epstein-Barr virus (a common human virus in the herpes family). Symptoms include headache, seizures, vision problems, dizziness, speech disturbance, paralysis, and mental deterioration. AIDS patients may develop one or more CNS lymphomas. Prognosis is poor due to advanced and increasing immunodeficiency.

Cryptococcal meningitis is seen in about 10 percent of untreated AIDS patients and in other persons whose immune systems have been severely suppressed by disease or drugs. It is caused by the fungus

Cryptococcus neoformans, which is commonly found in dirt and bird droppings. The fungus first invades the lungs and spreads to the covering of the brain and spinal cord, causing inflammation. Symptoms include fatigue, fever, headache, nausea, memory loss, confusion, drowsiness, and vomiting. If left untreated, patients with cryptococcal meningitis may lapse into a coma and die.

Cytomegalovirus (CMV) infections can occur concurrently with other infections. Symptoms of CMV encephalitis include weakness in the arms and legs, problems with hearing and balance, altered mental states, dementia, peripheral neuropathy, coma, and retinal disease that may lead to blindness. CMV infection of the spinal cord and nerves can result in weakness in the lower limbs and some paralysis, severe lower back pain, and loss of bladder function. It can also cause pneumonia and gastrointestinal disease.

Herpesvirus infections are often seen in AIDS patients. The herpes zoster virus, which causes chickenpox and shingles, can infect the brain and produce encephalitis and myelitis (inflammation of the spinal cord). It commonly produces shingles, which is an eruption of blisters and intense pain along an area of skin supplied by an infected nerve. In people exposed to herpes zoster, the virus can lay dormant in the nerve tissue for years until it is reactivated as shingles. This reactivation is common in persons with AIDS because of their weakened immune systems. Signs of shingles include painful blisters (like those seen in chickenpox), itching, tingling, and pain in the nerves.

Neuropathy: AIDS patients may suffer from several different forms of neuropathy, or nerve pain, each strongly associated with a specific stage of active immunodeficiency disease.

- Peripheral neuropathy describes damage to the peripheral nerves, the vast communications network that transmits information from the brain and spinal cord to every other part of the body. Peripheral nerves also send sensory information back to the brain and spinal cord. HIV damages the nerve fibers that help conduct signals and can cause several different forms of neuropathy.

- Distal sensory polyneuropathy causes either a numbing feeling or a mild to painful burning or tingling sensation that normally begins in the legs and feet. These sensations may be particularly strong at night and may spread to the hands. Affected persons have a heightened sensitivity to pain, touch, or other stimuli. Onset usually occurs in the later stages of the HIV infection and may affect the majority of advanced-stage HIV patients.

Neurosyphilis, the result of an insufficiently treated syphilis infection, seems more frequent and more rapidly progressive in people with HIV infection. It may cause slow degeneration of the nerve cells and nerve fibers that carry sensory information to the brain. Symptoms, which may not appear for some decades after the initial infection and vary from patient to patient, include weakness, diminished reflexes, unsteady gait, progressive degeneration of the joints, loss of coordination, episodes of intense pain and disturbed sensation, personality changes, dementia, deafness, visual impairment, and impaired response to light. The disease is more frequent in men than in women. Onset is common during mid-life.

Progressive multifocal leukoencephalopathy (PML) primarily affects individuals with suppressed immune systems (including nearly 5 percent of people with AIDS). PML is caused by the JC virus [a human polyomavirus], which travels to the brain, infects multiple sites, and destroys the cells that make myelin—the fatty protective covering for many of the body's nerve and brain cells. Symptoms include various types of mental deterioration, vision loss, speech disturbances, ataxia (inability to coordinate movements), paralysis, brain lesions, and, ultimately, coma. Some patients may also have compromised memory and cognition, and seizures may occur. PML is relentlessly progressive and death usually occurs within six months of initial symptoms.

Psychological and neuropsychiatric disorders can occur in different phases of the HIV infection and AIDS and may take various and complex forms. Some illnesses, such as AIDS dementia complex, are caused directly by HIV infection of the brain, while other conditions may be triggered by the drugs used to combat the infection. Patients may experience anxiety disorder, depressive disorders, increased thoughts of suicide, paranoia, dementia, delirium, cognitive impairment, confusion, hallucinations, behavioral abnormalities, malaise, and acute mania.

Stroke brought on by cerebrovascular disease has been considered a somewhat rare complication of AIDS, although the association between

AIDS and stroke may be much larger than previously thought. Researchers at the University of Maryland conducted the first population-based study to quantify an AIDS-associated stroke risk and found that AIDS increases the chances of suffering a stroke by as much as ten-fold. Researchers caution that additional studies are needed to confirm this association. Earlier studies have indicated that the HIV infection, other infections, or the body's immune system reaction to HIV may cause vascular abnormalities and/or make the blood vessels less responsive to changes in blood pressure, which could lead to rupture and hemorrhagic stroke.

Toxoplasma encephalitis, also called cerebral toxoplasmosis, occurs in about 10 percent of untreated AIDS patients. It is caused by the parasite *Toxoplasma gondii*, which is carried by cats, birds, and other animals and can be found in soil contaminated by cat feces and sometimes in raw or undercooked meat. Once the parasite invades the immune system, it remains there; however, the immune system in a healthy person can fight off the parasite, preventing disease. Symptoms include encephalitis, fever, severe headache that does not respond to treatment, weakness on one side of the body, seizures, lethargy, increased confusion, vision problems, dizziness, problems with speaking and walking, vomiting, and personality changes. Not all patients show signs of the infection.

Vacuolar myelopathy causes the protective myelin sheath to pull away from nerve cells of the spinal cord, forming small holes called vacuoles in nerve fibers. Symptoms include weak and stiff legs and unsteadiness when walking. Walking becomes more difficult as the disease progresses and many patients eventually require a wheelchair. Some patients also develop AIDS dementia. Vacuolar myelopathy may affect up to 30 percent of untreated adults with AIDS and its incidence may be even higher in HIV-infected children.

How are these disorders diagnosed?

Based on the results of the patient's medical history and a general physical exam, the physician will conduct a thorough neurological exam to assess various functions: motor and sensory skills, nerve function, hearing and speech, vision, coordination and balance, mental status, and changes in mood or behavior. The physician may order laboratory tests and one or more of the following procedures to help diagnose neurological complications of AIDS.

Computer-assisted imaging can reveal signs of brain inflammation, tumors and CNS lymphomas, nerve damage, internal bleeding or hemorrhage, white matter irregularities, and other brain abnormalities. Several painless imaging procedures are used to help diagnose neurological complications of AIDS.

- Computed tomography (also called a CT scan) uses x-rays and a computer to produce two-dimensional images of bone and tissue, including inflammation, certain brain tumors and cysts, brain damage from head injury, and other disorders. It provides more details than an x-ray alone.

- Magnetic resonance imaging (MRI) uses a computer, radio waves, and a powerful magnetic field to produce either a detailed three-dimensional picture or a two-dimensional "slice" of body structures, including tissues, organs, bones, and nerves. It does not use ionizing radiation (as does an x-ray) and gives physicians a better look at tissue located near bone.

- Functional MRI (fMRI) uses the blood's magnetic properties to pinpoint areas of the brain that are active and to note how long they stay active. It can assess brain damage from head injury or degenerative disorders such as Alzheimer's disease and can identify and monitor other neurological disorders, including AIDS dementia complex.

- Magnetic resonance spectroscopy (MRS) uses a strong magnetic field to study the biochemical composition and concentration of hydrogen-based molecules, some of which are very specific to nerve cells, in various brain regions. MRS is being used experimentally to identify brain lesions in people with AIDS.

Electromyography, or EMG, is used to diagnose nerve and muscle dysfunction (such as neuropathy and nerve fiber damage caused by the HIV virus) and spinal cord disease. It records spontaneous muscle activity and muscle activity driven by the peripheral nerves.

Biopsy is the removal and examination of tissue from the body. A brain biopsy, which involves the surgical removal of a small piece of the brain or tumor, is used to determine intracranial disorders and tumor type. Unlike most other biopsies, it requires hospitalization. Muscle or nerve biopsies can help diagnose neuromuscular problems, while a brain biopsy can help diagnose a tumor, inflammation, or other irregularity.

Cerebrospinal fluid analysis can detect any bleeding or brain hemorrhage, infections of the brain or spinal cord (such as neurosyphilis), and any harmful buildup of fluid. A sample of the fluid is removed by needle, under local anesthesia, and studied to detect any irregularities.

How are these disorders treated?

No single treatment can cure the neurological complications of AIDS. Some disorders require aggressive therapy while others are treated symptomatically.

Neuropathic pain is often difficult to control. Medicines range from analgesics sold over the counter to antiepileptic drugs, opiates, and some classes of antidepressants. Inflamed tissue can press on nerves, causing pain. Inflammatory and autoimmune conditions leading to neuropathy may be treated with corticosteroids, and procedures such as plasmapheresis (or plasma exchange) can clear the blood of harmful substances that cause inflammation.

Treatment options for AIDS- and HIV-related neuropsychiatric or psychotic disorders include antidepressants and anticonvulsants. Psychostimulants may also improve depressive symptoms and combat lethargy. Antidementia drugs may relieve confusion and slow mental decline, and benzodiazepines may be prescribed to treat anxiety. Psychotherapy may also help some patients.

Aggressive antiretroviral therapy is used to treat AIDS dementia complex, vacuolar myopathy, progressive multifocal leukoencephalopathy, and cytomegalovirus encephalitis. HAART, or highly active antiretroviral therapy, combines at least three drugs to reduce the amount of virus circulating in the blood and may also delay the start of some infections.

Other neuro-AIDS treatment options include physical therapy and rehabilitation, radiation therapy and/or chemotherapy to kill or shrink cancerous brain tumors that may be caused by the HIV virus, antifungal or antimalarial drugs to combat certain bacterial infections associated with the disorder, and penicillin to treat neurosyphilis.

What research is being done?

National Institute of Neurological Disorders and Stroke (NINDS)-funded projects are studying the role of virally infected brain macrophages (cells that normally work to protect against infection) in causing disease in the central nervous system of adult macaques. The focus of these projects includes gene analyses and the study of key neuroimmune regulatory molecules that are turned on in the brain during the course of viral infection at levels that have been shown to be toxic.

Several animal-based models of HIV (including mouse, rat, and simian models) are used by scientists to study disease mechanisms and the course of AIDS, and NINDS grantees are working to develop new models of HIV. The NINDS also supports research into the mechanisms of neurological illnesses related to immunodeficiency in AIDS patients. Several different investigators are studying the JC virus, which can reproduce in the brains of immunosuppressed patients and cause PML, and one study identified a novel receptor for the JC virus. Other studies of infectious agents include an investigation of the interaction of the fungal agent *Cryptococcus* with the blood vessels of the brain, and an analysis of neurosyphilis in people with AIDS. Scientists are also studying the effect of neurotoxic proteins and antiviral therapies directly on nerve cells as the cause for distal sensory peripheral neuropathy.

Several researchers are studying AIDS dementia and cognitive changes in HIV. NINDS-sponsored scientists are using fMRI and MRS to assess brain function and any behavioral deficits in HIV-affected individuals. Investigators hope to better understand how progressive neuronal cell death contributes to cognitive dysfunction and AIDS dementia. The National NeuroAIDS Tissue Consortium, a project supported jointly by the NINDS and its sister agency, the National Institute of Mental Health, is collecting tissues from people with AIDS who have suffered from dementia and other neurological complications of HIV infection for distribution to researchers around the globe.

The Neurological AIDS Research Consortium was established by the NINDS in 1993 to design and conduct clinical trials on HIV-associated neurologic disease. To date, the Consortium has supported studies of neurological function in advanced AIDS and the treatment of HIV-associated peripheral neuropathy, PML, and CMV infection. Consortium researchers are studying the drug selegiline as an add-on to antiretroviral therapy for HIV dementia, as well as the natural history of neurological disease in advanced HIV. Clinical studies have included a double-blind controlled study of prosaptide for the treatment of HIV-associated peripheral neuropathy, and trials of acetyl-L-carnitine and erythropoietin as treatments for toxic neuropathy in HIV infection.

Chapter 43

Pain Syndromes and HIV/AIDS

The advent of highly active antiretroviral treatment (HAART) has not diminished the need for palliative care for people living with HIV/AIDS. In fact, because of new treatments, fewer patients are dying from HIV/AIDS in the U.S. and the total number of people living with HIV/AIDS is increasing. New treatments, particularly HAART, are also responsible for additional symptoms and complications, including pain that must be understood and managed. Additionally, as the epidemiology of the AIDS epidemic changes in the United States, the challenge of managing pain in AIDS patients who have a history of substance abuse is a growing issue.

Several studies have documented that pain in individuals with HIV infection or AIDS is: highly prevalent, diverse, and varied in syndromal presentation; associated with significant psychological and functional morbidity; and alarmingly under treated.

Moreover, pain has a profound negative impact both on physical and psychological functioning and overall quality of life. It is important, therefore, that pain management be more integrated into the total care of patients with HIV disease. This chapter describes the types and prevalence of pain syndromes encountered in patients with HIV disease and reviews the psychological and functional impact of pain.

This chapter contains excerpts from "Pain" by William Breitbart, MD, in *A Clinical Guide to Supportive and Palliative Care for HIV/AIDS, 2003 Edition*, U.S. Department of Health and Human Services, 2003. The complete document, including references, is available online at http://www.hab.hrsa.gov/tools/palliative/chap4.html.

Pain is classified in two major categories, nociceptive and neuropathic pain. Nociceptive pain derives from the stimulation of intact "nociceptors" or pain receptors in afferent nerves and is further subdivided into somatic pain (involving skin, soft tissue, muscle, and bone) and visceral pain (involving internal organs and hollow viscera). Nociceptive pain may be well-localized (common in somatic pain) or more diffuse (common in visceral pain), and may be sharp, dull, aching, gnawing, throbbing, constant, or spasmodic, with varying intensity. Neuropathic pain involves stimulation of damaged or compromised nerve tissue, and may be burning, tingling, stabbing, shooting, with a sensation of electric shock, or allodynia (the sensation of pain or discomfort produced by a minimal stimulus such as light touch to the skin). The differentiation of pain into one of these subtypes (particularly nociceptive versus neuropathic) can help in determining appropriate therapy.

Summary of Pain Syndromes in HIV/AIDS

Pain syndromes encountered in AIDS are diverse in nature and etiology. The most common pain syndromes reported in studies to date include painful sensory peripheral neuropathy, pain due to extensive Kaposi sarcoma, headache, oral and pharyngeal pain, abdominal pain, chest pain, arthralgias and myalgias, and painful dermatologic conditions.

In 1997 it was demonstrated that while pains of a neuropathic nature (e.g., polyneuropathies, radiculopathies) certainly comprise a large proportion of pain syndromes encountered in AIDS patients, pains of a somatic and/or visceral nature are also extremely common clinical problems.

The etiology of pain syndromes seen in HIV disease can be categorized into three types: those directly related to HIV infection or consequences of immunosuppression; those due to AIDS therapies; and those unrelated to AIDS or AIDS therapies.

In studies to date, approximately 45 percent of pain syndromes encountered are directly related to HIV infection or consequences of immunosuppression; 15 percent to 30 percent are due to therapies for HIV- or AIDS-related conditions and to diagnostic procedures; and the remaining 25 percent to 40 percent are unrelated to HIV or its therapies.

Pain in Women with HIV/AIDS

One study has suggested that women with HIV disease experience pain more frequently than men with HIV disease and report somewhat higher levels of pain intensity. This may in part reflect the fact that women with AIDS-related pain are twice as likely as men to be under treated for their pain. Women with HIV disease have unique pain syndromes of a gynecologic nature specifically related to opportunistic infectious processes and cancers of the pelvis and genitourinary tract, and in one survey women with AIDS were significantly more likely to be diagnosed with radiculopathy and headache.

Pain in Children with HIV/AIDS

Children with HIV infection also experience pain. HIV-related conditions in children that are observed to cause pain include the following:

- meningitis and sinusitis (headaches)
- otitis media [inflammation of the middle ear]
- shingles
- cellulitis and abscesses
- severe candida dermatitis
- dental caries
- intestinal infections, such as *Mycobacterium avium-intracellulare* (MAI) and *Cryptosporidium*
- hepatosplenomegaly [enlargement of the liver and spleen]
- oral and esophageal candidiasis
- spasticity associated with encephalopathy that causes painful muscle spasms

Overview of Pain Management in HIV/AIDS

Optimal management of pain requires a multidisciplinary approach. The initial assessment should shed light on etiology and contributing factors as well as establish a baseline from which to monitor the impact of therapy. Clear communication between provider and patient/family is important to monitor the impact of any intervention.

Federal guidelines developed by the Agency for Health Care Policy and Research (now called Agency for Healthcare Research and Quality [AHRQ]) for the management of cancer pain also address the issue of pain management in AIDS. The guidelines state, the principles of pain assessment and treatment in the patient with HIV/AIDS are not fundamentally different from those in the patient with cancer and should be followed for patients with HIV/AIDS. In contrast to pain in cancer, pain in HIV disease more commonly may have an underlying treatable cause.

Optimal management of pain in AIDS is multimodal and requires pharmacologic, psychotherapeutic, cognitive-behavioral, anesthetic, neurosurgical and rehabilitative approaches. A multidimensional model of AIDS pain that recognizes the interaction of cognitive, emotional, socioenvironmental, and nociceptive aspects of pain suggests a model for multimodal intervention.

Pharmacologic Interventions for Pain

The World Health Organization (WHO) has devised guidelines for analgesic management of cancer pain which the AHRQ has endorsed for the management of pain related to cancer or AIDS. Theses guidelines, also known widely as WHO Analgesic Ladder, have been well validated. This approach advocates selection of analgesics based on the severity of pain as well as the type of pain (i.e., neuropathic versus non-neuropathic pain). For pain that is mild to moderate in severity, non-opioid analgesics such as NSAIDs (non-steroidal anti-inflammatory drugs) and acetaminophen are recommended. For pain that is persistent and moderate to severe in intensity, opioid analgesics of increasing potency (such as morphine) should be utilized.

Adjuvant agents, such as laxatives and psychostimulants, are useful in preventing as well as treating opioid side effects such as constipation or sedation respectively. Adjuvant analgesic drugs, such as the antidepressant analgesic, are suggested for considered use, along with opioids and NSAIDs, in all stages of the analgesic ladder (mild, moderate, or severe pain), but have their most important clinical application in the management of neuropathic pain.

The WHO approach, while not yet validated in AIDS, has been recommended by the AHRQ and clinical authorities in the fields of pain management and AIDS.

In addition, clinical reports have appeared in recent literature describing successful application of the WHO Analgesic Ladder principles to pain management in AIDS, with particular emphasis on the use of opioids.

Non-Pharmacologic Interventions

Physical interventions, psychological therapies, and neurosurgical procedures may also prove useful in the management of HIV-related pain.

Physical interventions range from bed rest and simple exercise programs to the application of cold packs or heat to affected sites. Other non-pharmacologic interventions include whirlpool baths, massage, the application of ultrasound and transcutaneous electrical nerve stimulation (TENS). Increasing numbers of AIDS patients have resorted to acupuncture to relieve their pain, with anecdotal reports of efficacy.

Several psychological interventions have demonstrated potential efficacy in alleviating HIV-related pain, including hypnosis, relaxation, and distraction techniques such as biofeedback and imagery, and cognitive behavioral techniques.

Where non-pharmacologic and standard pharmacologic treatments fail, anesthetic and even neurosurgical procedures (such as nerve block, cordotomy, and epidural delivery of analgesics) are additional options available to the patient who appreciates the risks and limitations of these procedures.

Additional points: Very likely some of the things you think of in answer to these questions can be recorded for you, such as your favorite music or a prayer. Then, you can listen to the tape whenever you wish. Or, if your memory is strong, you may simply close your eyes and recall the events or words.

Barriers to Pain Management in HIV/AIDS

A number of different factors have been identified as potential influences on the widespread under treatment of pain in AIDS, including patient-, clinician-, and health care system-related barriers. Sociodemographic factors that have been reported to be associated with under treatment of pain in AIDS patients include gender, education level, and substance abuse history. Women, less educated patients, minorities, and patients who reported injection drug use as their HIV risk transmission factor are significantly more likely to receive inadequate analgesic therapy for HIV-related pain.

Managing pain in AIDS patients with a history of substance use is a particularly challenging problem that HIV providers will face with increasing frequency.

Conclusion

Pain in AIDS, even in this era of protease inhibitors and decreased AIDS death rates, is a clinically significant problem contributing greatly to psychological and functional morbidity. Pain can be adequately treated and so must be a focus of palliative care of the person living with HIV/AIDS.

Chapter 44

Nutritional Problems and HIV/AIDS

Chapter Contents

Section 44.1

Nutrition and HIV/AIDS

"Nutrition," Fact Sheet 800, © 2007 AIDS InfoNet. Reprinted with permission. Fact sheets are regularly updated. Check http://www.aidsinfonet.org for the most recent information.

Why Is Nutrition Important?

Good nutrition means getting enough macronutrients and micronutrients. Macronutrients contain calories (energy): proteins, carbohydrates, and fats. They help you maintain your body weight. Micronutrients include vitamins and minerals. They keep your cells working properly, but will not prevent weight loss.

Good nutrition can be a problem for many people with HIV. When your body fights any infection, it uses more energy and you need to eat more than normal. But when you feel sick, you eat less than normal.

Some medications can upset your stomach, and some opportunistic infections can affect the mouth or throat. This makes it difficult to eat. Also, some medications and infections cause diarrhea. If you have diarrhea, your body actually uses less of what you eat.

When you lose weight, you might be losing fat, or you might be losing lean body weight like muscle. If you lose too much lean weight, your body chemistry changes. This condition is called wasting syndrome or cachexia. Wasting can kill you. If you lose more than 5 percent of your body weight, it could be a sign of wasting. Discuss it with your doctor.

Nutrition Guidelines for People with HIV

First, eat more. Extra muscle weight will help you fight HIV. This is very important. Many people want to lose weight, but for people with HIV, it can be dangerous.

Make sure you eat plenty of protein and starches, with moderate amounts of fat.

- Protein helps build and maintain your muscles. Meats, fish, beans, nuts, and seeds are good sources.

- Carbohydrates give you energy. Complex carbohydrates come from grains, cereals, vegetables, and fruits. They are a "time release" energy source and are a good source of fiber and nutrients. Simple carbohydrates, or sugars give you quick energy. You can get sugars in fresh or dried fruit, honey, jam, or syrups.

- Fat gives you extra energy. You need some—but not too much. The "monounsaturated" fats in nuts, seeds, canola and olive oils, and fish are considered "good" fats. The "saturated" fats in butter and animal products are "bad" fats.

A moderate exercise program will help your body turn your food into muscle. Take it easy, and work exercise into your daily activities.

Drinking enough liquids is very important when you have HIV. Extra water can reduce the side effects of medications. It can help you avoid a dry mouth and constipation. Remember that drinking tea, coffee, colas, chocolate, or alcohol can actually make you lose body liquid.

Practice Food Safety

It's very important to protect yourself against infections that can be carried by food or water.

Be sure to wash your hands before preparing food, and keep all of your kitchen tools and work areas clean. Wash all fruits and vegetables carefully. Don't eat raw or undercooked eggs or meat, and clean up juices from raw meat quickly. Keep leftovers refrigerated and eat them within three days. Check the expiration date on foods. Don't buy them or eat them if they're outdated.

Some germs are spread through tap water. If your public water supply isn't totally pure, drink bottled water.

What about Supplements?

Some people find it difficult to go shopping and prepare meals all the time. Supplements can help you maintain your body weight and get the vitamins and minerals you need. Don't use a product designed to help you lose weight, even if it says it contains everything needed for good nutrition. Your health care provider can help you choose a supplement that's right for you.

Vitamin and mineral supplements can be very helpful.

The Bottom Line

- Good nutrition is very important for people with HIV. When you are HIV-positive, you will need to increase the amount of food you eat and maintain your lean body weight.

- Be sure to eat a balanced diet, including plenty of protein and whole grain foods, with some sugar and fat. An exercise program will help build and maintain muscle.

- Drink plenty of liquids to help your body deal with any medications you are taking.

- Practice food safety. Keep your kitchen clean, wash foods, and be careful about food preparation and storage. If your tap water isn't pure, drink bottled water.

- If you feel you need to use nutritional supplements, be sure to get some expert advice from your health care provider.

Section 44.2

Mouth Problems and HIV/AIDS

"Mouth Problems and HIV," National Institute of Dental and Craniofacial Research (http://www.nidcr.nih.gov), National Institutes of Health (NIH), NIH Publication No. 04-5320, reviewed May 2005.

This information is for people who have mouth (oral) problems related to HIV infection. It explains the most common oral problems linked to HIV and describes what they look like. It also describes where in the mouth they occur and how they are treated.

They are common. Oral problems are very common in people with HIV. More than a third of people living with HIV have oral conditions that arise because of their weakened immune system. And even though combination antiretroviral therapy has made some oral problems less common, others are occurring more often with this type of treatment.

They can be painful, annoying, and lead to other problems. You may be told that oral problems are minor compared to other things you have to deal with. But you know that they can cause discomfort and embarrassment and really affect how you feel about yourself. Oral problems can also lead to trouble with eating. If mouth pain or tenderness makes it difficult to chew and swallow, or if you can't taste food as well as you used to, you may not eat enough. And, your doctor may tell you to eat more than normal so your body has enough energy to deal with HIV.

They can be treated. The most common oral problems linked with HIV can be treated. So talk with your doctor or dentist about what treatment might work for you.

Remember, with the right treatment, your mouth can feel better. And that's an important step toward living well, not just longer, with HIV.

If you have dry mouth: Dry mouth happens when you do not have enough saliva, or spit, to keep your mouth wet. Saliva helps you chew and digest food, protects teeth from decay, and prevents infections by controlling bacteria and fungi in the mouth. Without enough saliva you could develop tooth decay or other infections and might have trouble chewing and swallowing. Your mouth might also feel sticky, dry, and have a burning feeling. And you may have cracked, chapped lips.

To help with a dry mouth, try these things:

- Sip water or sugarless drinks often.
- Chew sugarless gum or suck on sugarless hard candy.
- Avoid tobacco.
- Avoid alcohol.
- Avoid salty foods.
- Use a humidifier at night.

Talk to your doctor or dentist about prescribing artificial saliva, which may help keep your mouth moist.

Table 44.1. Description and treatment of various mouth problems

Description	It Could Be:	What and Where?	Painful?	Contagious?	Treatment
Red sores (ulcers)	Aphthous (AF-thus) ulcers, also known as canker sores.	Red sores that might also have a yellow-gray film on top. They are usually on the moveable parts of the mouth such as the tongue or inside of the cheeks and lips.	Yes	No	Mild cases—over-the-counter cream or prescription mouthwash that contains corticosteroids. More severe cases—corticosterids in a pill form.
Red sores (ulcers)	Herpes (HER-peez), a viral infection.	Red sores usually on the roof of the mouth. They are sometimes on the outside of the lips, where they are called fever blisters.	Sometimes	Yes	Prescription pill can reduce healing time and frequency of outbreaks.
White hairlike growth	Hairy leukoplakia (Loo-ko-PLAY-key-uh) caused by the Epstein-Barr virus	White patches that do not wipe away; sometimes very thick and "hairlike." Usually appear on the side of the tongue or sometimes inside the cheeks and lower lip.	Not usually	No	Mild cases—not usually required. More severe cases—a prescription pill that may reduce severity of symptoms. In some severe cases, a pain reliever might also be required.

White creamy or bumpy patches (like cottage cheese)	Candidiasis (CAN-di-dye-uh-sis), a fungal (yeast) infection, also known as thrush	White or yellowish patches (or can sometimes be red). If wiped away, there will be redness or bleeding underneath. They can appear anywhere in the mouth.	Sometimes, a burning feeling	No	Mild cases—prescription antifungal lozenge or mouthwash. More severe cases—prescription antifungal pills.
Warts		Small, white, gray, or pinkish rough bumps that look like cauliflower. They can appear inside the lips and on other parts of the mouth.	Not usually	Possibly	Inside the mouth—a doctor can remove them surgically or use "cryosurgery"—a way of freezing them off; On the lips—a prescription cream that will wear away the wart. Warts can return after treatment.

Section 44.3

Wasting Syndrome

"Wasting Syndrome," Fact Sheet 519, © 2007 AIDS InfoNet. Reprinted with permission. Fact sheets are regularly updated. Check http://www.aidsinfonet.org for the most recent information.

What is AIDS wasting?

AIDS wasting is the involuntary loss of more than 10 percent of body weight, plus more than 30 days of either diarrhea, or weakness and fever. Wasting is linked to disease progression and death. Losing just 5 percent of body weight can have the same negative effects. Wasting is still a problem for people with AIDS, even people whose HIV is controlled by medications.

Part of the weight lost during wasting is fat. More important is the loss of muscle mass. This is also called "lean body mass," or "body cell mass." Lean body mass can be measured by bioelectrical impedance analysis (BIA.) This is a simple, painless office procedure.

AIDS wasting and lipodystrophy can both cause some body shape changes. Wasting is the loss of muscle. Lipodystrophy is a loss of fat. They are not the same thing. However, wasting in women can start with a loss of fat.

What causes AIDS wasting?

Several factors contribute to AIDS wasting syndrome.

- **Low food intake:** Low appetite is common with HIV. Also, some AIDS drugs have to be taken with an empty stomach, or with a meal. This can make it difficult for some people with AIDS to eat when they're hungry. Drug side effects such as nausea, changes in the sense of taste, or tingling around the mouth also decrease appetite. Opportunistic infections in the mouth or throat can make it painful to eat. Infections in the gut can make people feel full after eating just a little food. Finally, lack of money or energy may make it difficult to shop for food or prepare meals.

- **Poor nutrient absorption:** Healthy people absorb nutrients through the small intestine. In people with HIV disease, several infections (including parasites) interfere with this process. HIV may directly affect the intestinal lining and reduce nutrient absorption. Diarrhea, a frequent side effect of AIDS drugs, causes loss of calories and nutrients.

- **Altered metabolism:** Food processing and protein building are affected by HIV disease. Even before any symptoms show up, energy output is increased. This might be caused by the increased activity of the immune system. People with HIV need more calories just to maintain their body weight.

Hormone levels can affect the metabolism. HIV seems to change some hormone levels. Also, cytokines play a role in wasting. Cytokines are proteins that produce inflammation to help the body fight infections. People with HIV have very high levels of cytokines. This makes the body produce more fats and sugars, but less protein.

Unfortunately, these factors can work together to create a "downward spiral". For example, infections may increase the body's energy requirements. At the same time, they can interfere with nutrient absorption and cause fatigue. This can reduce appetite and make people less able to shop for or cook their meals. They eat less, which accelerates the process.

How is wasting treated?

There is no standard treatment for AIDS wasting. Treatments for wasting syndrome address each of the causes mentioned previously.

- **Reducing nausea and vomiting** helps increase food intake. Also, appetite stimulants including Megace and Marinol have been used. Megace, unfortunately, is associated with increases in body fat. Marinol (dronabinol) is sometimes used to increase appetite. It is a synthetic form of a substance found in marijuana. AIDS activists have long urged the legalization of marijuana. It reduces nausea and stimulates the appetite. In the late 1990s, several states legalized the medical use of marijuana.

- **Treating diarrhea and opportunistic infections in the intestines** helps alleviate poor nutrient absorption: There has been a lot of progress in this area. However, two parasitic infections—

cryptosporidiosis and microsporidiosis—are still extremely difficult to treat. Another approach is the use of nutritional supplements like Ensure and Advera. These have been specifically designed to provide easy-to-absorb nutrients. They have not been carefully studied yet.

- **Treating changes in metabolism:** Hormone treatments are being examined. Human growth hormone increases weight and lean body mass, while decreasing fat mass. However, it is extremely expensive and could cost over $40,000 per year to use. Testosterone and anabolic (muscle building) steroids might also help treat wasting. They are being studied alone and in combination with exercise. Also, thalidomide seems to reverse weight loss due to its ability to reduce levels of cytokines.

Progressive resistance training (PRT) is a form of exercise using small weights. A recent study found that PRT gave results like oxandrolone (an anabolic steroid) in increasing lean body mass. PRT was also more effective than oxandrolone in increasing physical functioning. It is less expensive, too.

The Bottom Line

- AIDS wasting is not well understood. However, it is clear that people with HIV disease need to avoid the loss of lean body mass. Various treatments for wasting are being studied.

- Be sure to monitor your weight. Maintain your intake of nutritious foods even if your appetite is low. Get treatment right away for serious diarrhea or any infection of your digestive system. These might cause problems with the absorption of nutrients.

Section 44.4

Scientists Find Key to Wasting Syndrome

"Scientists Find Key to 'Wasting Syndrome' Seen in Cancer, AIDS," U.S. Department of Veterans Affairs, reviewed/updated June 27, 2006.

Department of Veterans Affairs researchers and colleagues have discovered a biochemical mechanism that may explain wasting syndrome, a condition that causes severe weight loss and weakness in patients with chronic inflammatory diseases and often hastens their death. The findings, published in the EMBO (European Molecular Biology Organization) Journal, may lead to new drugs to ease the debilitating effects of cancer, AIDS, and other serious degenerative illnesses.

Scientists in San Diego pinpointed the biological chain of events that caused wasting in mice, then identified the same process in liver tissue from cancer patients. They said the striking similarity between the condition in mice and humans will expedite the development of new treatments.

"When we saw that it was virtually identical in animals and humans, we were ecstatic," said the study's senior author, Mario Chojkier, MD, of the Veterans Affairs (VA) San Diego Healthcare System and the University of California, San Diego (UCSD). "What we've described in animals has much greater relevance than we ever thought to human wasting syndrome. We're optimistic this will bring hope and relief very quickly to the bedside."

Dr. Chojkier and lead author Martina Buck, PhD, of VA, UCSD, and the Salk Institute for Biological Studies, described the steps by which tumor necrosis factor (TNF) alpha, an immune-system protein, prevents the production of albumin. Low levels of albumin, a critical protein made in the liver, is a keynote of wasting.

TNF-alpha and low albumin had for years been implicated in wasting, but the connection between the two was a mystery. Drs. Buck and Chojkier showed that TNF alpha causes oxidative stress in the liver cell and boosts the production of the free-radical gas nitric oxide. It also causes the addition of a phosphorous molecule to a protein called C/EBP beta, which normally joins DNA in the nucleus of the cell to make other proteins, such as albumin. Central to the researchers' finding

393

was that this extra phosphorous causes the C/EBP beta to shuttle out of the nucleus into the cytoplasm (the cell's external membrane), where transcription from the albumin gene can no longer take place.

"We found that this phosphorylation makes the C/EBP beta exit the nuclear area and go into the cytosol (the fluid in the cytoplasm), where there is no DNA for it to bind with. This means it can no longer produce the protein," said Dr. Chojkier.

The researchers found several ways of stopping the downward spiral caused by TNF-alpha. One way was to treat TNF-alpha-enhanced mice with vitamin E and other antioxidants. This blocked the chain of events leading to the "nuclear export" of C/EBP beta.

"If we block oxidative stress, we normalize everything," explained Dr. Chojkier. "C/EBP beta remains in the nucleus, it contacts the DNA, and proteins are produced. Or, if we block the nitric oxide synthase activity, this also blocks the downstream cascade, and everything normalizes."

According to Dr. Chojkier, a gastroenterologist and liver specialist, antioxidants such as vitamin E might halt wasting in humans if these supplements were delivered in very high amounts—or even better, if they were targeted to the liver.

"One solution will be to find a liver-specific antioxidant," he said. "With the technology we have today, this is very feasible. We believe this will provide an exciting avenue for intervention."

Dr. Chojkier also noted that there are already medications on the market, albeit for different conditions, that work by preventing phosphorylation, or the addition of a phosphorous molecule. These drugs could conceivably work in the liver to restore the normal production of albumin and treat wasting. Drs. Buck and Chojkier said they hope to test already-available compounds with the goal of finding one that is safe and effective for wasting.

Catabolic wasting, or cachexia (ka-kek'-sia), breaks down body tissue, regardless of how much nutrition the patient absorbs. "It's like a car that burns too much fuel," said Dr. Chojkier. The condition affects about half of all patients with cancer and AIDS and also affects patients with bacterial and parasitic diseases, rheumatoid arthritis, and chronic diseases of the bowel, liver, lungs, and heart. Infusions of albumin are occasionally used to treat the condition, but the treatment is expensive, complicated, and only suitable for certain patients.

Collaborating on the study with Drs. Buck and Chojkier were Lian Zhang and Nicholas A. Halasz of VA and UCSD, and Tony Hunter of the Salk Institute for Biological Studies. Funding for the study was provided by the Department of Veterans Affairs, the United States Public Health Service, and the American Liver Foundation.

Chapter 45

Using Marijuana for Pain and Nausea Associated with HIV/ AIDS Treatments

Chapter Contents

Section 45.1

Medical Marijuana and Dronabinol

"Medical Marijuana," From Project Inform, © 2005. For more information, contact the National HIV/AIDS Treatment Infoline, 1-800-822-7422, or visit our website at www.projectinform.org.

Introduction

Smoking marijuana has become a popular way to treat weight loss associated with HIV. Claims about its effectiveness are based largely on individual experience rather than data from studies. A synthetic form of the most active ingredient in marijuana, called dronabinol (Marinol), is approved by the U.S. Food and Drug Administration (FDA). It is available by prescription for treating HIV-related weight loss (anorexia), as well as treating nausea for people undergoing chemotherapy.

This section describes the different forms of marijuana that are currently available. Although many report that marijuana improves their appetite and weight, it's important to consider possible health risks before using it. Also, the only studies that have been conducted to assess the impact of medical marijuana in people with HIV have been very small and very brief. Much of the following information comes from research on people who do not have HIV disease.

Buyers' Clubs and the Law

Marijuana is an illegal substance, yet "buyers' clubs" have been established in some areas to provide the drug for people using marijuana for medical purposes. These clubs provide a safe place to buy marijuana. Even though they are illegal under federal law, some cities like San Francisco have local laws permitting them to operate. Some even have programs that provide medical marijuana free or at reduced cost to people with limited incomes.

Legislation was approved on a public vote in California that allows physicians to prescribe marijuana for some medical conditions. HIV-associated wasting is one of four conditions in the legislation. While some health care providers have voiced concern over the safety of marijuana smoking, many providers have also been impressed with positive results in weight gain, mood, and quality of life in their HIV-positive patients who use medical marijuana.

Safety Concerns

There are many possibly harmful effects from smoking marijuana, just as there would be from inhaling almost any other form of smoke. Most of the studies citing these effects were conducted many years ago, and conflicting reports can often be found among all of them. Many people question whether political motives may have influenced early studies of marijuana. For people living with HIV, the largest safety concerns when using marijuana are the affects on:

- immune function;

- lung complications (particularly with smoked marijuana);

- hormones; and

- mental state.

Immune Function

Marijuana and/or its psychoactive ingredient THC have been reported to suppress many immune functions. These include the function of cells important in controlling infections commonly seen among people living with HIV. Marijuana may also increase your risk for certain infections, including herpes and a variety of other bacterial, viral, and fungal infections. Some of these infections may result in increased HIV levels. None of this, however, has been clearly documented in HIV-positive people.

Some research suggests that marijuana has no significant effect—good or bad—on the immune system of people living with HIV. Studies from the Multicenter AIDS Cohort Study evaluating outcomes in 1,662 HIV-positive users of psychoactive drugs (marijuana, cocaine, LSD, etc.) found that none of the drugs were linked to a higher rate of HIV disease progression or loss of CD4+ cell counts. Of the men who took part in the study, 89 percent reported using marijuana in the preceding two years. A recent study, presented in 2000, examined the short-term impact of marijuana, dronabinol, or placebo on HIV levels, CD4+ cell count, and HIV levels. After 21 days, the use of marijuana did not appear to have harmful affects. Much longer-term studies are needed before concluding that marijuana use is either safe or unsafe for people living with HIV, however.

Lung Complications

Research comparing the effects of tobacco and marijuana smoking on the lungs shows that marijuana smoke can be harmful. Smoking marijuana increases the risks of lung complications, may worsen asthma, and may increase the risk of lung cancer over and above smoking tobacco.

Another possible harmful effect of smoking marijuana is that it may cause lung infections. In particular, a fungus sometimes found in marijuana called *Aspergillus* is thought to be the cause of possible infections. This infection has sometimes been seen in people with advanced HIV disease.

Some recommend putting marijuana in the microwave for ten seconds to kill any fungus that might be growing on it. The exact time needed to kill the fungus will vary depending on the oven settings, the quantity and moisture content of the marijuana, and the wattage of the microwave. There are no standards for this, but in general, smaller microwave ovens put out less power and would therefore require longer "cooking" times to kill a fungus.

Recent studies suggest that smoking marijuana may also decrease the ability of cells in the lung to destroy *Candida* and bacteria. *Candida* is the fungus responsible for candidiasis, a common condition in people living with HIV. People living with HIV who smoke marijuana may be at higher risk for lung complications. This particular effect might be minimized or eliminated by baking and eating marijuana (as in pot brownies and cakes)—rather than smoking it.

Impact on Hormones

Many men with HIV experience low testosterone levels during the course of HIV infection. Women may also experience lowered testosterone levels and changes in other hormones, both of which may be contributing factors in many menstrual irregularities seen in women living with HIV. Studies in animals and humans show that marijuana may further lower the levels of hormones, including testosterone. This information is important to people with HIV as lowered testosterone levels are associated with AIDS-related wasting. Marijuana could cause or worsen this condition, possibly leading to the necessity of testosterone replacement therapy.

Mental Status

The question of the neurological (change in mental status) effects of marijuana has been addressed by several studies in recent years. Marijuana use has been shown to have short-term impact on a person's ability to think, learn, judge, and perform tasks. Moreover, marijuana use has short-term effects on memory. It's less clear if marijuana has any long-term effects on mental status or mood. It is also less clear whether the effects noted are perceived as "good" or "bad" by those who experience them. Some people feel smoking marijuana offers relief from depression, while others say it increases their anxiety levels.

Marijuana's Impact on Appetite

Extensive research on how smoked marijuana affects appetite has been conducted, although much of it was published 20–50 years ago. Anecdotal accounts of increased food intake have always been reported by marijuana smokers—the so-called "munchies." The quality of the food (candy bars and chips versus vegetables, fruits, and protein) and quality of the weight gain (fat versus muscle) needs to be considered.

Overall, studies suggest that people using marijuana eat more but the food they eat is generally snack food, like cookies and junk food. They also exercise less and sleep more, all of which contributes to weight gain.

It's not at all clear that this kind of weight gain, that consists more of body fat than of lean muscle, will benefit the overall health and longevity of a person with HIV-related wasting. However, if medical marijuana is combined with a comprehensive nutritional and weight maintenance program, as well as exercise, it may prove useful. Because of these concerns, it is important that evaluating the medical effects of marijuana not be limited to measuring weight gain, as this may lead to false conclusions about its value.

When considering all the safety factors associated with marijuana use, it's important to weigh these factors against the harm being done by wasting. What may sound harmful to a healthy person may seem irrelevant to another when compared to the alternatives they face.

Oral THC Versus Marijuana

The oral drug, dronabinol (Marinol), was approved in 1992 for use in treating anorexia in people with HIV-related wasting. The active ingredient in dronabinol is THC, which is one of the main psychoactive agents in marijuana and the chemical that makes someone feel "stoned." For treating HIV-related weight loss, THC probably helps as an appetite stimulant, in the same way people who are "stoned" get the munchies.

People who use dronabinol have mixed experiences. Some report a minimal drug effect while others experience far too much euphoria or feeling stoned. This is because of the variability in how the oral drug gets into the bloodstream, or perhaps to an individuals' point of view and how they feel about such sensations. Smoking marijuana, or using edible forms of it, may be a more efficient way to get THC throughout the body. People who have tried both forms say that they are better able to control how stoned they get by smoking or eating marijuana and thus prefer it over the pill formulation.

Other Possible Uses for Medical Marijuana

For people living with HIV, marijuana may have other uses besides stimulating the appetite. Some research and reports of people's personal experiences support the notion that marijuana/THC can help treat nausea and vomiting. The exact reason why it works is unknown. Dronabinol is approved to ease nausea in people undergoing chemotherapy. Marijuana, therefore, may be a realistic alternative for people who don't benefit from standard anti-nausea medication. This could be an important benefit because so many people report difficulties with nausea when using anti-HIV therapies.

Marijuana has been shown to be an effective treatment for general pain associated with illness or serious injury. As with nausea, how marijuana relieves mild pain is not known. New studies suggest that marijuana may have anti-inflammatory effects.

The Future of Medical Marijuana

A recent report from the Institute of Medicine (IOM) of the U.S. National Academy of Sciences stated that certain chemicals found in marijuana may help manage certain conditions in some people, but that marijuana smoke, like tobacco smoke, is harmful. Though there is an oral medication (dronabinol) that is supposed to mimic the desired effects of smoking marijuana, many people prefer to smoke or eat marijuana in its natural form.

In an attempt to copy the effects of inhaling marijuana while eliminating the risks involved with smoking, some researchers are looking at the use of a vaporizer (or inhaler) for smokeless inhalation. Though not included in this IOM report, other sources indicate that a vaporizer is now readily available. This device heats marijuana to a certain temperature to release active chemicals without setting the dried plant on fire. Since this has only been around for a short time, it is not known how effective it is in delivering the drug. However, early results seem promising.

Overall, medical marijuana research will likely shift from study of the crude plant material to research and eventually drug development of chemicals derived from marijuana. This has already occurred with isolating THC and the development of dronabinol.

What currently holds back more studies of marijuana (or chemicals associated with marijuana) and its effects on the body is a complex matter. Aside from the obvious political concerns, research scientists are not given much incentive to work on marijuana and its derived chemicals. Namely, funding is scarce from government and private sources, and there is concern that the fruits of research will not be made public because of the controversial nature of the drug. Additionally, many researchers feel their reputations may be affected by working with marijuana because of its status as a street drug and controlled substance.

Nevertheless, more research related to marijuana could benefit many people, especially those living with HIV. There are indications that substances present in marijuana can stimulate appetite, relieve pain, and stop nausea. So, research that leads to uncovering the chemicals responsible for these effects and uncovering the best way to deliver them to the body could prove helpful. And though research may not eliminate all the safety concerns associated with medical marijuana, it may make this therapy a more realistic alternative for many people.

The Buying and Access of Medical Marijuana

- Dronabinol is available by prescription through hospitals and pharmacies.

- Medical marijuana buying, selling, and use is illegal in most of the United States.

- There are a limited number of buyers' clubs, providing a safe environment for people to buy medical marijuana. Some have programs that offer medical marijuana free or at reduced cost for people in need. The best buyers' clubs operate with the community oversight and accountability of a well-run non-profit agency.

- Not all buyers' clubs are ethical or conduct business in the best interest of people living with HIV. Buyer beware, and be aware of your options in your local area.

The Bottom Line on Medical Marijuana

- Medical marijuana may be useful in promoting appetite for people with HIV-related anorexia.

- Marijuana may also be useful in managing nausea and may help relieve pain.

- A synthetic form of an active ingredient in marijuana, dronabinol (Marinol), is approved by the FDA for treating HIV-related weight loss and for managing nausea associated with the use of chemotherapy.

Pros

- Dronabinol is FDA-approved and legally available by prescription through hospitals and pharmacies.

- People who have tried both dronabinol and medical marijuana contend that they are better able to control drug effects with medical marijuana.

- Some limited studies suggest that marijuana doesn't have negative long-term impact on HIV disease and measures of immune health, like CD4+ cell counts.

Cons

- Dronabinol has absorption problems and individuals claim difficulty in controlling the drug effect (feeling too "stoned").

- Medical marijuana is not legally available to many people. Third-party payers, like insurance and federal programs, do not cover its cost.

- Marijuana and its active ingredient THC has been shown in some studies to suppress immune function.

- Smoked marijuana increases the risk of lung infections and complications.

- Marijuana may be contaminated with insecticides, pesticides, fungus, and/or bacteria. Ingesting these could have mild to severe health consequences. (Some claim that microwaving marijuana for ten seconds on high may decrease risks associated with fungus contamination.)

- Marijuana/THC has short-term impact on mental status. Long-term effects are less clear.

- Some studies suggest that marijuana/THC may decrease testosterone levels.

- It is unknown if marijuana interacts with anti-HIV drug therapies, increases HIV replication or negatively impacts HIV disease progression.

Section 45.2

Studies Indicate Marijuana Use May Not Lead to Poor Adherence

Smoking marijuana does not lead to poorer adherence to HAART in patients with mild to severe nausea caused by anti-HIV drugs, according to a study published in the January 1st [2005] edition of the *Journal of Acquired Immune Deficiency Syndromes*. However, the U.S. investigators found that the use of other illicit drugs, and the smoking of marijuana by patients with no or mild nausea, was associated with non-adherence to HAART.

Marijuana is used by some HIV-positive individuals to stimulate appetite and to counter nausea caused by HAART. Nevertheless, there are concerns about the safety of marijuana use, not least the potential for use of the drug to decrease adherence to HAART due to its psychoactive effects.

It has been shown that the use of other illicit drugs, including heroin, cocaine, and speed decrease adherence to HAART, and two studies published in 2003 found that marijuana use had a similar affect. However, as marijuana is often used by HIV-positive patients to relieve symptoms or side effects, investigators postulated that use of the drug might not be associated with poor adherence in patients taking HAART who are experiencing adverse events, including nausea.

Investigators recruited 252 HIV-positive patients from three HIV clinics in northern California to their study in 2001. They were asked to report their adherence to HAART in the previous week. Patients who missed at least one dose were assessed as "non-adherent." Individuals were also asked to say if they had ever used marijuana and to report the use of marijuana, and any other illicit substances, in the past four weeks.

Of the 252 patients who completed the study questionnaire, 168 (67 percent) provided data about their adherence to HAART. In total, 41 individuals (24 percent) said that they had used marijuana in the previous four weeks.

A third of patients taking HAART (55 individuals) were assessed as non-adherent. In bivariate analysis, the investigators failed to find any positive or negative association between marijuana use and adherence (OR 0.92). Adherence was associated with a viral load below 50 copies/ml (p = 0.04) and having had mental distress about one's health (p = 0.04). Adherence was negatively associated with use of illicit drugs other than marijuana in the last four weeks (p = 0.02) and with alcohol use in the last four weeks (p = 0.04).

The investigators then looked at the subgroup of patients reporting moderate to severe nausea (43 individuals). Of the 20 patients who used marijuana, 75 percent were assessed as being adherent compared to 48 percent of the 23 patients who did not report use of the drug (p = 0.07).

However, when the investigators looked at the 125 patients with no or mild nausea, they found that marijuana users were significantly less likely to be adherent than non-users (p = 0.02).

"No crude association was found between marijuana use and adherence," write the investigators, who add, "our data do suggest that use of smoked marijuana specifically to ameliorate nausea may be associated with adherence to antiretroviral therapy...in addition, our data confirm previously reported findings that the use of other illicit drugs is associated with lower rates of adherence."

The investigators note that the use of marijuana for medical purposes remains controversial and "do not here advocate its widespread use...however, in certain circumstances, specifically when patients are using marijuana to relieve nausea, marijuana is not associated with lower rates of adherence."

Reference

de Jong, BC, et al. Marijuana use and its association with adherence to antiretroviral therapy among HIV-infected persons with moderate to severe nausea. J *Acquir Immune Defic Syndr* 38: 43–46, 2005.

Chapter 46

Tips for Managing the Side Effects of Anti-HIV Medicines

Almost all medicines have side effects, including medicines for HIV. Always let your doctor know if your side effects are severe, especially if you are finding it difficult to stay on your treatment plan.

The following is information on some common side effects and tips on how to deal with them.

Anemia

Anemia means you have a low red blood cell count. The red blood cells take oxygen to different parts of the body, and when your body is short of oxygen, you feel tired.

Many people with HIV have anemia at some point. HIV can cause it; so can some of the anti-HIV drugs.

To see if you have anemia (a symptom of anemia is feeling tired, fatigued, or short of breath), your health care provider can do a simple blood test. If you are anemic, food or other medicines can help.

Quick Tips: Anemia

- First, find out if you have anemia. If you are short of breath or tired and the tiredness doesn't go away after getting rest, ask your doctor whether you should get tested for anemia.

"Treatment Decisions: Side Effects Guide," U.S. Department of Veterans Affairs, National HIV/AIDS Program, updated October 16, 2006.

- If you find out you have anemia, your doctor will prescribe a treatment according to the cause of the anemia. Some of these treatments include the following:

  - changing medications

  - taking iron, folate, or vitamin B_{12}

  - changing your diet

Diarrhea

Diarrhea is common in people with HIV, and it can be caused by some anti-HIV medicines. Diarrhea can range from being a small hassle to being a serious medical problem. Talk to your health care provider if diarrhea goes on for a long time, if it is bloody, if it is accompanied by fever, or if it worries you.

When you have diarrhea, always be sure to replace the fluids you have lost by drinking ginger ale, broth, herbal tea, or water.

You can also ask your doctor about taking medicines to help with your diarrhea.

Quick Tips: Diarrhea

Following is what to try:

- Try the BRATT diet (bananas, rice, applesauce, tea, and toast).

- Eat foods high in soluble fiber. This kind of fiber can slow the diarrhea by soaking up liquid. Soluble fiber is found in oatmeal, grits, and soft bread (but not in whole grain).

- Try psyllium husk fiber bars (another source of soluble fiber). You can find these at health food stores. Eating two of these bars and drinking a big glass of water before bedtime may help your diarrhea.

- Ask your doctor about taking calcium pills.

- Drink plenty of clear liquids.

Following is what to avoid:

- Stay away from foods high in insoluble fiber, such as whole grains, brown rice, bran, or the skins of vegetables and fruits. These kinds of foods can make diarrhea worse.

- Avoid milk products.
- Don't eat too many greasy, high-fiber, or very sweet foods.
- Don't take in too much caffeine.
- Avoid raw or undercooked fish, chicken, and meat.

Dry Mouth

Certain HIV medicines can cause dry mouth, making it difficult to chew, swallow, and talk.

Treating dry mouth can be simple—start by drinking plenty of liquids during or between meals. If your dry mouth is severe or doesn't go away, talk to your doctor about prescribing a treatment for you.

Quick Tips: Dry mouth

- Rinse your mouth throughout the day with warm, salted water.
- Carry sugarless candies, lozenges, or crushed ice with you to cool the mouth and give it moisture.
- Try slippery elm or licorice tea (available in health food stores). They can moisten the mouth, and they taste great.
- Ask your doctor about mouth rinse and other products to treat your dry mouth.

Fatigue

Many people feel tired, especially when they are stressed or their lives are busier than usual. Symptoms of being tired can include: having a hard time getting out of bed, walking up stairs, or even concentrating on something for very long.

If the tiredness (or fatigue) doesn't go away, even after you have given your body and mind time to rest, this tiredness can become a problem. It can get worse if you don't deal with it.

Talk with your health care provider if your fatigue is not going away or is becoming too hard to deal with. The more information you can give your doctor about how you are feeling, the more likely the two of you will be able to come up with the right treatment for your fatigue.

Quick Tips: Fatigue

- Get plenty of rest.

- Go to sleep and wake up at the same time every day. Changing your sleeping habits too much can actually make you feel tired.

- Try to get some exercise.

- Keep prepackaged or easy-to-make food in the kitchen for times when you're too tired to cook.

- Follow a healthy, balanced diet. Your health care provider may be able to help you create a meal plan.

- Talk to your doctor about the possibility that you have anemia. Anemia means that you have a low red blood cell count, and it can make you feel tired.

Hair Loss

Many people lose their hair as they get older, or when they are going through a very stressful time in their lives.

You can also lose your hair from taking certain medications, including those used to treat HIV.

Quick Tips: Hair Loss

- To stop any more hair loss, stay away from doing such things as dyeing, perming, and straightening your hair.

- If losing your hair is very upsetting for you and causing anxiety, you may want to talk to you doctor about whether you can try something like Rogaine, which is a medicine that helps your hair to regrow.

- Since stress can make hair loss worse, try to reduce stress and anxiety in your life.

Headaches

The most common cause of headaches is tension or stress, something we all have from time to time. Medications, including anti-HIV drugs, can cause them, too.

Headaches usually can be taken care of with drugs you can buy without a prescription, such as aspirin. You can also help to prevent future headaches by reducing stress.

Quick Tips: Headaches

For on-the-spot headache relief, try some of these suggestions:

- Lie down and rest in a quiet, dark room.

- Take a hot, relaxing bath.

- Give yourself a "scalp massage"—massage the base of your skull with your thumbs and massage both temples gently.

- Check with your doctor about taking an over-the-counter pain reliever, such as aspirin.

To prevent headaches from happening again, try the following:

- Avoid things that can cause headaches, like chocolate, red wine, onions, hard cheese, and caffeine.

- Reduce your stress level.

Nausea and Vomiting

Certain medications used to treat HIV can cause nausea. They make you feel sick to your stomach and want to throw up. This usually goes away a few weeks after starting a new medication.

Call your doctor if you vomit repeatedly throughout the day, or if nausea or vomiting keeps you from taking your medication.

Quick Tips: Nausea and Vomiting

Following is what to try:

- Eat smaller meals and snack more often.

- The BRATT diet (bananas, rice, applesauce, tea, and toast) helps with nausea and diarrhea.

- Leave dry crackers by your bed. Before getting out of bed in the morning, eat a few and stay in bed for a few minutes. This can help reduce nausea.

- Try some herbal tea—such as peppermint or ginger tea.

- Sip cold, carbonated drinks such as ginger ale or Sprite.

- Open your windows when cooking so the smell of food won't be too strong.

- Talk with your health care provider about whether you should take medicine for your nausea.

- If you do vomit, be sure to "refuel" your body with fluids such as broth, carbonated beverages, juice, or popsicles.

Following is what to avoid:

- Avoid things that can upset the stomach, such as alcohol, aspirin, caffeine, and smoking.

- Avoid hot or spicy foods.

- Don't eat too many greasy or fried foods.

- Don't lie down immediately after eating.

Pain and Nerve Problems

HIV itself and some medications for HIV can cause damage to your nerves. This condition is called peripheral neuropathy. When these nerves are damaged, your feet, toes, and hands can feel like they're burning or stinging. It can also make them numb or stiff.

You should talk to your doctor if you have pain like this.

Quick Tips: Pain and Nerve Problems

- Massaging your feet can make the pain go away for a while.

- Soak your feet in ice water to help with the pain.

- Wear loose-fitting shoes and slippers.

- When you're in bed, don't cover your feet with blankets or sheets. The bedding can press down on your feet and toes and make the pain worse.

- Ask your doctor about taking an over-the-counter pain reliever to reduce the pain and swelling.

Rash

Some medications can cause skin problems, such as rashes. Most rashes come and go, but sometimes they signal that you are having a bad reaction to the medication.

It's important that you check your skin for changes, especially after you start a new medication. Be sure to report any changes to your health care provider.

Quick Tips: Rash

- Avoid extremely hot showers or baths. Water that is too hot can irritate the skin.

- Avoid being in the sun. Sun exposure can make your rash worse.

- Keep medications such as Benadryl on hand in case you develop a rash. Ask your doctor for suggestions.

- Try using unscented, non-soapy cleansers for the bath or shower.

- A rash that blisters, or involves your mouth, the palms of your hands, or the soles of your feet, or one that is accompanied by shortness of breath, can be dangerous: contact your doctor right away.

Weight Loss

Weight loss goes along with some of these other side effects. It can happen because of vomiting, nausea, fatigue, and other reasons.

Talk with your health care provider if you're losing weight without trying, meaning that you're not on a reducing diet.

Quick Tips: Weight Loss

- Be sure to keep track of your weight, by stepping on scales and writing down how much you weigh. Tell your doctor if there are any changes.

- Create your own high-protein drink by blending together yogurt, fruit (for sweetness), and powdered milk, whey protein, or soy protein.

- Between meals, try store-bought nutritional beverages or bars (such as Carnation Instant Breakfast, Benefit, Ensure, Scandishake, Boost High Protein, NuBasics). Look for ones that are high in proteins, not sugars or fats.

- Spread peanut butter on toast, crackers, fruit, or vegetables.

- Add cottage cheese to fruit and tomatoes.

- Add canned tuna to casseroles and salads.

- Add shredded cheese to sauces, soups, omelets, baked potatoes, and steamed vegetables.

- Eat yogurt on your cereal or fruit.

- Eat hard-boiled (hard-cooked) eggs. Use them in egg-salad sandwiches or slice and dice them for tossed salads.

- Add diced or chopped meats to soups, salads, and sauces.

- Add dried milk powder, whey protein, soy protein or egg white powder to foods (for example, scrambled eggs, casseroles, and milkshakes).

Part Six

Issues for Women, Children, and Adolescents with HIV/AIDS

Chapter 47

How HIV/AIDS Affects Women's Health

The number of women with HIV (human immunodeficiency virus) infection and AIDS (acquired immunodeficiency syndrome) has increased steadily worldwide. By the end of 2005, according to the World Health Organization (WHO), 17.5 million women worldwide were infected with HIV.

According to the Centers for Disease Control and Prevention (CDC), between 2000 through 2004, the estimated number of AIDS cases in the United States increased 10 percent among females and 7 percent among males. In 2004, women accounted for 27 percent of the 44,615 newly reported AIDS cases among adults and adolescents. HIV disproportionately affects African American and Hispanic women. Together they represent less than 25 percent of all U.S. women, yet they account for more than 79 percent of AIDS cases in women.

Worldwide, more than 90 percent of all adolescent and adult HIV infections have resulted from heterosexual intercourse. Women are particularly vulnerable to heterosexual transmission of HIV due to substantial mucosal exposure to seminal fluids. This biological fact amplifies the risk of HIV transmission when coupled with the high prevalence of non-consensual sex, sex without condom use, and the unknown and/or high-risk behaviors of their partners.

Women suffer from the same complications of AIDS that afflict men, but also suffer gender-specific manifestations of HIV disease,

Excerpted from "HIV Infection in Women," National Institute of Allergy and Infectious Diseases (http://www.niaid.gov), a component of the National Institutes of Health (NIH), updated May 18, 2006.

such as recurrent vaginal yeast infections, severe pelvic inflammatory disease (PID), and an increased risk of precancerous changes in the cervix including probable increased rates of cervical cancer. Women also exhibit different characteristics from men for many of the same complications of antiretroviral therapy, such as metabolic abnormalities.

Frequently, women with HIV infection have great difficulty accessing health care and carry a heavy burden of caring for children and other family members who may also be HIV-infected. They often lack social support and face other challenges that may interfere with their ability to obtain or adhere to treatment.

Current Research

The National Institute of Allergy and Infectious Diseases (NIAID) is studying the course of HIV/AIDS disease in women through the Women's Interagency HIV Study (WIHS) and supports clinical trials to investigate gender-specific differences in disease progression, complications, and treatment though the Adult AIDS Clinical Trials Group (AACTG), the Pediatric AIDS Clinical Trials Group (PACTG), and the Terry Beirn Community Programs for Clinical Research on AIDS (CPCRA). The HIV Prevention Trials Network (HPTN) investigates non-vaccine prevention strategies.

Natural History and Epidemiological Research

Women's Interagency HIV Study (WIHS) is a multi-site, prospective cohort of predominantly minority HIV-infected and uninfected women and is currently following 2,441 women. The study recently increased enrollment to evaluate clinical outcomes in the era of highly active antiretroviral therapy (HAART), including time to develop AIDS, impact of resistance to antiretroviral therapy, the effect of co-infections such as hepatitis C and human papillomavirus (HPV), the effects of metabolic abnormalities and toxicities, the impact of hormonal factors on HIV disease, and the impact of aging on HIV disease.

Recently, WIHS implemented an intensive protocol to evaluate cardiovascular manifestations of HIV among women. This study was the outgrowth of a workshop held in May 2003 that was co-sponsored by NIAID and the National Heart, Lung and Blood Institute. So that gender comparisons can be made, a similar investigation is taking place in the Multicenter AIDS Cohort Study, a cohort of men who have sex with men, and the Tri-Service AIDS Clinical Consortium, a cohort of HIV-infected U.S. military personnel.

Topical Microbicides

Because HIV is spread predominantly through sexual transmission, the development of chemical, biological, and physical barriers that can be used intravaginally or intrarectally to inactivate HIV and other sexually transmitted disease (STD) pathogens is critically important for controlling HIV infection.

Scientists are developing and testing new chemical and biological compounds that women could apply before intercourse to protect themselves against HIV and other sexually transmitted organisms. These include creams or gels, known as topical microbicides, that ideally would be non-irritating, inexpensive, and unobtrusive. The research effort for developing topical microbicides includes basic research, preclinical product development, and clinical evaluation.

At present, NIAID is supporting the development and evaluation of 23 compounds and/or combinations through its Integrated Preclinical/Clinical Program for HIV Topical Microbicides. Some of the new products in development include a combination product using dendrimer and BufferGel, both of which have entered into clinical testing separately and the use of bioengineered Lactobacillus expressing a broad range of protein-based microbicides.

In February 2005, NIAID initiated a multicenter clinical trial (HPTN 035) to examine the safety and preliminary effectiveness of BufferGel and PRO2000/5 Gel (P) to prevent HIV infection. The trial, which is the first microbicide safety and effectiveness trial of this magnitude to be supported by NIAID, is being conducted through the HPTN and represents a partnership among various research institutions in Africa and the United States. Women are currently being enrolled at sites in Philadelphia, Pennsylvania; Lilongwe and Blantrye, Malawi; and Durban and Hlabisa, South Africa, Harare and Chitungwiza, Zimbabwe, and Lusaka, Zambia.

Another study, the HIV Prevention Preparedness Study (HPTN 055) was conducted in Zambia, South Africa, and Tanzania to assess the ability of sites to recruit and retain participants for future efficacy trials of topical microbicides. This study has helped obtain reliable data on HIV seroprevalence and seroincidence in the target populations.

Recently, NIAID-funded investigators demonstrated that combination microbicides may be more efficient than single microbicides at preventing vaginal transmission of simian HIV (SHIV) in rhesus macaques. This has important implications for future microbicide research because it is highly possible that first generation microbicides may at best be only 30 to 50 percent effective, given the complexity of HIV transmission. Thus, combinations resulting in additive or synergistic inhibition of HIV transmission could offer the potential to reduce individual microbicide concentrations resulting in a more potent and cost effective microbicide strategy.

Another finding recently released provided proof that disrupting how the virus attaches itself to cells completely protected monkeys that were vaginally exposed to SHIV. This was done with the use of PSC-RANTES, a chemically modified form of a protein called RANTES, that works by targeting a protein in the body called C-C chemokine receptor 5 (CCR5), a receptor on human cells to which HIV binds. In addition to CD4, there are co-receptors, such as CCR5 and CXCR4. Sexual transmission of HIV is thought to predominantly involve CCR5. HIV needs CCR5 to achieve infection of any given cell.

For the virus to be transmitted during heterosexual intercourse— the primary method the virus is spread in many parts of the world— the virus must attach to CCR5 in cells within the vaginal mucosa. When these cells were protected with a topical microbicide containing a high enough concentration of PSC-RANTES, however, the virus could not attach to them, thus preventing transmission. This work represents the first demonstration of significant protection through a range of doses for any protein-based microbicide and demonstrated that it was possible to achieve in vivo concentrations of protein microbicides that could afford 100 percent protection of exposed individuals. To further develop vaginal microbicides, NIAID entered into an agreement with the International Partnership for Microbicides (IPM) in 2006 to share information and expertise.

NIAID's Topical Microbicide Strategic Plan, which details long-range plans for advancing microbicide concepts from the laboratory to clinical trials, is available on NIAID's website at http://www.niaid.nih.gov/publications/topical_microbicide_strategic_plan.pdf.

Transmission

Transmission of HIV to Women

In the United States, most women are infected with HIV during sex with an HIV-infected man or while using HIV-contaminated syringes for the injection of drugs such as heroin, cocaine, and amphetamines. Of the new HIV infections diagnosed among women in the United States in 2004, CDC estimated 70 percent were attributed to heterosexual contact and 28 percent to injection drug use.

In this country, studies have shown that during unprotected heterosexual intercourse with an HIV-infected partner, women have a greater risk of becoming infected than uninfected men who have heterosexual intercourse with an HIV-infected woman. In other parts of the world, however, this is not necessarily true. In Uganda, for example, one study demonstrated that the risk of HIV transmission from woman to man was the same as from man to woman. This difference may be due to the lack of circumcision in Ugandan men.

Studies in both the United States and abroad have demonstrated that STDs, particularly infections that cause ulcerations of the vagina (for example, genital herpes, syphilis, and chancroid), greatly increase a woman's risk of becoming infected with HIV. NIAID-sponsored cohort studies in the United States have also found a number of other factors to be associated with an increased risk of heterosexual HIV transmission, including alcohol use, history of childhood sexual abuse, current domestic abuse, and use of crack/cocaine.

Consistent and correct use of male latex condoms greatly reduces the risk of becoming infected with HIV. In studies of heterosexual couples, in which one individual was HIV-positive and the other uninfected and regular condom use was reported, the rate of HIV transmission was extremely low.

Studies examining the use of antiretroviral drugs to try to prevent transmission are also underway. For example, the HPTN (HPTN 052) has a study examining serodiscordant couples with CD4 counts above 300 cells to determine whether HAART, when given to the infected partner along with prevention counseling and interventions like condoms, prevents HIV transmission to the uninfected partner better than prevention counseling and prevention services alone.

Mother-to-Child Transmission (MTCT) of HIV

In the United States, approximately 25 percent of pregnant HIV-infected women who do not receive AZT or a combination of antiretroviral therapies pass the virus to their babies. If women do receive a combination of antiretroviral therapies during pregnancy, however, the risk of HIV transmission to the newborn drops below 2 percent. (There were 111 infected infants born in the U.S. in 2005. For more information, go to http://www.cdc.gov/hiv/topics/surveillance/resources/reports/2005report/table23.htm.)

The risk of MTCT is significantly increased if the mother has advanced HIV disease, high amounts of HIV in her bloodstream, or fewer-than-normal amounts of the CD4+ T cells.

419

Other factors that may increase the risk include: drug use, such as heroin or crack/cocaine; severe inflammation of fetal membranes; or prolonged period between membrane rupture and delivery

Most MTCT, an estimated 50 to 70 percent, probably occurs late in pregnancy or during birth. Although the exact ways the virus is transmitted are unknown, scientists think it may happen when the mother's blood enters fetal circulation or by mucosal exposure to the virus during labor and delivery. One NIAID-sponsored study also found that HIV-infected women who gave birth more than four hours after rupture of the fetal membranes were nearly twice as likely to transmit HIV to their babies, as compared to women who delivered within four hours of membrane rupture. In the same study, HIV-infected women who used heroin or crack/cocaine during pregnancy were also twice as likely to transmit HIV to their babies as compared to HIV-infected women who did not use drugs.

NIAID supports research on MTCT through the PACTG, AACTG, and HPTN, and until recently, through the Women and Infants Transmission Study (WITS), a prospective cohort study that has followed HIV-infected mothers and their children since 1988. Since that time, WITS researchers have examined factors that contribute to perinatal transmission, evaluated disease progression and contributing factors during pregnancy and postpartum in HIV-infected women and their infants, and evaluated diagnostic tools for determining HIV status in infants. Sponsored by NIAID, the National Institute of Child Health and Human Development, and the National Institute on Drug Abuse, WITS will be phasing out in 2007.

The first regimen to prevent MTCT was identified in a landmark study conducted in 1994 by the PACTG. A specific regimen of AZT (azidothymidine) given to an HIV-infected woman during pregnancy and to her baby after birth was shown to reduce mother-to-child HIV transmission by two-thirds.

In another NIAID-sponsored study (HIVNET 012) in Uganda, researchers identified a highly effective and safe drug regimen for preventing transmission of HIV from an infected mother to her newborn that is more affordable and practical than any other course of therapy examined to date. The study demonstrated that a single oral dose of the antiretroviral drug, nevirapine (NVP), given to an HIV-infected woman in labor and another dose given to her baby within three days of birth reduces the transmission rate by about half compared with a course of AZT given only during labor and delivery. Additional data from this study demonstrated the continued benefit and safety of NVP in reducing MTCT up to 18 months, even in a breastfeeding population.

This study suggests that women in the United States who are identified as HIV-infected very late in pregnancy or at the time of labor and delivery could lower the rates of HIV transmission to their babies by following a NVP-containing regimen.

Data from HIVNET 012 also showed that resistance to NVP was present in approximately 19 percent of women six to eight weeks after the single dose of NVP. After 12 to 24 months, there was no NVP resistance detectable in these women using standard methods of HIV resistance testing. Nevertheless, these data are of concern because preliminary data from a small, uncontrolled trial presented at the 2004 Retrovirus Conference in San Francisco by Jourdain, et al. showed that women who had received previous single dose NVP had poorer virologic outcome when treated with HAART than women who had never received NVP.

Studies are now underway to examine the effects of exposure to single dose nevirapine (SD NVP) on future treatment options for women and children. One study currently open to enrollment in Africa is evaluating the effect of previous exposure to SD NVP on the mother's future treatment options (Optimal Combined Therapy after Nevirapine Exposure, AACTG 5208). A similar trial for infants is in development (PACTG 1060). Strategies to minimize viral resistance after SD NVP are also being explored in two other studies. The first study will compare the impact of three antiretroviral strategies administered on reducing NVP resistance following SD NVP, and the second will examine the pharmacokinetics and incidence of NVP resistance in women who receive SD NVP alone or in combination with one of two other regimens.

The HPTN is also conducting a study to compare three antiretroviral regimens for post-exposure prophylaxis of HIV-uninfected infants born to HIV-infected women whose HIV status was unknown at the time of delivery and who were therefore not exposed to a prenatal or perinatal antiretroviral regimen (HPTN 040).

HIV may also be transmitted from a nursing mother to her child. A series of studies have determined that breastfeeding increases the risk of HIV transmission by about 14 percent. Currently, the Joint United Nations Programme on HIV/AIDS (UNAIDS) recommends that HIV-positive women be educated and counseled so they can make an informed decision about how to best feed their children.

Research to identify effective strategies for reducing the risk of transmission through breastfeeding is underway in areas of the world where the benefits of breastfeeding outweigh the risks. This includes early weaning strategies as well as evaluating drugs or vaccines to reduce the risk of transmission from breastfeeding.

To further evaluate ways to prevent HIV transmission during breastfeeding, the HPTN is initiating a study of NVP for breast-feeding infants of HIV-infected mothers (HPTN 046). Similarly, an investigator-initiated study for preventing MTCT is underway in Ethiopia and Uganda to evaluate a six-week regimen of NVP administered to HIV-uninfected infants born to HIV-infected breastfeeding mothers. In Uganda, another component of the study will be added to passively immunize the breastfeeding children with HIV immunoglobulin (HIV-Ig).

Signs and Symptoms of HIV Infection

Many manifestations of HIV infection are similar in men and women. Both men and women with HIV may have non-specific symptoms even early in disease, including low-grade fevers, night sweats, fatigue, and weight loss. Anti-HIV therapies, as well as treatments for other infections associated with HIV, appear to be similarly effective in men and women. Other conditions, however, occur in different frequencies in men and women. HIV-infected men, for instance, are eight times more likely than HIV-infected women to develop a skin cancer known as Kaposi sarcoma. In some studies, women had higher rates of herpes simplex infections than men.

Data from several studies conducted by the Community Programs for Clinical Research on AIDS (CPCRA) found that HIV-infected women were also more likely than HIV-infected men to develop bacterial pneumonia. This finding may be explained by factors such as a delay in seeking care among HIV-infected women as compared to men, and less access to anti-HIV therapies or preventive therapies for *Pneumocystis carinii/jiroveci* pneumonia, or PCP.

Woman-Specific Symptoms of HIV Infection

Women also experience HIV-associated gynecologic problems, many of which occur in uninfected women but with less frequency or severity.

Vaginal yeast infections, common and easily treated in most women, often are particularly persistent and difficult to treat in HIV-infected women. Data from WIHS suggest that these infections are considerably more frequent in HIV-infected women. Health care providers commonly treat yeast infections with fluconazole. A CPCRA study demonstrated that weekly doses of fluconazole can also safely prevent oropharyngeal and vaginal, but not esophageal, yeast infections, without resulting in drug resistance.

Other vaginal infections may occur more frequently and with greater severity in HIV-infected women, including bacterial vaginosis and common STDs such as gonorrhea, chlamydia, and trichomoniasis.

Severe herpes simplex virus ulcerations, which are sometimes unresponsive to therapy with the standard drug acyclovir, can severely compromise a woman's quality of life.

Idiopathic genital ulcers, with no evidence of an infectious organism or cancerous cells in the lesion, are a unique manifestation of HIV infection. These ulcers, for which there is no proven treatment, are sometimes confused with those caused by herpes simplex virus.

HPV infections, which cause genital warts and can lead to cervical cancer, occur more frequently in HIV-infected women. A precancerous condition associated with HPV, called cervical dysplasia, is also more common and more severe in HIV-infected women and more apt to recur after treatment.

PID appears to be more common and more aggressive in HIV-infected women than in uninfected women. PID may become a chronic and relapsing condition as a woman's immune system deteriorates.

Menstrual irregularities frequently are reported by HIV-infected women and are being actively studied by NIAID-supported scientists. Although menstrual irregularities were equally common in HIV-infected women and at-risk HIV-negative women in a WIHS survey, women with CD4+ T-cell counts below 50 per cubic millimeter (mm^3) of blood were more likely to report no periods than were uninfected women, or HIV-infected women with higher CD4+ T-cell counts.

Gynecologic Screening

CDC currently recommends that HIV-positive women have a complete gynecologic evaluation, including a Pap smear, as part of their initial HIV evaluations, or upon entry to prenatal care, and another Pap smear six months later. If both smears are negative, annual screening is recommended thereafter in asymptomatic women. The agency also recommends more frequent screenings—every six months—for women with symptomatic HIV infection, prior abnormal Pap smears, or signs of HPV infection.

Early Diagnosis

Some women in the United States have poor access to health care. In addition, women may not think they are at risk for HIV infection. They may not heed symptoms that could serve as warning signals of

HIV infection, such as recurrent yeast infections. PID and the other symptoms discussed previously should signal health care providers to offer women HIV testing with counseling.

Early diagnosis of HIV infection allows women to take full advantage of antiretroviral treatments and preventive medicines for opportunistic infections when their health care providers think it is appropriate. Both appropriate therapy and preventive drugs can forestall the development of AIDS-related symptoms and prolong life in HIV-infected women as well as men. Early diagnosis also allows women to make informed reproductive choices. Health care providers should be alert to early signs of HIV infection in women. In addition, all women should consider HIV testing if they have engaged in behaviors that put them at risk of infection.

Survival among HIV-Infected Women

Women whose HIV infections are detected early and receive appropriate treatment survive as long as HIV-infected men. Although several studies have shown HIV-infected women to have shorter survival times than men, this may be because women are less likely than men to be diagnosed early.

In an analysis of several studies involving more than 4,500 people with HIV infection, women were 33 percent more likely than men to die within the study period. The investigators could not definitively identify the reasons for excess mortality among women in this study, but they speculated that poorer access to or use of health care resources among HIV-infected women as compared to men, domestic violence, homelessness, and lack of social supports may have been important factors.

Chapter 48

HIV during Pregnancy, Labor and Delivery, and after Birth

This text is intended for women who are HIV positive and pregnant or have recently given birth. It describes the steps an HIV-positive pregnant woman can take to preserve her health and prevent transmission of HIV to her baby. The information in this chapter is based on the U.S. Public Health Service's Recommendations for Use of Antiretroviral Drugs in Pregnant HIV-1-Infected Women for Maternal Health and Interventions to Reduce Perinatal HIV-1 Transmission in the United States and Guidelines for the Use of Antiretroviral Agents in Pediatric HIV Infection (available at http://aidsinfo.nih.gov/guidelines).

I am pregnant, and I may have HIV. Will I be tested for HIV when I visit a doctor?

In most cases, health care providers cannot test you for HIV without your permission. However, the U.S. Public Health Service recommends that all pregnant women be tested. If you are thinking about being tested, it is important to understand the different ways perinatal HIV testing is done. There are two main approaches to HIV testing in pregnant women: opt-in and opt-out testing.

In opt-in testing, a woman cannot be given an HIV test unless she specifically requests to be tested. Often, she must put this request in writing.

"HIV during Pregnancy, Labor and Delivery, and after Birth: Health Information for HIV Positive Pregnant Women," AIDSinfo (http://www.aidsinfo.nih.gov), a service of the U.S. Department of Health and Human Services, August 2006.

In opt-out testing, health care providers must inform pregnant women that an HIV test will be included in the standard group of tests pregnant women receive. A woman will receive that HIV test unless she specifically refuses. The CDC currently recommends that health care providers adopt an opt-out approach to perinatal HIV testing.

What are the benefits of being tested?

By knowing your HIV status, you and your doctor can decide on the best treatment for you and your baby and can take steps to prevent mother-to-child transmission of HIV. It is also important to know your HIV status so that you can take the appropriate steps to avoid infecting others.

What happens if I agree to be tested?

If you agree to be tested, your doctor should counsel you before the test about the way your life may change after you receive the test results. If the test indicates that you have HIV, you should be given a second test to confirm the results. If your second test is positive for HIV, you and your doctor will decide which treatment options are best for you and your baby. If the test indicates that you do not have HIV, you may receive counseling on HIV prevention.

What happens if I refuse to be tested?

If you decide that you do not want to be tested for HIV, your doctor may offer you counseling about the way HIV is transmitted and the importance of taking steps to prevent HIV transmission. He or she may also talk to you about the importance of finding out your HIV status so that you can take steps to prevent your baby from becoming infected.

Will my baby be tested for HIV?

Health care providers recommend that all babies born to HIV-positive mothers be tested for HIV. However, states differ in the ways they approach HIV testing for babies.

- Some states require that babies receive a mandatory HIV test if the status of the mother is unknown.

- Some states require that health care providers test babies for HIV unless the mother refuses.

- Some states are only required to offer an HIV test to pregnant women (not their babies), which they can either accept or refuse.

How can I find out the testing policies of my state?

The U.S. Department of Health and Human Services (HHS) can provide you with HIV testing information for your state. Contact HHS at 877-696-6775 or 202-619-0257.

Should I take anti-HIV medications if I am HIV positive and pregnant?

You should take anti-HIV medications if the following apply to you:

- You are experiencing severe symptoms of HIV or have been diagnosed with AIDS.
- Your CD4 count is 200 cells/mm^3 or less (treatment should be considered at 350 cells/mm^3 or less).
- Your viral load is greater than 1,000 copies/ml.

You should also take anti-HIV medications to prevent your baby from becoming infected with HIV. Specific treatment to prevent mother-to-child transmission of HIV is discussed in the following sections.

How do I find out what treatment regimen is best for me?

HIV treatment is an important part of maintaining your health and preventing your baby from becoming infected with HIV. Decisions about when to start HIV treatment and which medications to take should be based on many of the same factors that women who are not pregnant must consider. These factors include the following:

- risk that the HIV infection may become worse
- risks and benefits of delaying treatment
- potential drug toxicities and interactions with other drugs you are taking
- the need to adhere to a treatment regimen closely
- the results of drug resistance testing

In addition to these factors, pregnant women must consider the following issues:

- benefit of lowering viral load and reducing the risk of mother-to-child transmission of HIV

- unknown long-term effects on your baby if you take anti-HIV medications during your pregnancy

- information available about the use of anti-HIV medications during pregnancy

You should discuss your treatment options with your doctor so that together you can decide which treatment regimen is best for you and your baby.

What treatment regimen should I follow during my pregnancy if I have never taken anti-HIV medications?

Your best treatment options depend on when you were diagnosed with HIV, when you found out you were pregnant, and at what point you sought medical treatment during your pregnancy. Women who are in the first trimester of pregnancy and who do not have symptoms of HIV disease may consider delaying treatment until after ten to twelve weeks into their pregnancies. After the first trimester, pregnant women with HIV should receive at least AZT (Retrovir, zidovudine, or ZDV); your doctor may recommend additional medications depending on your CD4 count, viral load, and drug resistance testing.

I am taking anti-HIV medications, and I just learned that I am pregnant. Should I stop taking my medications?

Do not stop taking any of your medications without consulting your doctor first. Stopping HIV treatment could lead to problems for you and your baby. If you are taking anti-HIV medications and your pregnancy is identified during the first trimester, talk with your doctor about the risks and benefits of continuing your current regimen. He or she may recommend that you stop your anti-HIV medications or change the medications you take. If your pregnancy is identified after the first trimester, it is recommended that you continue with your current treatment. No matter what HIV treatment regimen you were on before your pregnancy, it is generally recommended that AZT become part of your regimen.

Will I need treatment during labor and delivery?

Most mother-to-child transmission of HIV occurs around the time of labor and delivery. Therefore, HIV treatment during this time is very important for protecting your baby from HIV infection. Several treatment regimens are available to reduce the risk of transmission to your baby. The most common regimen is the three-part AZT regimen:

1. HIV infected pregnant women should take AZT starting at 14 to 34 weeks of pregnancy. You can take either 100 mg five times a day, 200 mg three times a day, or 300 mg twice a day.

2. During labor and delivery, you should receive intravenous (IV) AZT.

3. Your baby should take AZT (in liquid form) every six hours for six weeks after he or she is born.

If you have been taking any other anti-HIV medications during your pregnancy, your doctor will probably recommend that you continue to take them on schedule during labor.

Better understanding of HIV transmission has contributed to dramatically reduced rates of mother-to-child transmission of HIV. Discuss the benefits of HIV treatment during pregnancy with your doctor; these benefits should be weighed against the risks to you and to your baby.

Are there any anti-HIV medications that may be dangerous to me or my baby during my pregnancy?

Although information on anti-HIV medications in pregnant women is limited compared to information for non-pregnant adults, enough is known to make recommendations about which medications are appropriate for you and your baby. However, the long-term consequences of babies' exposure to anti-HIV medications in utero are unknown. Talk to your doctor about which medications may be harmful during your pregnancy and what medication substitutions and dose changes are possible.

The non-nucleoside reverse transcriptase inhibitor (NNRTI) nevirapine (Viramune or NVP) may be part of your HIV treatment regimen. Long-term use of NVP may cause negative side effects, such as exhaustion or weakness; nausea or lack of appetite; yellowing of eyes or skin; or signs of liver toxicity, such as liver tenderness or enlargement or elevated liver enzyme levels. These negative side effects have not been observed with short-term use (one or two doses) of NVP during pregnancy. However, because pregnancy can mimic some of the early symptoms of liver toxicity, your doctor should monitor your condition closely while you are taking NVP. Also, NVP should be used with caution in women who have never received HIV treatment and who have CD4 counts greater than 250 cells/mm^3. Liver toxicity has occurred more frequently in these patients.

Note: Delavirdine (Rescriptor or DLV) and efavirenz (Sustiva or EFV), the two other FDA-approved NNRTIs, are not recommended for the treatment of HIV-positive pregnant women. Use of these medications during pregnancy may lead to birth defects.

Nucleoside reverse transcriptase inhibitors (NRTIs) may cause mitochondrial toxicity, which may lead to a buildup of lactic acid in the blood. This buildup is known as hyperlactatemia or lactic acidosis. This toxicity may be of particular concern for pregnant women and babies exposed to NRTIs in utero.

Protease inhibitors (PIs) are associated with increased levels of blood sugar (hyperglycemia), development of diabetes mellitus or a worsening of diabetes mellitus symptoms, and diabetic ketoacidosis. Pregnancy is also a risk factor for hyperglycemia, but it is not known whether PI use increases the risk for pregnancy-associated hyperglycemia or gestational diabetes.

Note: Enfuvirtide (Fuzeon or T-20) is the only FDA-approved fusion inhibitor; very little is known about use of this drug during pregnancy.

What delivery options are available to me when I give birth?

Depending on your health and treatment status, you may plan to have either a cesarean (also called C-section) or a vaginal delivery. The decision of whether to have a cesarean or a vaginal delivery is something that you should discuss with your doctor during your pregnancy.

How do I decide which delivery option is best for my baby and me?

It is important that you discuss your delivery options with your doctor as early as possible in your pregnancy so that he or she can help you decide which delivery method is most appropriate for you.

Cesarean delivery is recommended for an HIV-positive mother when the following occur:

- her viral load is unknown or is greater than 1,000 copies/ml at 36 weeks of pregnancy

- she has not taken any anti-HIV medications or has only taken AZT (Retrovir, zidovudine, or ZDV) during her pregnancy

- she has not received prenatal care until 36 weeks into her pregnancy or later

To be most effective in preventing transmission, the cesarean should be scheduled at 38 weeks or should be done before the rupture of membranes (also called water breaking).

Vaginal delivery is an option for an HIV-positive mother when the following occur:

- she has been receiving prenatal care throughout her pregnancy

- she has a viral load less than 1,000 copies/ml at 36 weeks, and

- she is taking AZT with or without other anti-HIV medications

Vaginal delivery may also be recommended if a mother has ruptured membranes and labor is progressing rapidly.

What are the risks involved with these delivery options?

All deliveries have risks. The risk of mother-to-child transmission of HIV may be higher for vaginal delivery than for a scheduled cesarean. For the mother, cesarean delivery has an increased risk of infection, anesthesia-related problems, and other risks associated with any type of surgery. For the infant, cesarean delivery has an increased risk of infant respiratory distress.

What else I should know about labor and delivery?

Intravenous (IV) AZT should be started three hours before a scheduled cesarean delivery and should be continued until delivery. Intravenous AZT should be given throughout labor and delivery for a vaginal delivery. It is also important to minimize the baby's exposure to the mother's blood. This can be done by avoiding any invasive monitoring and forceps- or vacuum-assisted delivery.

All babies born to HIV-positive mothers should receive anti-HIV medication to prevent mother-to-child transmission of HIV. The usual treatment for infants is six weeks of AZT; sometimes, additional medications are also given.

I am an HIV-positive pregnant woman, and I am currently on an HIV regimen. Will my regimen change after I give birth?

Many women who are on an HIV treatment regimen during pregnancy decide to stop or change their regimens after they give birth. You and your doctor should discuss your postpartum treatment options during your pregnancy or shortly after delivery. Don't stop taking any of your medications without consulting your doctor first. Stopping HIV treatment could lead to problems.

How will I know if my baby is infected with HIV?

Babies born to HIV-positive mothers are tested for HIV differently than adults. Adults are tested by looking for antibodies to HIV in their blood. A baby keeps antibodies from its mother, including antibodies to HIV, for many months after birth. Therefore, an antibody test given before the baby is one year old may be positive even if the baby does NOT have HIV infection. For the first year, babies are tested for HIV directly, and not by looking for antibodies to HIV. When babies are more than one year old, they no longer have their mother's antibodies and can be tested for HIV using the antibody test.

Preliminary HIV tests for babies are usually performed at three time points:

- within 48 hours of birth

- at one to two months of age

- at three to six months of age

Babies are considered HIV positive if they test positive on two of these preliminary HIV tests.

At 12 months, babies who test positive to the preliminary tests should have an HIV antibody test to confirm infection. Babies who test negative for HIV antibodies at this time are not HIV infected. Babies who test positive for HIV antibodies will need to be retested at 15 to 18 months. A positive HIV antibody test given after 18 months of age confirms HIV infection in children.

Are there any other tests my baby will receive after birth?

Babies born to HIV-positive mothers should have a complete blood count (CBC) after birth. They should also be monitored for signs of anemia, which is the main negative side effect caused by the six-week AZT (also known as Retrovir, zidovudine, or ZDV) regimen infants should take to reduce the risk of HIV infection. They may also undergo other routine blood tests and vaccinations for babies.

Will my baby receive anti-HIV medication?

It is recommended that all babies born to HIV-positive mothers receive a six-week course of oral AZT to help prevent mother-to-child transmission of HIV. This oral AZT regimen should begin within six to twelve hours after your baby is born. Some doctors may recommend that AZT be given in combination with other anti-HIV medications. You and your doctor should discuss the options to decide which treatment is best for your baby.

In addition to HIV treatment, your baby should also receive treatment to prevent *Pneumocystis carinii/jiroveci* pneumonia (PCP). The recommended treatment is a combination of the medications sulfamethoxazole and trimethoprim. This treatment should be started when your baby is four to six weeks old and should continue until your baby is confirmed to be HIV negative. If your baby is HIV positive, he or she will need to take this treatment indefinitely.

What type of medical follow-up should I consider for my baby and me after I give birth?

Seeking the right medical and supportive care services is important for your and your baby's health. These services may include the following:

- routine medical care
- HIV specialty care
- family planning services
- mental health services
- substance abuse treatment
- case management

Talk to your doctor about these services and any others you may need. He or she should be able to help you locate appropriate resources.

What else should I think about after I give birth?

The CDC recommends that in areas where safe drinking water and infant formula are available (such as the United States), women should not breastfeed in order to avoid transmission of HIV to their infants through breast milk.

Physical and emotional changes during the postpartum period, along with the stresses and demands of caring for a new baby, can make it difficult to follow your HIV treatment regimen. Adherence to your regimen is important for you to stay healthy. Other issues you may want to discuss with your doctor include the following:

- concerns you may have about your regimen and treatment adherence

- feelings of depression (many women have these feelings after giving birth)

- long-term plans for continuing medical care and HIV treatment for you and your baby

If you are interested in joining a pregnancy registry that monitors HIV-positive women during their pregnancies and after giving birth, please visit the Food and Drug Administration's Guide to Pregnancy Registries at http://www.fda.gov/womens/registries. Researchers are especially interested in learning more about the effects of anti-HIV drugs during pregnancy. HIV-positive pregnant women are therefore encouraged to register with the Antiretroviral Pregnancy Registry at http://www.APRegistry.com.

For more information, contact your doctor or an AIDSinfo Health Information Specialist at 800-448-0440 or http://aidsinfo.nih.gov.

Chapter 49

Prevention of Mother-to-Child Transmission of HIV

Chapter Contents

Section 49.1

Reducing Mother-to-Child Transmission of HIV

"Mother-to-Child (Perinatal) HIV Transmission and Prevention," Centers for Disease Control and Prevention (CDC), March 8, 2007. References and examples of prevention programs are available online at http://www.cdc.gov/hiv/resources/factsheets/perinatl.htm.

HIV transmission from mother to child during pregnancy, labor, delivery, or breastfeeding is called perinatal transmission. Research published in 1994 showed that zidovudine (ZDV) given to pregnant HIV-infected women reduced this type of HIV transmission. Since then, the testing of pregnant women and treatment for those who are infected have resulted in a dramatic decline in the number of children perinatally infected with HIV.

Perinatal HIV transmission is the most common route of HIV infection in children and is now the source of almost all AIDS cases in children in the United States. Most of the children with AIDS are members of minority races/ethnicities.

Statistics

HIV/AIDS in 2004

The following are based on data from the 35 areas with long-term, confidential name-based HIV reporting.

- HIV/AIDS was diagnosed for an estimated 145 children who had been infected with HIV perinatally.

- Approximately 6,100 persons who had been infected with HIV perinatally were living with HIV/AIDS at the end of 2004.

- Of the perinatally infected persons living with HIV/AIDS, 66 percent were African American.

AIDS in 2004

- Of the 48 children for whom AIDS was diagnosed during 2004, 47 had been infected with HIV perinatally.

- An estimated 57 persons with AIDS who died had been infected with HIV perinatally.

- Since the beginning of the epidemic, AIDS had been diagnosed for an estimated 8,779 children who had been infected perinatally. Of those, an estimated 4,982 had died.

- Over the course of the epidemic, the number of perinatally transmitted AIDS cases has decreased dramatically. The number of infants infected with HIV through mother-to-child transmission decreased from an estimated peak of 1,750 HIV-infected infants born each year during the early to mid-1990s to 280–370 infants in 2000 (CDC, unpublished data, 2000). This decrease is largely due to the use of antiretroviral therapy during pregnancy and labor.

Risk Factors and Barriers to Prevention

Lack of Awareness of HIV Serostatus

The main risk factor, which is also a barrier to the prevention of mother-to-child HIV transmission, is lack of awareness of HIV serostatus.

Of the estimated 120,000 to 160,000 HIV-infected women in the United States, 80 percent are of childbearing age. Because approximately 25 percent of all people infected with HIV do not know their HIV status, many of these women may not know they are infected.

Without antiretroviral therapy, approximately 25 percent of pregnant HIV-infected women will transmit the virus to their child.

Sexual Contact with HIV-Infected Men

The risk factors for women have changed. Earlier in the epidemic, more women were exposed to HIV through injection drug use. During the 1990s, women's exposure through sexual contact with HIV-infected men played a larger role in HIV infection than did injection drug use. This is why women should know their own, and their partners', HIV serostatus and risk factors.

Uneven HIV Testing Rates

Recent CDC studies found that HIV testing rates for pregnant women varied widely and that a relatively high proportion of women of childbearing age were unaware that treatment is available to reduce the risk of perinatal transmission. However, in a 2002 study of HIV testing in the United States, 69 percent of the 748 women who had recently been pregnant reported that they had been tested during prenatal care.

Because of prenatal testing, most HIV-infected women know they are infected before they give birth. Still, testing rates in the United States remain uneven: 18 percent of the women in another study were not tested until after childbirth.

State HIV testing rates differ, depending on the testing approach used. For example, rates for states using the opt-in approach (women are provided pretest counseling and must specifically consent to an HIV test) ranged from 25 percent to 69 percent The opt-out approach (women are told that an HIV test will be included in the standard group of prenatal tests but that they may decline testing) results in higher testing rates. CDC recommends the opt-out approach, but in many prenatal settings, it has not been implemented. CDC is working with state public health departments and national organizations to increase the rates of HIV testing among pregnant women.

Prevention

The annual number of new HIV infections in the United States has declined from a peak of more than 150,000 during the mid-1980s and has stabilized at approximately 40,000 since the late 1990s. Persons of minority races/ethnicities are disproportionately affected by the HIV epidemic. To reduce further the incidence of HIV, CDC announced a new initiative, Advancing HIV Prevention (AHP), in 2003. This initiative comprises four strategies: making HIV testing a routine part of medical care, implementing new models for diagnosing HIV infections outside medical settings, preventing new infections by working with HIV-infected persons and their partners, and further decreasing perinatal HIV transmission.

With regard to perinatal HIV transmission, AHP recommends the routine voluntary testing of all pregnant women to further reduce the number of children who are infected. In addition, voluntary rapid HIV testing, which has been shown to be feasible and accurate, should be offered to women in labor whose HIV serostatus is unknown.

AHP builds on the widespread success of the U.S. Public Health Service recommendations for the HIV counseling and testing of pregnant women and for the use of antiretroviral therapy during pregnancy.

Already, perinatal HIV prevention has saved lives and resources.

- The number of children with a diagnosis of AIDS who had been perinatally exposed to HIV declined from 122 in 2000 to 47 in 2004.

- Antiretroviral therapy administered during pregnancy, labor, and delivery and then to the newborn, as well as elective cesarean section for women with high viral loads (more than 1,000 copies/ml), can reduce the rate of perinatal HIV transmission to 2 percent or less. If medications are started during labor, decreased rate of perinatal transmission can still be achieved (less than 10 percent).

- The estimated annual cost of perinatal HIV prevention in the United States is $67.6 million. This investment prevents 656 HIV infections and saves $105.6 million in medical care costs alone—a net savings of $38.1 million annually.

CDC funds 15 state and local health departments to conduct perinatal HIV prevention programs.

Section 49.2

Mother-to-Child Transmission Programs to Prevent HIV Worldwide

"Prevention of Mother-to-Child Transmission of HIV," U.S. Agency for International Development (http://www.usaid.gov), July 2005.

One of the tragic consequences of the HIV/AIDS pandemic is mother-to-child transmission (MTCT) of HIV. Transmission of the virus can occur during pregnancy, at the time of delivery, or through breastfeeding. Approximately 630,000 babies became infected with HIV in 2004 and Africa bears 90 percent of this burden. Worldwide, more than 4 million children are estimated to have died from AIDS, primarily contracted through MTCT.

The best way to avoid MTCT is to prevent HIV infection among women of reproductive age. However, for the close to 20 million women already infected, the U.S. Agency for International Development is committed to helping reduce the likelihood of transmitting the virus to their infants.

USAID has been working to prevent MTCT since 1999. These programs expanded significantly with the announcement of President Bush's International Mother and Child HIV Prevention Initiative in June of 2002. The primary objectives of this plan are expanding voluntary HIV counseling and testing for pregnant women, administering single dose antiretroviral drugs to mother and infant, supporting safe infant feeding options, and starting women and their spouses on full antiretroviral therapy, where capacity of health care systems allow.

Six months after the announcement of this initiative, President Bush reinforced his dedication to combating global HIV/AIDS with the President's Emergency Plan for AIDS Relief. The Emergency Plan aims to support treatment for at least 2 million people living with HIV/AIDS, prevent 7 million new infections, and support care for 10 million people infected with and affected by HIV, including orphans and vulnerable children.

What are USAID's primary MTCT interventions?

Improvement of antenatal services: USAID-supported sites are improving antenatal services—including voluntary counseling and testing—by training health workers and counselors, upgrading medical facilities, and providing HIV test kits. Community outreach workers are integral to reaching women and their families in areas underserved by traditional medical facilities.

Short-course antiretroviral prophylaxis for HIV-infected pregnant women: USAID currently funds the provision of antiretroviral drugs to reduce mother-to-child transmission, which studies have shown can reduce infection rates in newborn babies by 20 to 50 percent.

Support for safe infant feeding practices: Safe infant feeding is one of the most complex aspects of MTCT prevention. In most developing countries, the majority of women do not know their HIV status and safe, affordable, and culturally acceptable alternatives to breastfeeding are limited. USAID funded MTCT programs provide HIV-positive women with information and support to help them make informed decisions about how to feed their babies.

Strengthening health, family planning, and safe motherhood programs: Over the past 20 years USAID family planning programs have strengthened health systems to support safe motherhood. This includes improving obstetrical practices in order to reduce MTCT during delivery. Additionally, health counseling and safe, effective contraception can help women practice safer sex and prevent unintended pregnancies, potentially reducing the number of HIV-infected children.

What is MTCT plus?

Existing MTCT programs may provide a good foundation for the wider introduction of care and treatment. MTCT Plus programs strive to expand focus from the health of the infant to also include mother, father, and siblings—thereby maintaining the family unit. This approach is advantageous because clients are already identified and at least a basic level of health care infrastructure exists. MTCT Plus programs should include nutritional, medical, and psychosocial support as well as antiretroviral therapy for mothers and family members, where clinically appropriate.

USAID has programs to prevent mother-to-child transmission of HIV in 26 countries in every region of the world: Bolivia, Cambodia, Democratic Republic of the Congo, El Salvador, Eritrea, Ethiopia, Ghana, Guinea, Guyana, Haiti, Indonesia, Kenya, Malawi, Mozambique, Namibia, Nigeria, Peru, Rwanda, Senegal, South Africa, Tanzania, Russia, Uganda, Ukraine, Zambia, and Zimbabwe.

Section 49.3

Pasteurizing Breast Milk May Prevent HIV Transmission

"Pasteurizing Breast Milk May Prevent HIV Transmission," Voice of America (http://www.voanews.com), November 20, 2006.

Every day, thousands of infants in the developing world are infected with HIV. Many get the virus that causes AIDS through breastfeeding from their HIV-positive mothers. Now some researchers think they may be able to prevent some of that transmission by having mothers pasteurize their breast milk.

According to researcher Kiersten Israel-Ballard, "We have found that [the technique] is able to kill HIV." She explains that HIV can come in two forms, one that is attached to the cell and one that is cell-free. "We've been able to show that this method can kill the cell-free HIV. We're still working on proving that the other form is destroyed, although that seems very promising."

Israel-Ballard says data show that most of the good things in breast milk, such as antibodies, proteins, and vitamins, are preserved in the process, which she calls "flash pasteurization." She says women can do it at home with simple tools. "It involves the mother expressing her milk into a glass jar and then putting it into a pan that is full of water and she brings that to a boil. So when the water boils, she removes the milk and the milk has actually been flash pasteurized."

Working with a joint team from the University of California at Davis and at Berkeley, Israel-Ballard surveyed women in several African countries. She reports they overwhelmingly told her they'd be willing to perform the extra steps to keep their children from becoming infected.

"In developing countries ... most of the transmission happens from breastfeeding," the researcher points out, adding, "We need to really focus on safe ways that these babies can eat. They need breast milk in these countries because breast milk is protective. It prevents them from getting sick and dying from diarrheal diseases, respiratory illnesses. These babies die from these things. They don't only die from HIV."

Israel-Ballard says her team will look at doing a full trial of the method in several African countries in the near future. She was in Boston, Massachusetts, this month [November 2006] at the American Public Health Association annual meeting.

—by Rose Hoban

Section 49.4

Breast Milk Banks Offer Options for New Mothers with HIV

"Human Milk Banks," National Women's Health Information Center (NWHIC), Office on Women's Health, U.S. Department of Health and Human Services, October 2005. Further reading and resources are available online at http://www.4woman.gov/breastfeeding/index.cfm?page=359.

Ideally, breast milk comes from a baby's own mother. But when this is not possible, you can give your baby breast milk from donors (other women's breast milk), which provides the same precious nutrition and disease fighting properties as your own breast milk. If your baby has special needs, such as intolerance to formula, severe allergies, is failing to thrive on formula, is premature or has other health problems, he or she may need donated human milk not only for health, but also for survival.

There are several reasons why a mother may not be able to breastfeed her own baby:

- In a premature delivery, a mother's milk supply may not become established enough to provide milk for her baby. Sometimes the stress of caring for a very ill infant prevents the milk supply from developing.

- A mother who delivers twins or triplets might not have enough milk supply to nourish all of the babies.

- Some medicines taken by the mother for a health problem, such as chemotherapy for cancer, can harm a baby.

- A mother might have an infection that could be spread to her baby through breastfeeding, such as HIV or hepatitis.

- A mother might have a health problem that prevents her from breastfeeding or makes it impossible for her to produce milk.

Breast milk from donors is stored in human milk banks. At this time, there are only six human milk banks in the United States. While the number of infants and children who depend upon donor milk for health or survival is small, their numbers are greater than is the supply available from these milk banks.

Human milk banks screen the donors, and collect, screen, process, and dispense donor human milk. Because babies who use donor milk are not related to the donors, every possible step is taken to ensure the milk is safe. And the milk is only dispensed by a prescription from your health care provider. The prescription must show how many ounces of processed milk are needed per day, and for how many weeks or months. The milk bank also needs your name, the baby's name, and your address and phone number. Then, you or your health care provider can contact a milk bank to order the milk. If the milk bank is close to you, you can pick up the milk there. If you live out of the area, the milk bank can ship the frozen milk in coolers every few days.

The cost of donor milk is about $3 per ounce. Sometimes there is another fee for shipping. Most health insurance companies cover the cost of donor milk if it is medically necessary. To find out if your insurance will cover the cost of the milk, call your insurance company or ask your health care provider. If your insurance company does not cover the cost of the milk, talk with the milk bank to find out how payment can be made later on, or how to get help with the payments. A milk bank will never deny donor milk to a baby in need.

Chapter 50

HIV Infection in Infants and Children

The National Institute of Allergy and Infectious Diseases (NIAID) has a lead role in research devoted to children infected with HIV (human immunodeficiency virus), the virus that causes AIDS (acquired immunodeficiency syndrome). NIAID-supported researchers are developing and refining treatments to prolong the survival and improve the quality of life of HIV-infected infants and children through the Pediatric AIDS Clinical Trials Group (PACTG). The PACTG is a nationwide clinical trials network jointly sponsored by NIAID and the National Institute of Child Health and Human Development (NICHD). NIAID also supports research on ways to prevent mother-to-child transmission (MTCT) of HIV through the PACTG and its HIV Prevention Trials Network (HPTN), a global clinical trials network designed to test promising non-vaccine strategies to prevent the spread of HIV/AIDS.

In this era of antiretroviral therapy, epidemiologic studies such as NIAID's Women and Infant's Transmission Study (WITS) are examining risk factors for transmission as well as the course of HIV disease in pregnant women and their babies. Researchers have helped illuminate the mechanisms of HIV transmission, the distinct features of pediatric HIV infection, and how the course of disease and the usefulness of therapies can differ in children and adults.

"HIV Infection in Infants and Children: NIAID Fact Sheet," National Institute of Allergy and Infectious Diseases (http://www.niaid.nih.gov), a component of the National Institutes of Health (NIH), updated July 16, 2004.

A Global Problem

According to UNAIDS (The Joint United Nations Programme on HIV/AIDS) at the end of 2003, an estimated 2.5 million children worldwide under age 15 were living with HIV/AIDS. Approximately 500,000 children under 15 had died from the virus or associated causes in that year alone. As HIV infection rates rise in the general population, new infections are increasingly concentrating in younger age groups.

December 2003 UNAIDS/World Health Organization (WHO) worldwide statistics show the following:

- Children under age 15 who were newly infected with HIV—700,000.

- Thirteen percent of all new HIV infections were in children under age 15.

- Three million children in sub-Saharan Africa, the region with the highest number of cases, are living with HIV.

More than 95 percent of all HIV-infected people now live in developing countries, which have also suffered 95 percent of all deaths from AIDS. In those countries with the highest prevalence, UNAIDS predicts that, between 2000 and 2020, 68 million people will die prematurely as a result of AIDS. In seven sub-Saharan African countries, mortality due to HIV/AIDS in children under age five has increased by 20 to 40 percent. Life expectancy for a child born in Botswana, the country with the highest HIV prevalence in the world, has dropped below 40 years—a level not seen in that country since before 1950.

The United States has a relatively small percentage of the world's children living with HIV/AIDS. From the beginning of the epidemic through the end of 2002, 9,300 American children under age 13 had been reported to the Centers for Disease Control and Prevention (CDC) as living with HIV/AIDS. The vast majority of HIV-infected children acquire the virus from their mothers before or during birth or through breastfeeding. Because of the widespread use of AZT and other highly active antiretroviral therapy (HAART) in HIV-infected pregnant women in the United States, only 92 new cases of pediatric AIDS were reported in 2002. More than three times that number are infected with HIV but have not yet developed AIDS.

- The U.S. city with the highest rate of pediatric AIDS through 2002 was New York City, followed by Miami, FL, and Washington, DC.

- The disease disproportionately affects children in minority groups, especially African Americans. Out of 9,300 cases in children under 13 reported to the CDC through December 2002, 59 percent were black/non-Hispanic, 23 percent were Hispanic, 17 percent were white/non-Hispanic, and less than 1 percent were in other minority groups.

New anti-HIV drug therapies and promotion of voluntary testing continue to positively affect the death rate. CDC reported a drop of 68 percent from 1998 to 2002 in the estimated number of children who died from AIDS.

Transmission

Almost all HIV-infected children acquire the virus from their mothers before or during birth or through breastfeeding. In the United States, approximately 25 percent of pregnant HIV-infected women not receiving AZT therapy have passed on the virus to their babies. The rate is significantly higher in developing countries.

Prior to 1985 when screening of the nation's blood supply for HIV began, some children as well as adults were infected through transfusions with blood or blood products contaminated with HIV. A small number of children also have been infected through sexual or physical abuse by HIV-infected adults.

Pregnancy and Birth

Most MTCT, estimated to cause more than 90 percent of infections worldwide in infants and children, probably occurs late in pregnancy or during birth. Although the precise mechanisms are unknown, scientists think HIV may be transmitted when maternal blood enters the fetal circulation or by mucosal exposure to virus during labor and delivery. The role of the placenta in maternal-fetal transmission is unclear and the focus of ongoing research.

The risk of MTCT is significantly increased if the mother has advanced HIV disease, increased levels of HIV in her bloodstream, or fewer numbers of the immune system cells—CD4+ T cells—that are the main targets of HIV.

Other factors that may increase the risk are maternal drug use, severe inflammation of fetal membranes, or a prolonged period between membrane rupture and delivery. A study sponsored by NIAID and others found that HIV-infected women who gave birth more than four hours after the rupture of the fetal membranes were nearly twice as likely to transmit HIV to their infants, as compared to women who delivered within four hours of membrane rupture.

Breastfeeding

HIV also may be transmitted from a nursing mother to her infant. Studies have suggested that breastfeeding introduces an additional risk of HIV transmission of approximately 10 to 14 percent among women with chronic HIV infection. In developing countries, an estimated one-third to one-half of all HIV infections are transmitted through breastfeeding.

WHO recommends that all HIV-infected women be advised about both the risks and benefits of breastfeeding for their infants so they can make informed decisions. In countries where safe alternatives to breastfeeding are readily available and economically feasible, this alternative should be encouraged. In general, in developing countries where safe alternatives to breastfeeding are not readily available, the benefits of breastfeeding in terms of decreased illness and death due to other infectious diseases greatly outweigh the potential risk of HIV transmission.

Preventing Mother-to-Child Transmission

In 1994, a landmark study conducted by the PACTG demonstrated that AZT, given to HIV-infected women who had very little or no prior antiretroviral therapy and CD4+ T-cell counts above 200/mm^3, reduced the risk of MTCT by two-thirds, from 25 percent to 8 percent. In the study, AZT therapy was initiated in the second or third trimester and continued during labor, and infants were treated for six weeks following birth. AZT produced no serious side effects in mothers or infants. Long-term follow up of the infants and mothers is ongoing.

A few years later, another PACTG study found that the risk of transmitting HIV from an HIV-positive mother to her newborn infant could be reduced to 1.5 percent in those women who received antiretroviral treatment and appropriate medical and obstetrical care during pregnancy.

Combination therapies have been shown to be beneficial in treating HIV-infected adults, and current guidelines have been designed accordingly. In HIV-infected pregnant women, the safety and pharmacology of these potent drug combinations need to be better understood, and NIAID is conducting studies in this area.

The AZT regimen is not available in much of the world because of its high cost and logistical requirements. The cost of a short-course

AZT regimen is substantially lower, but is still prohibitive in many countries. International agencies are studying whether there may be innovative ways to provide AZT at lower cost, for example, through reductions in drug prices to developing countries or partnerships with industry. As a result, NIAID continues to evaluate other strategies that may be simpler and less costly to prevent MTCT in various settings. In September 1999, one such study demonstrated that short-course therapy with nevirapine lowered the risk of HIV-1 transmission during the first 14 to 16 weeks of life by nearly 50 percent compared to AZT in a breastfeeding population. As a follow up, NIAID released a final report on additional data showing that the results of nevirapine were sustained after 18 months. These findings have significant implications because this simple, inexpensive regimen offers a potential cost-effective alternative for decreasing MTCT in developing countries.

In addition, in April 1999 the International Perinatal HIV Group reported that elective cesarean section delivery can help reduce vertical transmission of HIV, though it is not without risk to certain women. When AZT treatment is combined with elective caesarian delivery, a transmission rate of 2 percent has been reported.

Because a significant amount of MTCT occurs around the time of birth, and the risk of maternal-fetal transmission depends, in part, on the amount of HIV in the mother's blood, it may be possible to reduce transmission using drug therapy only around the time of birth. NIAID has planned other studies that will assess the effectiveness of this approach as well as the role of new antiretrovirals, microbicides, and other innovative strategies in reducing the risk of MTCT of HIV.

Diagnosis

HIV infection is often difficult to diagnose in very young children. Infected babies, especially in the first few months of life, often appear normal and may show no telltale signs allowing for a definitive diagnosis of HIV infection. Moreover, all children born to infected mothers have antibodies to HIV, made by the mother's immune system, that cross the placenta to the baby's bloodstream before birth and persist for up to 18 months. Because these maternal antibodies reflect the mother's but not the infant's infection status, the test for HIV infection is not useful in newborns or young infants.

In recent years, investigators have demonstrated the utility of highly accurate blood tests in diagnosing HIV infection in children six months of age and younger. One laboratory technique, called polymerase chain reaction (PCR), can detect minute quantities of the virus in an infant's blood. Another procedure allows physicians to culture a sample of an infant's blood and test it for the presence of HIV.

Currently, PCR assays or HIV culture techniques can identify at birth about one-third of infants who finally and ultimately prove to be HIV infected. With these techniques, approximately 90 percent of HIV-infected infants are identifiable by two months of age, and 95 percent by three months of age. One innovative new approach to both RNA and DNA PCR testing uses dried blood spot specimens, which should make it much simpler to gather and store specimens in field settings.

Progression of HIV Disease in Children

Researchers have observed two general patterns of illness in HIV-infected children. About 20 percent of children develop serious disease in the first year of life; most of these children die by age four. The remaining 80 percent of infected children have a slower rate of disease progression, many not developing the most serious symptoms of AIDS until school entry or even adolescence. A report from a large European registry of HIV-infected children indicated that half of the children with perinatally acquired HIV disease were alive at age nine. Another study of 42 perinatally HIV-infected children, who survived beyond nine years of age, found about one-quarter of the children to be asymptomatic with relatively intact immune systems.

The factors responsible for the wide variation observed in the rate of disease progression in HIV-infected children are a major focus of the NIAID pediatric AIDS research effort. WITS is a multi-site perinatal HIV study. It has found that maternal factors, including vitamin A level and CD4+ T-cell counts during pregnancy, as well as infant viral load and CD4+ T-cell counts in the first several months of life, can help identify those infants at risk for rapid disease progression who may benefit from early aggressive therapy.

Signs and Symptoms

Many children with HIV infection do not gain weight or grow normally. HIV-infected children frequently are slow to reach important milestones in motor skills and mental development such as crawling, walking, and talking. As the disease progresses, many children develop neurologic problems and other symptoms of HIV encephalopathy (a brain disorder).

Like adults with HIV infection, children with HIV develop life-threatening opportunistic infections (OIs), although the incidence of various OIs differs in adults and children.

- Toxoplasmosis (a parasitic disease) is seen less frequently in HIV-infected children than in HIV-infected adults, while serious bacterial infections occur more commonly in children than in adults.

- *Pneumocystis carinii/jiroveci* pneumonia (PCP) is the leading cause of death in HIV-infected children with AIDS. PCP, as well as cytomegalovirus (CMV) disease, usually are primary infections in children, whereas in adults these diseases result from the reactivation of latent infections.

- A lung disease called lymphocytic interstitial pneumonitis (LIP), rarely seen in adults, occurs more frequently in HIV-infected children. This condition, like PCP, can make breathing progressively more difficult and often results in hospitalization.

- Severe candidiasis, a yeast infection that can cause unrelenting diaper rash and infections in the mouth and throat that make eating difficult, is found frequently in HIV-infected children.

- As children with HIV become sicker, they may suffer from chronic diarrhea due to opportunistic pathogens.

Children with HIV suffer the usual childhood infections more frequently and more severely than uninfected children. These infections can cause seizures, fever, pneumonia, recurrent colds, diarrhea, dehydration, and other problems that often result in extended hospital stays and nutritional problems.

Treatment

While the basic principles that guide treatment of pediatric HIV infection are the same as for an HIV-infected adult, there are a number of unique scientific and medical concerns that are important to consider in treating children with HIV infection. These range from differences in age-related issues such as CD4+ T-cell counts and drug metabolism to requirements for special formulations and treatment regimens that are appropriate for infants through adolescents. As in adults, treating HIV-infected children today is a complex task of using potent combinations of antiretroviral agents to maximally suppress viral replication. NIAID investigators are defining the best treatments for pediatric patients.

NIAID-supported researchers are focusing not only on the development of new antiretroviral products but also on the critical question of how to best use the treatments that are currently available, especially in resource-poor nations. Treatment strategy questions should be designed to identify, for example, the best initial therapy, when failing regimens should be modified, and strategies to address the antiretroviral needs of children with advanced disease. Another high priority is the long-term assessment of these strategies to determine sustained antiretroviral benefits as well as to monitor for potential adverse consequences of treatment. Current guidelines for the use of antiretroviral agents in pediatric HIV infection is available at http://www.aidsinfo.nih.gov/guidelines.

Problems in Families

A mother and child with HIV usually are not the only family members with the disease. Often, the mother's sexual partner is infected, and other children in the family may be infected as well. Frequently, a parent with AIDS does not survive to care for his or her HIV-infected child.

In the countries hardest hit by the AIDS epidemic, some 14 million children under 15 around the world have been orphaned by AIDS—80 percent of them (11 million) in sub-Saharan Africa alone. The rate is expected to increase. One in three of these orphans is under age five. Communities and extended families are struggling with and often overwhelmed by the vast number of children orphaned by AIDS. Many orphans and other children from families devastated by AIDS face multiple risks, such as forced relocation, violence, living on the streets, drug use, and even commercial sex. Other children suffer because sexuality education and services are not available to them or not effectively communicated to them. Living in a country undergoing political turmoil or can also raise the risk of a child becoming HIV-infected.

In the United States, most children living with HIV/AIDS live in inner cities, where poverty, illicit drug use, poor housing, and limited access to and use of medical care and social services add to the challenges of HIV disease.

One encouraging note is, according to UNAIDS, that where information, training, and services to help prevent HIV infection are made available and affordable, young people are more likely to make use of them than their elders.

Management of the complex medical and social problems of families affected by HIV requires a multidisciplinary case management team, integrating medical, social, mental health, and educational services. NIAID provides special funding to many of its clinical research sites to provide for services, such as transportation, day care, and the expertise of social workers, crucial to families devastated by HIV.

Chapter 51

Pediatric AIDS

Chapter Contents

Section 51.1

AIDS in Children:
Symptoms, Diagnosis, and Treatment

Symptoms in Children

HIV-infected children get sick frequently and severely. When a child's number of CD4 cells is low, the immune system does not work as it should. HIV-infected children can get the same infections as uninfected children. Because a child with HIV has a weakened immune system, these infections can be more frequent, more severe, and harder to cure. Examples of common infections include infections of the ears, sinuses, lungs (pneumonia), blood (sepsis), urinary tract, bladder, intestines, and skin, as well as fluid around the brain (meningitis). HIV-infected children can also demonstrate swollen glands, breathing problems, fever, poor weight gain, and slow development.

If the immune system is weakened beyond a certain point, children may also get infected with germs that would not cause disease in children with normal immune systems, or they may get sicker and have more extensive illness. They may develop opportunistic infections such as: *Pneumocystis carinii* [also called *jiroveci*] pneumonia (PCP), Candida (thrush), herpes simplex (HSV), *Mycobacterium avium* complex (MAC), *Cryptosporidium*, Cytomegalovirus, Cryptococcus, toxoplasmosis, herpes zoster, or chickenpox (which is much worse in children with HIV).

In addition, tuberculosis, diarrhea, and respiratory illnesses are more frequent in children living with HIV in developing countries.

Diagnosis

ELISA Test

There are different ways to diagnose HIV, depending on the age of the person. When HIV gets into the body, the immune system makes a substance called an HIV antibody. HIV infection can be detected by an HIV antibody test, which is used for children over 12 to 18 months of age, adolescents, and adults in the U.S. This antibody test is called an enzyme-linked immunosorbent assay (ELISA)—a laboratory test used to detect the presence of antibodies in the blood. The ELISA is used to screen for HIV infection and a positive result indicates antibodies are present.

False Positive

After the ELISA test, a second or confirmatory test is necessary to rule out a "false-positive" test. The second test may be another ELISA, a rapid test (third generation ELISA), or a Western blot. A rapid HIV test is also an antibody test. The advantage of a rapid test is patients do not have to return at another time to get their test results—the results are usually available in approximately 30 minutes. Rapid tests are single-use and do not require laboratory facilities or highly trained staff, which makes them particularly suitable for use in developing countries.

The amount of time it takes for a person to develop antibodies after becoming infected with HIV varies. The majority of people with HIV will produce antibodies by about 45 days after infection. In a small proportion of people, it may take up to six months for antibodies to develop, and it may take even longer for a very few people. This is one reason why a lack of HIV antibodies does not always mean a person is free from infection, and repeat testing may be necessary.

Confirmed Positive

A confirmed positive test indicates a person has been infected with HIV. It is important to bear in mind that the HIV antibody test is not an "AIDS test"; there is no such thing.

Babies born to women infected with HIV will test positive for the HIV antibody at birth. This is because the mother's antibody to HIV is passed to the baby in the womb. These babies are considered to be HIV-exposed. A newborn with HIV antibodies is not necessarily infected with HIV.

Other Tests

There are also tests that can look for the virus itself or parts of the virus (antigen testing and RNA viral load testing), damage to the immune system, or other aspects of the body's response to the effects of the virus. The best way to diagnose HIV infection in an infant younger than 12 to 18 months is to look for the virus itself in the infant's blood. The most common test in the U.S. is HIV DNA PCR (polymerase chain reaction), which looks for the DNA (genetic material) of the virus. PCR can identify the virus in more than 90 percent of infants infected before birth and during delivery by the time they are one month of age, and in almost all infants infected before or during delivery by the time they are three to six months of age.

Testing has been shown to be part of an effective means of preventing HIV transmission. People who are aware of their HIV status are in a position to gain access to treatment, counseling, and education to prevent further transmission.

Treatment

The goals of HIV treatment include the following:

- decreasing the amount of HIV in the blood or controlling the virus itself so it cannot destroy the immune system

- preventing the infections resulting from a weakened immune system caused by HIV, and

- treating the problems caused by HIV

There is no cure. Currently, there is no treatment that cures HIV infection, but drugs are available to help decrease and control the virus. Antiretroviral therapy (ART) can keep HIV from replicating (making copies of itself) and causing more damage to the immune system; however, it does not cure HIV or AIDS.

In the developing world, antiretrovirals are not available to the majority of infected persons. But the tide is beginning to change and treatments are becoming available to HIV-infected children and their families.

Formulations to facilitate pediatric dosing of ART are lacking. There are no fixed-dosed combinations (FDCs) of triple therapy (a combination of three antiretroviral drugs) for children. Liquid medication is more expensive than adult pills, is bulky and costly, and may require refrigeration. But pediatric doses require the flexibility to give the right amount of medication based on weight. Formulations that can be administered safely, in appropriate doses for children, are greatly needed.

Section 51.2

Oral Generic AIDS Drug Offers Hope for Pediatric Patients with HIV

"FDA Tentatively Approves a Generic AIDS Drug in Association with the President's Emergency Plan for AIDS Relief," U.S. Food and Drug Administration (http://www.fda.gov), December 21, 2005.

The Food and Drug Administration (FDA) today [December 21, 2005] announced the tentative approval of Stavudine (stav' yoo deen) for Oral Solution, 1 mg/ml to be manufactured by Aurobindo Pharma LTD. of Hyderabad, India. This product is the first generic version of the already approved Zerit for oral solution manufactured by Bristol-Myers Squibb. This child-friendly product is indicated for use in pediatric patients with HIV, from birth through adolescence. This product will now be available for consideration for purchase under the President's Emergency Plan for AIDS Relief (PEPFAR).

"All patients who depend on FDA-approved medicines are of great importance for our agency, but none more so than infants and children," said Dr. Murray Lumpkin, the FDA Deputy Commissioner for International and Special Programs. "We take deep satisfaction in approving products that can bring much-needed relief to children infected with HIV."

The Emergency Plan for AIDS Relief, which President Bush first announced in his 2003 State of the Union Address, is currently providing $15 billion to fight the HIV/AIDS pandemic over five years, with a special focus on 15 of the hardest hit countries. The president's plan is designed to prevent 7 million new HIV infections, treat at least 2 million HIV-infected people, and care for 10 million HIV-affected individuals, AIDS orphans and vulnerable children. It targets three specific areas related to HIV/AIDS:

- prevention of HIV transmission
- treatment of AIDS and associated conditions
- care, including palliative care for HIV infected-individuals, and care for orphans and vulnerable children

In support of the president's plan, the Office of Generic Drugs (OGD), within the FDA's Center for Drug Evaluation and Research (CDER), has approved or tentatively approved over a dozen applications for a number of products to treat HIV/AIDS through an innovative product development and expedited application review process. FDA staff, including members of CDER's OGD, Division of Antiviral Drug Products, and FDA's Office of Regulatory Affairs developed a focused, interactive approach to the product development and application review process to diligently resolve any issues that would delay the submission of and the completion of the review of a quality marketing application. The success of this process has been demonstrated by the number of quality, safe and effective generic products available for consideration for purchase by the president's plan.

"We are very pleased to be able to make this important pediatric formulation of Stavudine available to the patients being helped by President Bush's Emergency Plan for AIDS Relief," said Gary J. Buehler, Director of CDER's Office of Generic Drugs. "FDA's action on this application adds another critical product to the arsenal of drugs available for the global fight against HIV/AIDS."

Stavudine (d4T) is active against the human immunodeficiency virus (HIV) that causes AIDS. It is in the class of drugs called nucleoside reverse transcriptase inhibitors (NRTIs), which help keep the AIDS virus from reproducing. This antiretroviral drug is used in combination with other antiretroviral agents for the treatment of HIV-1 infection.

The agency's tentative approval means that although existing patents and/or exclusivity prevent marketing of this product in the United States, it meets all of FDA's manufacturing quality and clinical safety and efficacy standards required for marketing in the United States. As with all generic applications before granting approval or tentative approval, FDA conducts an on-site inspection of each manufacturing facility and the facilities performing the bioequivalence studies. The inspection assesses the ability of the manufacturer to produce a quality product, and the quality of the bioequivalence data supporting the application.

More information on HIV and AIDS is available online at FDA's website: http://www.fda.gov/oashi/aids/hiv.html.

Section 51.3

HIV Treatment May Help Reduce Severity of Mental Impairment in Children with HIV Infection

National Institute of Mental Health (http://www.nimh.nih.gov),
National Institutes of Health (NIH), March 3, 2007.

During the first few years of life, children born with HIV infection are most susceptible to central nervous system (CNS) disease, and can develop impaired cognitive, language, motor, and behavioral functioning. However, National Institutes of Health (NIH)-funded researchers have found that among children with HIV infection, treatment with a protease inhibitor-(PI) based highly active antiretroviral therapy (HAART) helped protect against cognitive and motor difficulties compared to a control group of age-matched children who were born to HIV-infected mothers but who did not contract the virus themselves (e.g., HIV-exposed).

The findings are part of the large-scale, longitudinal study conducted within the Pediatric AIDS Clinical Trials Group (PACTG) Network and are published in the March 2007 issue of *Pediatrics*. This particular protocol within PACTG is designed to follow HIV-exposed and infected infants, children, and adolescents from birth to age 24 and tracks long-term benefits or any harmful effects of medications or vaccines developed to prevent or treat HIV. Jane C. Lindsey, ScD, of Harvard School of Public Health and colleagues examined the effects of HIV infection and the impact of PI-based HAART on the neurodevelopment of infants and children during the first three years of life. They compared infants and children infected with HIV who were born after June 1997—when PI-based HAART became available for use in children—with a control group of children who were exposed but did not contract the virus from their infected mothers.

Before one year of age, children with HIV infection had lower mental and motor skills than their HIV-exposed but uninfected counterparts. However, using standardized tests, the researchers found that the mental and motor skills of uninfected children appeared to decline with age—likely resulting from the complex interplay between genetic and environmental factors. In contrast, test scores of the children with HIV infection for mental skills declined less than expected, and their scores for motor skills actually improved slightly. HIV-infected children who were born prior to 1997 and therefore did not receive PI-based HAART continued to decline in mental and motor skills.

The results offer encouragement for treating infants and young children with HIV infection, who are at the highest risk for neurodevelopmental difficulties. However, more research is needed to better understand how PI-based HAART intersects with genetic, health, and environmental factors to affect neurodevelopment in these children.

Chapter 52

HIV Infection in Adolescents and Young Adults in the United States

There is a rising concern about the effects of HIV/AIDS among adolescents and young adults between the ages of 13 to 24 in the United States. The Centers for Disease Control and Prevention (CDC) reported 40,049 cumulative cases of AIDS among people ages 13 to 24 through 2004. Since the epidemic began, an estimated 10,129 adolescents and young adults with AIDS have died and the proportion diagnosed with AIDS has also increased. Likewise, the proportion of adolescents and young adults with an AIDS diagnosis has increased from 3.9 percent in 1999 to 4.2 percent in 2004.

Moreover, African American and Hispanic adolescents have been disproportionately affected by the HIV/AIDS epidemic. Between the ages of 13 and 19, African Americans and Hispanics accounted for 66 percent and 21 percent, respectively, of the reported AIDS cases in 2003.

Because the average duration from HIV infection to the development of AIDS is ten years, most adults with AIDS were likely infected as adolescents or young adults. In 2004, an estimated 4,883 were diagnosed with HIV/AIDS, while an estimated 18,293 were living with HIV/AIDS. However, health experts estimate the number of adolescents and adults living with HIV infection to be much higher.

"HIV Infection in Adolescents and Young Adults in the U.S.: NIAID Fact Sheet," National Institute of Allergy and Infectious Diseases (http://www.niaid .nih.gov), a component of the National Institutes of Health (NIH), updated May 18, 2006.

Transmission

Modes of Transmission

Most HIV-infected adolescents and young adults are exposed to the virus through sexual intercourse. Recent HIV surveillance data suggest that the majority of HIV-infected adolescent and young adult males are infected through sex with men. Only a small percentage of males appear to be exposed by injection drug use and/or heterosexual contact. These data also suggest that adolescent and young adult females infected with HIV were exposed through heterosexual contact, with a very small percentage through injection drug use. In addition, there is an increasing number of children who were infected as infants that are now surviving to adolescence.

Sexually Transmitted Diseases (STDs) and HIV

Approximately 25 percent of cases of STDs reported in the United States each year are among teenagers. This is particularly significant because the risk of HIV transmission increases substantially if either partner is infected with an STD. Discharge of pus and mucus as a result of STDs, such as gonorrhea or chlamydia, also increase the risk of HIV transmission three- to five-fold. Likewise, STD-induced ulcers from syphilis or genital herpes increase the risk of HIV transmission nine-fold.

Care and Treatment

Because many adolescents and young adults tend to think they are invincible, this belief may cause them to engage in risky behavior, delay HIV testing, and if they test positive, delay or refuse treatment. The inability to link them to medical care can lead to increased transmission of HIV. Health care providers report that many young people, when they learn they are HIV-positive, take several months to accept their diagnosis and return for treatment.

Health care providers may be able to help young people understand their situation during visits by doing the following:

- ensuring confidentiality

- explaining the information clearly

- eliciting questions

- emphasizing the success of newly available treatments

The U.S. Department of Health and Human Services has also developed documents that address the standard of care for the treatment of HIV, including information about how to treat HIV in adolescents. The documents *Guidelines for the Use of Antiretroviral Agents in HIV-Infected Adults and Adolescents* and *Guidelines for the Use of Antiretroviral Agents in Pediatric HIV Infection* are available from AIDSinfo (http://www.aidsinfo.nih.gov).

According to the *Guidelines for the Use of Antiretroviral Agents in HIV-Infected Adults and Adolescents,* adolescents exposed to HIV sexually or via injection drug use appear to follow a clinical course that is more similar to HIV disease in adults than in children. Most adolescents with sexually acquired HIV are in a relatively early stage of infection and are ideal candidates for early intervention that includes education and counseling, identifying high-risk behaviors, and recommended therapies and behavioral changes.

Adolescents who were infected at birth or via blood products as young children, however, follow a unique clinical course that may differ from that of other adolescents and adults. Health care providers should refer to the treatment guidelines for detailed information about treating HIV-infected adolescents.

Current Research

The National Institute of Allergy and Infectious Diseases (NIAID) supports research in adolescents and young adults through studies conducted by clinical trial networks and sites within the United States. These studies help evaluate promising therapies to do the following:

- prevent HIV infection

- discover new therapies to improve control of viral replication in people with HIV/AIDS

- prevent and treat co-infections and cancers associated with AIDS

- prevent and treat complications of HIV therapies

- reconstitute HIV-damaged immune systems

In response to the growing epidemic among adolescents and young adults in the United States, NIAID supports the Pediatric AIDS Clinical Trials Group (PACTG) (http://pactg.s-3.com), a clinical trial network co-funded with the National Institute of Child Health and Human Development (NICHD). The PACTG's adolescent treatment research agenda focuses on the following:

- studying the safety and use of new and existing drugs and treatment management to prevent perinatal transmission and pediatric infection

- studying the effects of treatment on acute and early infection

- increasing commitment to long-term studies of safety and clinical effectiveness of antiretroviral therapies

- engaging youth in treatment research opportunities

- restoring immune function

- promoting domestic and international collaborations, including prevention and behavioral research

- expanding and enhancing adolescent research at all PACTG sites

In addition, NICHD supports the Adolescent Medicine Trials Network (ATN) (http://www.atnonline.org) for HIV/AIDS Interventions. Its mission is to conduct research, both independently and in collaboration with existing research networks supported by NIAID, on promising behavioral, microbicidal, prophylactic, therapeutic, and vaccine modalities in HIV-infected and HIV-at-risk adolescents between the ages 12 to 24 years old.

As such, recruiting adolescents and young adults into clinical trials is important to ensure that research results will be applicable to therapy for that age group. Most clinical trials are open to adolescents and young adults, but in reality very few enroll. Of the approximately 9,500 participants in studies conducted by the NIAID-supported Adult and Pediatric AIDS Clinical Trials Groups in FY 2005, only 5.4 percent of the participants were adolescents (ages 13 to 19).

For information specifically about clinical trials conducted by the NIAID Intramural AIDS Research Program, go to their website at http://www.clinicaltrials.gov.

Chapter 53

Why Women and Girls Need Better HIV/AIDS Prevention Options

The Increasing Impact of AIDS on Women

Two and a half decades into the HIV/AIDS pandemic, the disease continues to outpace the global response. According to new data released by the Joint United Nations Programme on HIV/AIDS (UNAIDS), an estimated 38.6 million people are now living with HIV worldwide, and the rates of infection among women have been rising in almost every region of the world. In 2005, women represented 48 percent of HIV-infected adults worldwide and 59 percent in sub-Saharan Africa.[1] Among young people ages 15 to 24 in sub-Saharan Africa, the difference in rates of infection is even more striking: HIV-infected young women outnumber their male counterparts three to one.[2]

Women's and girls' increased biological vulnerability to HIV infection, coupled with social and economic inequities, fuel the epidemic in resource-poor nations. Entrenched gender norms and inequalities result in power imbalances in relationships, affecting women's ability to control or negotiate the terms of sexual relations and condom use. Poverty and reliance on men for economic support also limit women's power to protect themselves and force some to turn to transactional sex for survival. Also, cultural norms that preclude women's access to knowledge about sexuality and the threat of violence or loss of economic support can impede women's ability to communicate with their partners about HIV prevention.

In addition to the impact of the disease itself on HIV-positive women, the burden of caring for those with HIV-related illnesses and for children orphaned by AIDS typically falls on women and girls. HIV-affected women and families are increasingly impoverished, further increasing their vulnerability to infectious diseases. Additionally, women who are infected or affected by HIV often face stigma and discrimination, at times leading to ostracism, abuse, and destitution.

The Effect of AIDS on Women and Girls[3]

- Worldwide 17.3 million women aged 15 years and older are living with HIV.

- Seventy-six percent of all HIV-positive women live in sub-Saharan Africa.

- Seventy-four percent of young people living with HIV in sub-Saharan Africa are women.

- Female infections are on the rise in Southeast Asia, Eastern Europe, the U.S., and Latin America.

- In 2005, fewer than 10 percent of women living in low- and middle-income countries received antiretroviral treatment to prevent HIV transmission to newborns.

Women Need a Range of Prevention Options and Approaches

Given the complex web of physiological and socioeconomic factors increasing women's vulnerability to infection, a comprehensive response to HIV/AIDS today requires a scaling up and strengthening of a range of prevention approaches. Such interventions include access to HIV and sexual and reproductive health education, particularly for young people; efforts to positively shift gender norms and combat sexual coercion and violence; initiatives to increase access and availability of male and female condoms; promotion of mutual fidelity and abstinence, where feasible; increasing access to voluntary HIV counseling and testing with referrals to appropriate treatment, care, and support; and programs for the prevention of mother-to-child transmission.

Currently available approaches to HIV prevention, however, are insufficient. New and better long-term prevention tools—especially methods that women can initiate or control—are needed. Vaccines and microbicides, currently under development, are promising new technologies. Microbicides, for use by women to prevent or reduce the risk of HIV infection during sexual intercourse, could increase women's level of control and ability to protect themselves. An effective AIDS vaccine offers a long-term solution to the epidemic. Women would be able to access and use a vaccine with or without their partners' knowledge. Adolescent girls, who are particularly vulnerable to infection, could potentially be vaccinated as pre-adolescents before the onset of sexual activity or other potentially high-risk behaviors.

Vaccines or microbicides would be significant options alone or could be used as dual protection with other new HIV prevention methods, such as cervical barriers, or existing technologies, such as the female condom, to augment their effectiveness. Together, these tools provide a range of choices that must be available to meet women's and girls' needs and preferences. A wider range of options would also increase the likelihood of use and thus reduce HIV infection rates.

The Global Effort to Find an AIDS Vaccine

Today, scientists think that an AIDS vaccine is possible. As of June 2006, there are about 30 ongoing clinical trials of preventive AIDS vaccine candidates in approximately two dozen countries around the world.[4] To support research and development to discover a vaccine, sustained and strategically-targeted funding and political commitment are critical.

Resources for research and development have risen from around $535 million in 2002 to $759 million in 2005.[5] Scientific consortia comprising leading HIV researchers are now tackling the most critical questions. However, the effort still is not commensurate with the challenge. In the past 30 years, we have not been able to develop a licensed vaccine without private-sector involvement, and to date, industry engagement in vaccine research and development has been minimal. Currently, pharmaceutical and biotechnology companies contribute less than 10 percent of total investment in preventive AIDS vaccine research and development.

Conclusion

Vaccines and microbicides hold the promise of being among the most powerful health and equity tools in the world. For this reason, the international community must ensure the inclusion of AIDS vaccine and microbicide research and development within broader HIV/AIDS, development, and poverty reduction agendas.

Accelerated vaccine and microbicide research must be among the top global health—and women's health—priorities. Women's advocates, policy makers, researchers, development organizations, and others committed to improving women's lives around the world should advocate for AIDS vaccine research, become actively involved in the vaccine development process, and thereby help ensure women's future access to critical AIDS preventive technology.

The International AIDS Vaccine Initiative (IAVI) is a global not-for-profit organization whose mission is to ensure the development of safe, effective, accessible, preventive HIV vaccines for use throughout the world. Founded in 1996 and operational in 23 countries, IAVI and its network of collaborators research and develop vaccine candidates. IAVI's financial and in-kind supporters include the Alfred P. Sloan Foundation, the Bill and Melinda Gates Foundation, The New York Community Trust, The Rockefeller Foundation, and The Starr Foundation; the governments of the Basque Country, Canada, Denmark, European Union, Ireland, The Netherlands, Norway, Sweden, United Kingdom, and the United States; multilateral organizations such as The World Bank; corporate donors including BD (Becton, Dickinson and Co.), Continental Airlines, DHL, Merck and Co. Inc., and Pfizer Inc.; leading AIDS charities such as Broadway Cares/Equity Fights AIDS, Crusaid, Deutsche AIDS-Stiftung, and Until There's A Cure Foundation; other private donors such as the Haas Charitable Trusts; and many generous individuals from around the world. For more information, see http://www.iavi.org.

References

1. UNAIDS, *2006 Report on the Global AIDS Epidemic,* 30 May 2006, available from http://www.unaids.org/en/HIV_data/2006GlobalReport/default.asp.

2. UNAIDS, *The Female AIDS Epidemic: 2005 Statistics* (Geneva: UNAIDS, November 2005).

3. UNAIDS, 2006.

4. International AIDS Vaccine Initiative, *IAVI Database of AIDS Vaccines in Human Trials,* June 2006, available from http://www.iavireport.org/trialsdb.

5. HIV Vaccines and Microbicides Resource Tracking Working Group, *Adding It All Up: Funding for HIV Vaccine and Microbicide Development,* 2000-2006 (New York: IAVI, August 2006).

Part Seven

Living with HIV/AIDS

Chapter 54

Staying Healthy If You Have HIV/AIDS

This chapter is for people who are infected with the human immunodeficiency virus (HIV) and for their friends and families. HIV is the virus that causes acquired immunodeficiency syndrome (AIDS).

Although infection with HIV is serious, people with HIV and AIDS are living longer, healthier lives today, thanks to new and effective treatments. This chapter will help you understand how you can live with HIV and keep yourself healthy.

How long does it take to go from HIV infection to a diagnosis of AIDS?

There is no one answer to this question because everyone is different. Estimates of the average length of time for progression from HIV to AIDS are being developed. Before antiretroviral therapy became available in 1996, scientists estimated that AIDS would develop within ten years in about half the people with HIV. Since 1996, new medical treatments have been developed that can prevent or cure some of the illnesses associated with AIDS, though they cannot cure AIDS itself.

Various factors, including your genetic makeup, can influence the time between HIV infection and the development of AIDS:

Excerpted from "Living with HIV/AIDS," Centers for Disease Control and Prevention (http://www.cdc.gov); National Center for HIV, STD, and TB Prevention; September 2005.

471

Time between HIV Infection and AIDS: Shorter

- older age
- infection with more than one type of HIV
- poor nutrition
- severe stress

Time between HIV Infection and AIDS: Longer

- closely adhering to your doctor's recommendations
- eating healthy foods
- taking care of yourself

What is clear is that you have some control over the progression of HIV infection.

How can I stay healthy longer?

There are many things you can do for yourself to stay healthy. Here are a few.

- Make sure you have a health care provider who knows how to treat HIV. Begin treatment promptly once your doctor tells you to.

- Keep your appointments. Follow your doctor's instructions. If your doctor prescribes medicine for you, take the medicine just the way he or she tells you to because taking only some of your medicine gives your HIV infection more chance to fight back.

- If you get sick from your medicine, call your doctor for advice; don't make changes to your medicine on your own or because of advice from friends.

- Get immunizations (shots) to prevent infections such as pneumonia and flu. Your doctor will tell you when to get these shots. Practice safe sex to reduce your risk of getting a sexually transmitted disease (STD) or another strain of HIV.

- If you smoke or use drugs not prescribed by your doctor, quit.

- Eat healthy foods. This will help keep you strong, keep your energy and weight up, and help your body protect itself.

- Exercise regularly.

- Get enough sleep and rest.

- Take time to relax. Many people find that meditation or prayer, along with exercise and rest, help them cope with the stress of having HIV or AIDS.

There are also many things you can do to protect your health when you prepare food or eat, when you travel, and when you're around pets and other animals. You can read more about these things in [other chapters in this book] or in the brochures in the Centers for Disease Control and Prevention (CDC)'s Opportunistic Infection series. You can get these brochures and other information about HIV by calling CDC-INFO at 800-232-4636 or by going to the CDC internet address, http://www.cdc.gov/hiv/dhap.htm.

What can I expect when I go to the doctor?

During your first appointment your doctor will ask you questions, examine you, take a blood sample, and do some other tests. Your doctor also may do a skin test for tuberculosis and give you some immunizations (shots).

Tell your doctor about any health problems you are having so that you can get treatment. You also should ask your doctor any questions you have about HIV or AIDS, such as the following:

- what to do if your medicine makes you sick

- where to get help for quitting smoking or using drugs

- how to create a healthier diet

- how to minimize the chance that you will spread HIV to your partners

Your blood sample is used for many tests, including the CD4 cell count and viral load. Your CD4 cell count tells you how many CD4 cells you have in your blood. If you are getting treatment, your CD4 cell counts indicate how well it is working. If your CD4 cell count rises, your body is better able to fight infection. Viral load testing measures the amount of HIV in your blood. Your viral load helps predict what will happen next with your HIV infection if you don't get treatment.

Keep your follow-up appointments with your doctor. At these appointments you and your doctor will talk about your test results, and he or she may prescribe medicine for you.

What is the treatment for HIV or AIDS?

Antiretroviral medicines: Because HIV is a certain type of virus called a retrovirus, the drugs used to treat it are called antiretroviral medicines. These powerful medicines control the virus and slow progression of HIV infection, but they do not cure it. You need to take these medicines exactly as your doctor prescribes.

HAART: The current recommended treatment for HIV is a combination of three or more medicines. This regimen of medicines is called highly active antiretroviral therapy (HAART). How many pills you will need to take and how often you will take them depends on which medicines your doctor chooses for you. Remember, each HAART regimen is tailored to each individual patient. There is no one best regimen.

HAART may cause some side effects. You and your doctor should discuss potential side effects so that you will know if they occur. If you experience any side effects, even those that may seem minor, you should talk about them with your doctor.

Other medicines: Your doctor may also prescribe other medicines for you, depending on your CD4 cell count. Always discuss any side effects with your doctor. Never change the way you are taking any of the medicines without first talking with your doctor. If you don't take your medicines the right way, they may not be as effective as they should be.

Treating other infections: If your HIV infection gets worse and your CD4 cell count falls below 200, you are more likely to get other infections. Your doctor may prescribe medicines to prevent particular infections, such as PCP.

The most important thing you can do after you learn that you have HIV is to work closely with your doctor. Because HIV and HIV-related illnesses vary from person to person, your doctor will design a medical care plan specifically for you. To help your doctor make the best choices for you, you must tell your doctor about any side effects or symptoms you have.

What are some of the other diseases I could get?

Because HIV damages your immune system, you may have a higher chance of getting certain diseases, called opportunistic infections. They are so named because an HIV-infected person's weakened immune system gives these diseases the opportunity to develop. Fortunately, people with HIV who are taking HAART can go a long time before their immune system is damaged enough to allow an opportunistic infection to occur. That's why it is so important to get tested and start treatment early. Many people may not know they have HIV until AIDS and an opportunistic infection develop. Many germs can cause opportunistic infections.

Certain symptoms can occur with opportunistic infections.

- breathing problems
- mouth problems, such as thrush (white spots), sores, change in taste, dryness, trouble swallowing, or loose teeth
- fever for more than two days
- weight loss
- change in vision or floaters (moving lines or spots in your vision)
- diarrhea
- skin rashes or itching

Tell your doctor right away if you have any of these problems. Your doctor can treat most of your HIV-related problems, but sometimes you may need to go to a specialist. Visit a dentist at least twice a year, more often if you have mouth problems.

Table 54.1. Examples of common opportunistic infections

Common Name	Full Name	Pronunciation
PCP	*Pneumocystis carinii*[1] pneumonia	NEW-mo-SIStis CA-RIN nee-eye
MAC	*Mycobacterium avium* complex	my-ko-bakavium TEER-i-um AYE-vee-um
CMV	Cytomegalovirus	si-to-MEG-ehlo-vi-res
TB	Tuberculosis	too-burr-qu-LOsis
Toxo	Toxoplasmosis	tok-so-plaz-MOsis
Crypto	Cryptosporidiosis	krip-to-spo-ride-O-sis
Hep C	Hepatitis C	hep-a-TI-tis C
HPV	Human papillomavirus	HU-man PAP-i-LO-ma VI-res

1. Also called *Pneumocystis jiroveci*

How do I protect other people from my HIV?

Things you should do:

- **Abstain from sex.** The surest way to avoid transmission of STDs, including a different strain of HIV, is to not have sexual intercourse.

- **Use condoms correctly and consistently.** Correct and consistent use of the male latex condom can reduce the risk for STD transmission. However, no protective method is 100 percent effective. Condom use cannot guarantee absolute protection against any STD.

    - If you are allergic to latex, you can use polyurethane condoms.

    - Condoms lubricated with spermicides are no more effective than other lubricated condoms in protecting against the transmission of HIV and other STDs.

    - If you use condoms incorrectly, they can slip off or break, which reduces their protective effects. Inconsistent use, such as not using condoms with every act of intercourse, can lead to STD transmission because transmission can occur with just one act of intercourse.

- **Use protection during oral sex.** A condom or dental dam (a square piece of latex used by dentists) can be used. Do not reuse these items.

- **Tell others that you have HIV.**

    - Tell people you've had sex with. This can be difficult, but they need to know so they can get the help they need. Your local public health department may help you find these people and tell them they have been exposed to HIV. If they have HIV, this may help them get care and avoid spreading HIV to others.

    - Tell people you are planning on having sex with. Practicing safe sex will help protect your health and that of your partners.

    - If you are a man and had sex with a woman who became pregnant, you need to tell the woman that you have HIV, even if you are not the father of the baby. If she has HIV, she needs to get early medical care for her own health and her baby's health.

Things you should not do:

- **Don't share sex toys.** Keep sex toys for your own use only.

- **Don't share drug needles or drug works.** Use a needle exchange program if one is available. Seek help if you inject drugs. You can fight HIV much better if you don't have a drug habit.

- **Don't donate blood, plasma, or organs.**

- **Don't share razors or toothbrushes.** HIV can be spread through fresh blood on such items.

Is there special advice for women with HIV?

Yes. If you are a woman with HIV, your doctor should check you for STDs and perform a Pap test at least once a year.

As a woman with HIV, you are more likely to have abnormal Pap test results. Infection with HIV means your body is less effective in controlling all types of viruses. The human papillomavirus (HPV) is a specific virus that can infect cervical cells (the cells that the Pap test looks at). Your doctor may recommend a special test that can look for HPV as part of your exam. If your Pap test result is abnormal, your doctor may need to repeat it or do other tests. If you have had an abnormal Pap test result in the past, tell your doctor.

If you are thinking about avoiding pregnancy or becoming pregnant, talk with your doctor. You might ask some of the following questions:

- What birth control methods are best for me?

- Will HIV cause problems for me during pregnancy or delivery?

- Will my baby have HIV?

- Will treatment for my HIV infection cause problems for my baby?

- If I choose to get pregnant, what medical and community programs and support groups can help me and my baby?

If you become pregnant, talk to your doctor right away about medical care for you and your baby. You also need to plan for your child's future in case you get sick.

Your HIV treatment will not change very much from what it was before you became pregnant. You should have a Pap test and tests for

STDs during your pregnancy. Your doctor will order tests and suggest medicines for you to take. Talk with him or her about all the pros and cons of taking medicine while you are pregnant.

Talk with your doctor about how you can prevent giving HIV to your baby. It is very important that you get good care early in your pregnancy. The chances of passing HIV to your baby before or during birth are about one in four, or 25 percent, but treatment with antiretroviral medicines has been shown to greatly lower this risk. Your doctor will want you to take these medicines to increase your baby's chance of not getting HIV.

Although you are pregnant, to avoid catching other diseases and to avoid spreading HIV, you should still use condoms each time you have sex. Even if your partner already has HIV, he should still use condoms.

After birth, your baby will need to be tested for HIV, even if you took antiretroviral medicines while you were pregnant. Your baby will need to take medicine to prevent HIV infection and PCP. Talk with your doctor about your baby's special medical needs. Because HIV infection can be passed through breast milk, you should not breastfeed your baby.

Where can I find help in dealing with HIV?

If you are living with HIV or AIDS, you may need many kinds of support: medical, emotional, psychological, and financial. Your doctor, your local health and social services departments, local AIDS service organizations, and libraries can help you in finding all kinds of help, such as the following:

- answers to your questions about HIV and AIDS

- doctors, insurance, and help in making health care decisions

- food, housing, and transportation

- planning to meet financial and daily needs

- support groups for you and your loved ones

- home nursing care

- help in legal matters, including Americans with Disabilities Act (ADA) claims

- confidential help in applying for Social Security disability benefits

You can also get help by calling CDC-INFO at 800-232-4636.

Many people living with HIV feel better if they can talk with other people who also have HIV. Here are some ways to find support.

- Contact your local AIDS service organization. Look under "AIDS" or "Social Service Organizations" in the yellow pages of your telephone book.

- Contact a local hospital, church, or American Red Cross chapter for referrals.

- Read HIV newsletters or magazines.

- Join support groups or internet forums.

- Volunteer to help others with HIV.

- Be an HIV educator or public speaker, or work on a newsletter.

- Attend social events to meet other people who have HIV.

Today, thousands of people are living with HIV or AIDS. Many are leading full, happy, and productive lives. You can too if you work with your doctor and others and take the steps outlined in this chapter to stay healthy.

Chapter 55

Eating Right
when You Have HIV/AIDS

Why is nutrition important?

Nutrition is important for everyone because food gives our bodies the nutrients they need to stay healthy, grow, and work properly. Foods are made up of six classes of nutrients, each with its own special role in the body:

- Protein builds muscles and a strong immune system.
- Carbohydrates (including starches and sugars) give you energy.
- Fat gives you extra energy.
- Vitamins regulate body processes.
- Minerals regulate body processes and also make up body tissues.
- Water gives cells shape and acts as a medium where body processes can occur.

Having good nutrition means eating the right types of foods in the right amounts so you get these important nutrients.

Do I need a special diet?

There are no special diets, or particular foods, that will boost your immune system. But there are things you can do to keep your immunity up.

"Diet and Nutrition," U.S. Department of Veterans Affairs, National HIV/AIDS Program (http://www.hiv.va.gov), updated May 2, 2007.

When you are infected with HIV, your immune system has to work very hard to fight off infections—and this takes energy (measured in calories). This means you may need to eat more food than you used to.

If you are underweight—or you have advanced disease, high viral loads, or opportunistic infections—you should include more protein as well as extra calories (in the form of carbohydrates and fats). You'll find tips for doing this in the next section.

If you are overweight, you should follow a well-balanced meal plan such as the U.S. Government's Food Pyramid guide at http://www.mypyramid.gov. Keep in mind, you may need to eat more food to meet your extra needs.

How do I keep from losing weight?

Weight loss is a common problem for people infected with HIV, and it should be taken very seriously. Losing weight can be dangerous because it makes it harder for your body to fight infections and to get well after you're sick.

People with HIV often do not eat enough because of the following:

- HIV and HIV medicines may reduce your appetite, make food taste bad, and prevent the body from absorbing food in the right way.

- Symptoms like a sore mouth, nausea, and vomiting make it difficult to eat.

- Fatigue from HIV or the medicines may make it hard to prepare food and eat regularly.

- To keep your weight up, you will need to take in more protein and calories. What follows are ways to do that.

To Add Protein to Your Diet

Protein-rich foods include meats, fish, beans, dairy products, and nuts. To boost the protein in your meals do the following:

- Spread nut butter on toast, crackers, fruit, or vegetables.

- Add cottage cheese to fruit and tomatoes.

- Add canned tuna to casseroles and salads.

- Add shredded cheese to sauces, soups, omelets, baked potatoes, and steamed vegetables.

- Eat yogurt on your cereal or fruit.

- Eat hard-boiled (hard-cooked) eggs. Use them in egg-salad sandwiches or slice and dice them for tossed salads.

- Add diced or chopped meats to soups, salads, and sauces.

- Add dried milk powder or egg white powder to foods (like scrambled eggs, casseroles, and milkshakes).

To Add Calories to Your Diet

The best way to increase calories is to add carbohydrates and some extra fat to your meals. Carbohydrates include both starches and simple sugars. Starches are in the following: breads, muffins, biscuits, crackers; oatmeal and cold cereals; pasta; potatoes; and rice.

Simple sugars are in the following:

- fresh or dried fruit (raisins, dates, apricots, etc.)

- jelly, honey, and maple syrup added to cereal, pancakes, and waffles

Fats are more concentrated sources of calories. Add moderate amounts of the following to your meals:

- butter, margarine, sour cream, cream cheese, peanut butter

- gravy, sour cream, cream cheese, grated cheese

- avocados, olives, salad dressing

How can I maintain my appetite?

When you become ill, you often lose your appetite. This can lead to weight loss, which can make it harder for your body to fight infection. Here are some tips for increasing your appetite:

- Try a little exercise, like walking or doing yoga. This can often stimulate your appetite and make you feel like eating more.

- Eat smaller meals more often. For instance, try to snack between meals.

- Eat whenever your appetite is good.

- Do not drink too much right before or during meals. This can make you feel full.

- Avoid carbonated (fizzy) drinks and foods such as cabbage, broccoli, and beans. These foods and drinks can create gas in your stomach and make you feel full and bloated.

- Eat with your family or friends.
- Choose your favorite foods, and make meals as attractive to you as possible. Try to eat in a pleasant location.

How much water do I need?

Drinking enough liquids is very important when you have HIV. Fluids transport the nutrients you need through your body. Extra water can do the following:

- reduce the side effects of medications
- help flush out the medicines that have already been used by your body
- help you avoid dehydration (fluid loss), dry mouth, and constipation
- make you feel less tired

Many of us don't drink enough water every day. You should be getting at least eight to ten glasses of water (or other fluids, such as juices or soups) a day.

Here are some tips on getting the extra fluids you need:

- Drink more water than usual. Try other fluids, too, like Gatorade or Sprite.
- Avoid colas, coffee, tea, and cocoa. These may contain caffeine and can actually dehydrate you. Read the labels on drinks to see if they have caffeine in them.
- Avoid alcohol.
- Begin and end each day by drinking a glass of water.
- Suck on ice cubes and popsicles.

Note: If you have diarrhea or are vomiting, you will lose a lot of fluids and will need to drink more than usual.

Do I need supplements?

Our bodies need vitamins and minerals, in small amounts, to keep our cells working properly. They are essential to our staying healthy. People with HIV need extra vitamins and minerals to help repair and heal cells that have been damaged.

Even though vitamins and minerals are present in many foods, your health care provider may recommend a vitamin and mineral supplement (a pill or other form of concentrated vitamins and minerals). While vitamin and mineral supplements can be useful, they can in no way replace eating a healthy diet. If you are taking a supplement, here are some things to remember:

- Always take vitamin pills on a full stomach. Take them regularly.

- Some vitamins and minerals, if taken in high doses, can be harmful. Talk with your health care provider before taking high doses of any supplement.

Table 55.1 lists some nutrients that affect the immune system.

What should I know about food safety?

Paying attention to food and water safety is important when you have HIV, because your immune system is already weakened and working hard to fight off infections. If food is not handled or prepared in a safe way, germs from the food can be passed on to you. These germs can make you sick. You need to handle and cook food properly to keep those germs from getting to you. Here are some food safety guidelines:

- Keep everything clean. Clean your counters and utensils often.

- Wash your hands with soap and warm water before and after preparing and eating food.

- Check expiration dates on food packaging. Do not eat foods that have a past expiration date.

- Rinse all fresh fruits and vegetables with clean water.

- Thaw frozen meats and other frozen foods in the refrigerator or in a microwave. Never thaw foods at room temperature. Germs that grow at room temperature can make you very sick.

- Clean all cutting boards and knives (especially those that touch chicken and meat) with soap and hot water before using them again.

- Make sure you cook all meat, fish, and poultry "well-done." You might want to buy a meat thermometer to help you know for sure that it is done. Put the thermometer in the thickest part of the meat and not touching a bone. Cook the meat until it reaches 165 to 212° F on your thermometer.

Table 55.1. Vitamins and minerals that affect the immune system (Adapted from the Food and Agriculture Organization of the United Nations, http://www.fao.org.)

Name	What It Does	Where to Get It	About Supplements
Vitamin A and beta-carotene	Keeps skin, lungs, and stomach healthy.	liver, whole eggs, milk, dark green, yellow, orange, and red vegetables and fruit (like spinach, pumpkin, green peppers, squash, carrots, papaya, and mangoes)—also found in orange and yellow sweet potatoes	It's best to get vitamin A from food. Vitamin A supplements are toxic in high doses. Supplements of beta-carotene (the form of vitamin A in fruits and vegetables) have been shown to increase cancer risk in smokers.
Vitamin B-group, (B_1, B_2, B_6, B_{12}, folate)	Keeps the immune and nervous system healthy.	white beans, potatoes, meat, fish, chicken, watermelon, grains, nuts, avocados, broccoli, and green leafy vegetables	
Vitamin C	Helps protect the body from infection and aids in recovery.	citrus fruits (like oranges, grapefruit, and lemons), tomatoes, and potatoes	
Vitamin E	Protects cells and helps fight off infection.	green leafy vegetables, vegetable oils, and peanuts	Limit to 400 IU per day.
Iron	Not having enough iron can cause anemia.	green leafy vegetables, whole grain breads and pastas, dried fruit, beans, red meat, chicken, liver, fish, and eggs	Limit to 45 mg per day unless otherwise instructed by your doctor. Iron may be a problem for people with HIV because it can increase the activity of some bacteria. Supplements that do not contain iron may be better. Ask your doctor.
Selenium	Important for the immune system.	whole grains, meat, fish, poultry, eggs, peanut butter, and nuts	Limit to 400 mcg per day.
Zinc	Important for the immune system.	meat, fish, poultry, beans, peanuts, and milk and dairy products	Limit to 40 mg per day.

- Do not eat raw, soft-boiled, or "over easy" eggs, or Caesar salads with raw egg in the dressing.

- Do not eat sushi, raw seafood, or raw meats, or unpasteurized milk or dairy products.

- Keep your refrigerator cold, set no higher than 40° F. Your freezer should be at 0° F.

- Refrigerate leftovers at temperatures below 40° F. Do not eat leftovers that have been sitting in the refrigerator for more than three days.

- Keep hot items heated to over 140° F, and completely reheat leftovers before eating.

- Throw away any foods (like fruit, vegetables, and cheese) that you think might be old. If food has a moldy or rotten spot, throw it out. When in doubt, throw it out.

- Some germs are spread through tap water. If your public water supply isn't totally pure, drink bottled water.

Can diet help ease side effects and symptoms?

Many symptoms of HIV, as well as the side effects caused by HIV medicines, can be helped by using (or avoiding) certain types of foods and drinks.

Below are some tips for dealing with common problems people with HIV face. You should also look in the side effects section for more information.

Nausea

- Try the BRATT diet (bananas, rice, applesauce, tea, and toast).

- Try some ginger—in tea, ginger ale, or ginger snaps.

- Don't drink liquids at the same time you eat your meals.

- Eat something small, like crackers, before getting out of bed.

- Keep something in your stomach; eat a small snack every one to two hours.

- Avoid foods like fatty, greasy, or fried foods; very sweet foods (candy, cookies, or cake); spicy foods; foods with strong odors.

Mouth and Swallowing Problems

- Avoid hard or crunchy foods such as raw vegetables.

- Try eating cooked vegetables and soft fruits (like bananas and pears).

- Avoid very hot foods and beverages. Cold and room temperature foods will be more comfortable to your mouth.

- Do not eat spicy foods. They can sting your mouth.

- Try soft foods like mashed potatoes, yogurt, and oatmeal.

- Also try scrambled eggs, cottage cheese, macaroni and cheese, and canned fruits.

- Rinse your mouth with water. This can moisten your mouth, remove bits of food, and make food taste better to you.

- Stay away from oranges, grapefruit, and tomatoes. They have a lot of acid and can sting your mouth.

Diarrhea

- Try the BRATT diet (bananas, rice, applesauce, tea, and toast).

- Keep your body's fluids up (hydrated) with water, Gatorade, or other fluids (those that don't have caffeine).

- Limit sodas and other sugary drinks.

- Avoid greasy and spicy foods.

- Avoid milk and other dairy products.

- Eat small meals and snacks every hour or two.

- Try taking Glutamine protein powder to help repair the intestinal lining.

Remember, there is no one "right" way to eat. Eating well means getting the right amount of nutrients for your particular needs. Your health care provider can refer you to a dietitian or nutritionist who can help design a good diet for you.

For general guidelines on good nutrition, you can follow the U.S. Government's Food Pyramid guide. Check it out here: http://www.mypyramid.gov.

Chapter 56

Protecting Yourself from Foodborne Illness

Tips for Safe Food Handling

Wash Your Hands

- Wash hands with soap and warm water before handling food, after using the toilet, after changing a baby's diaper, coughing or sneezing, and after touching animals.

Cook Foods Adequately

- Use a food thermometer to make sure meat and poultry (including ground) are cooked to safe temperatures.

- Use a food thermometer to make sure leftovers are reheated to 165° F (74° C).

- Cook shellfish until the shell opens and the flesh is fully cooked; cook fish until the flesh is firm and flakes easily with a fork.

- Cook eggs until the white and yolk are firm.

"Tips for Safe Food Handling: A Guide for the Persons Living with HIV/AIDS" and "Foodborne Pathogens: Information for Immune-Compromised People," © Washington State University Department of Food Science and Human Nutrition. Reprinted with permission. Available online at http://foodsafety.wsu.edu/consumers/specialprecautions/hiv.html; accessed May 24, 2007.

Avoid Cross Contamination

- Wash knives, cutting boards, and food preparation areas with hot, soapy water after touching poultry, meat, and seafood.

- Wash hands with soap and warm water before and after handling foods.

- Rinse fresh fruits and vegetables well before eating.

Keep Foods at Safe Temperatures

- Refrigerator temperature should be less than 40° F (4.4° C) (check with a thermometer) and only store refrigerated perishable foods for four days or less.

- Store eggs and poultry in the refrigerator.

- Thaw foods in the refrigerator or in the microwave; do not defrost at room temperature.

- Discard or freeze leftovers and uneaten ready-to-eat foods after four days.

Avoid Risky Foods

- Drink only pasteurized milk and fruit juices.

- Use water from a safe water supply for drinking and food preparation.

- Avoid eating raw sprouts (like alfalfa, bean, or any other raw sprout).

- Avoid hot dogs, deli meats, and pâté if served without reheating to steaming hot.

- Avoid eating raw or undercooked seafood.

- Avoid eating raw or undercooked meat and poultry.

- Avoid refrigerated smoked fish and seafood.

- Avoid eating foods containing raw eggs; use pasteurized eggs or egg products in uncooked foods containing eggs.

- Use cheese and yogurt made from pasteurized milk.

- Obtain shellfish from approved sources.

Raw or undercooked animal products are the foods that are most likely to contain pathogens. These foods should be avoided by everyone and should never be consumed by immunocompromised persons.

Foodborne Pathogens: Information for Immunocompromised People

Listeria

Listeria (lis-ter'e'ah) is a bacteria that causes listeriosis. *Listeria* are most often found in foods such as raw milk, soft cheeses (especially if made with raw milk), raw meats, raw and smoked fish, raw sprouts, and some ready-to-eat foods including hot dogs, deli meats, lunch meats, refrigerated smoked fish, and seafood.

There are many sources of *Listeria* on foods, including soil and animals. The bacteria are killed by cooking or pasteurization, but can grow in food stored in the refrigerator. Foods that have a risk of contamination with *Listeria* are ready-to-eat foods that were re-contaminated in the processing plant after cooking or pasteurization.

What Is My Risk of Getting a Listeria *Infection?*

Listeria infections are rare with around 2,500 cases and 500 deaths a year in the United States. An outbreak of *Listeria* infections in 2002 caused 23 deaths. The outbreak was linked to deli turkey. A study in 1991 found listeriosis is 300 times more frequent in people with AIDS than in the general population. Symptoms include fever, muscle aches, nausea, diarrhea, or meningitis. Occasionally, *Listeria* infections occur in the blood or the brain of people who are pregnant or immunocompromised. When this happens, serious illness and even death can result.

How Can I Prevent Listeriosis?

Never eat these foods because they may contain *Listeria*, *Salmonella*, and many other foodborne pathogens.

- raw (unpasteurized) milk
- raw-milk fresh cheese and yogurt (aged hard cheeses made from raw milk are safe)
- raw or undercooked seafood
- raw or undercooked meat and poultry

For an added margin of safety from listeriosis, do not eat the following:

- soft cheese (Brie, feta, Camembert, queso fresco, and similar soft Mexican-style cheeses) unless it is labeled as made with pasteurized milk

- refrigerated cooked or smoked seafood and fish (may be labeled as nova-style, kippered, lox, or jerky) unless it is contained in a cooked dish

- hot dogs, deli meats, and pâté or meat spreads unless they are reheated to steaming hot

- unwashed fruits and vegetables

Hot dogs should be reheated according to package directions or brought to a boil and cooked for five minutes. Heating lunchmeat and hot dogs kills *Listeria* that may be present on these foods.

Lunchmeats should be reheated to steaming hot before eating. If you prefer cold lunchmeats, they can be reheated and then cooled in the refrigerator before eating. Some companies that make hot dogs and lunchmeats now produce meats that are low risk for *Listeria*. You can contact companies to learn if the product is formulated to prevent *Listeria* growth.

Perishable foods may be kept for four days if temperature of refrigerator is less than 40° F. Check your refrigerator temperature with a thermometer. It should be between 35° F–40° F. Freeze or discard ready-to-eat perishable food after four days.

Toxoplasma

Where Are Toxoplasma *Found?*

Cats are carriers of the *Toxoplasma* (tox'o-plasma) parasite, and can pass it through their feces to people, food, and animals. *Toxoplasma* can be found in raw or undercooked meat.

What Is My Risk of Getting a Toxoplasma *Infection?*

About 35 percent of the U.S. population has been infected with *Toxoplasma*. A *Toxoplasma* infection (toxoplasmosis or toxo for short) generally does not cause illness.

The Centers for Disease Control (CDC) estimates 225,000 cases and 750 deaths occur in the U.S. each year from *Toxoplasma* infections.

Symptoms include flu-like symptoms, central nervous system disease, and inflammation of the heart or pneumonia.

What If I Test Positive for Toxoplasma*?*

Testing for prior exposure to *Toxoplasma* is frequently conducted for HIV infected individuals because a *Toxoplasma* infection can result in very serious illness when a person is immunocompromised (CD4 count below 100). If you test positive for *Toxoplasma* (seropositive), then, depending on your CD4 count, you may be put on a treatment regimen.

What If I Test Negative for Toxoplasma*?*

The following recommendations will help prevent becoming infected with *Toxoplasma*:

- Use a food thermometer to make sure meat and poultry are cooked to safe temperatures.

- Wash hands often, especially after handling pets and before handling food.

- Do not handle pets while preparing or eating food.

- Have another person clean the cat litter box. If you must clean the box yourself, wear vinyl or household cleaning gloves and immediately wash your hands well with soap and water right after changing the litter.

- Thoroughly rinse fresh fruits and vegetables under running water before eating.

Cryptosporidium

Where Are Cryptosporidium *Found?*

Cryptosporidium (krip'to-spo-rid'e-um) is a parasite that infects many types of animals and humans. You can be exposed to *Cryptosporidium* from the feces of an infected person or animal, or by eating contaminated food or drinking contaminated water. *Cryptosporidium* causes the infection cryptosporidiosis (crypto).

What Is My Risk of Getting Cryptosporidiosis?

The CDC estimates 300,000 cases and 66 deaths occur in the U.S. each year. Symptoms include diarrhea, stomach cramps, and fever.

For persons with a weakened immune system, cryptosporidiosis can be a very serious infection. If you are immunocompromised, the illness may last for weeks or months.

If your CD4 count is below 200, cryptosporidiosis may give symptoms for a long time. If your CD4 count is above 200, your symptoms may last only one to three weeks. Symptoms may come back if your CD4 count later drops below 200.

How Can I Prevent Crypto?

To keep yourself safe from crypto, use these tips:

- Wash hands often with soap and water.

- Avoid touching farm animals.

- Avoid touching the feces of pets or humans.

- Avoid swallowing water when swimming in the ocean, lakes, rivers, or pools, and when using hot tubs.

- Wash fruits and vegetables thoroughly.

- Cook food to safe temperatures. Use a food thermometer

- Drink safe water. (The CDC recommends that persons who are immunocompromised boil drinking water for one minute, drink distilled water, or use a water purifier that uses reverse osmosis or filters water at less than 1 micron. Links to water purifiers include: http://www.cdc.gov/ncidod/dpd/healthywater/ immuno.htm; http://www.fhcrc.org/clinical/ltfu/patient/ water_safety.html; http://www.NSF.org.)

Salmonella *and* Campylobacter

Where are Salmonella *and* Campylobacter *found?*

Salmonella (sal'mo-nel'ah) and *Campylobacter* (campy'lo-bacter) are most often found in protein foods like raw (unpasteurized) milk, raw or undercooked poultry, meat, eggs, salads (chicken, tuna, potato), and cream desserts and fillings made with uncooked eggs. Fresh fruits and vegetables may also have *Salmonella* and *Campylobacter*.

What Is My Risk of Getting a Salmonella *or* Campylobacter *Infection?*

The CDC estimates 1.4 million cases of *Salmonella* infection and 582 deaths occur in the U.S. each year. It has been estimated that the person with AIDS is 12–20 times more likely to get a *Salmonella* infection than the general population. Symptoms include diarrhea, fever, abdominal cramps, and vomiting.

The CDC estimates 2.4 million cases of *Campylobacter* and 124 deaths occur in the U.S. each year. Symptoms include diarrhea, cramps, fever, and vomiting.

How Can I Prevent a Salmonella *or* Campylobacter *Infection?*

To keep yourself safe from *Salmonella* and *Campylobacter* infections follow these tips:

- Do not eat raw or undercooked eggs.

- Use pasteurized eggs or egg products or pasteurize your eggs in uncooked foods containing eggs. (To pasteurize your own eggs, stir together eggs and either one-quarter cup sugar, water or other liquid from the recipe in a saucepan. Cook over low heat, stirring constantly until the mixture reaches 160° F. These eggs can be safely used in recipes and require no further cooking.)

- Use only pasteurized milk, cheese, and yogurt.

- Use only pasteurized fruit juices.

- Use a food thermometer to make sure meat and poultry are cooked to safe temperatures.

- Do not eat raw sprouts (like alfalfa).

- Thoroughly rinse fresh fruits and vegetables under running water before eating.

- Wash hands, knives, cutting boards, and food preparation areas with hot soapy water after handling foods to avoid cross contamination.

Escherichia coli (E. coli) O157

Where Are E. coli *Found?*

E. coli are common bacteria that are found in animals and in the soil. A few types of *E. coli,* including O157, can cause serious illness. Food sources of *E. coli* include raw or undercooked meat, dry-cured salami, raw sprouts, raw (unpasteurized) milk, fruits, vegetables, unpasteurized fruit juice, and fresh cider.

What Is My Risk of Getting an E. coli *Infection?*

The CDC estimates that 73,000 cases of *E. coli* O157 infection and 61 deaths occur in the U.S. each year. Symptoms include severe diarrhea that is often bloody, abdominal pain, and vomiting.

How Can I Prevent an E. coli *Infection?*

To keep yourself safe from *E. coli* O157, follow these tips:

- Use a food thermometer to make sure meat is cooked to safe temperatures.
- Use only pasteurized milk, cheese, and yogurt.
- Use only pasteurized fruit juices.
- Do not eat raw sprouts (like alfalfa, bean, or any other raw sprout).
- Thoroughly rinse fresh fruits and vegetables under running water before eating.
- Use water from a safe source for drinking and food preparation.

Chapter 57

Exercise when You Have HIV

Being HIV positive is no different from being HIV negative when it comes to exercise. Regular exercise is part of a healthy lifestyle.

Early in the AIDS epidemic, HIV-positive persons had many health problems. They often had trouble keeping their normal weight and muscle mass. People wasted away and died.

Now that anti-HIV drugs have become available, many long-term survivors have stronger immune systems. Newly infected persons have hope for a normal lifespan, if they take care of their bodies. And that includes getting regular exercise.

Benefits of Exercise

Following are some of the benefits of exercise:

- Maintains or builds muscle mass
- Reduces cholesterol and triglyceride levels (less risk of heart disease)
- Increases energy
- Regulates bowel function
- Strengthens bones (less risk of osteoporosis)
- Improves blood circulation
- Increases lung capacity

"Exercise," U.S. Department of Veterans Affairs, National HIV/AIDS Program (http://www.hiv.va.gov), updated May 2, 2007.

497

- Helps with sound, restful sleep
- Lowers stress
- Improves appetite

Before Starting

Before starting an exercise program, talk to your doctor about what you have done in the past for exercise; mention any problems that you had. Consider your current health status and other medical conditions that may affect the type of exercise you can do.

Make sure you can set aside time for your exercise program. The Surgeon General's report on exercise suggests 30 to 45 minutes a day of brisk walking, bicycling, or working around the house. This amount of exercise can reduce risks of developing coronary heart disease, high blood pressure, colon cancer, and diabetes.

If this amount of time seems too much, consider starting with three times a week. The important thing is consistency. This is an ongoing program and you will not benefit without consistency.

Types of Exercise

Two types of exercise are resistance training and aerobic exercise. Resistance training—sometimes called strength training—helps to build muscle mass. Aerobic exercise is important because it strengthens your lungs and your heart. You can read more about these in the following sections.

Resistance Training

Resistance or strength training is important for people with HIV because it can help offset the loss of muscle sometimes caused by the disease. This form of exercise involves exertion of force by moving (pushing or pulling) objects of weight. They can be barbells, dumbbells, or machines in gyms. You can also use safe, common household objects such as plastic milk containers filled with water or sand, or you can use your own body weight in exercises such as push-ups or pull-ups. The purpose of resistance training is to build muscle mass.

Use the correct amount of weight for the exercise you are performing. You should not feel pain during the exercise. When starting a resistance training program, you should feel a little sore for a day or two, but not enough to limit your regular activities. If you do feel very sore, you have used too much weight or have done too many repetitions. Rest an extra day and start again using less weight.

Aerobic Exercise

Aerobic exercise strengthens your lungs and heart. Walking, jogging, running, swimming, hiking, and cycling are forms of this exercise.

This movement increases the rate and depth of your breathing, which in turn increases how much blood and oxygen your heart pumps to your muscles. To achieve the maximum benefit of this kind of exercise, your heart rate should reach the target rate for at least 20 minutes. It may take you weeks to reach this level if you haven't been exercising much.

Your target heart rate is the rate (the number of times your heart beats per minute) at which you receive the maximum benefit from exercise. At your target heart rate, you're working hard but not too hard. To find your target heart rate, you have to measure your pulse at different times while you exercise. Table 57.1 gives target heart rates for different ages. If you're just starting out, aim for the lower end of your range. To measure your heart rate while you're exercising, find your pulse (usually easiest to find at your wrist near the base of your thumb, or on the side of your neck), and count how many times you feel your pulse beat in a minute. You can also count how many times you feel your pulse beat in ten seconds, and then multiply this number by six.

If you don't want to take your pulse while you are exercising, here are some other ways to tell if your workout is too hard or too easy:

- If you can talk while you exercise, you are not working too hard.

- If you can sing while you exercise, you are not working hard enough.

- If you get out of breath quickly, you are working too hard.

Table 57.1. Target heart rate zones

Age	Target Heart Rate Zone 50–75 percent
20 years	100–150 beats per minute
25 years	98–146 beats per minute
30 years	95–142 beats per minute
35 years	93–138 beats per minute
40 years	90–135 beats per minute
45 years	88–131 beats per minute
50 years	85–127 beats per minute
55 years	83–123 beats per minute
60 years	80–120 beats per minute
65 years	78–116 beats per minute
70 years	75–113 beats per minute

Remember, if you are walking, jogging, or running outdoors, make sure you save enough energy for the return trip. Don't overdo it.

Designing a Program

When beginning an exercise program, start slow and build. Start any exercise session with a warmup. This can be as short as a few stretches, if you are working out later in the day when your muscles and joints are already loose, or a short ten-minute stretch session if you are working out first thing in the morning, when your muscles and joints are still tight. Your warmup should not tire you out, but invigorate you and decrease the risk of joint or muscle injury.

If you join a gym, ask about what comes with the membership. Many gyms offer a free evaluation, weighing and measuring you and asking what your goals are. Some gym memberships come with a free workout with a personal trainer and program to help you achieve your goals.

Finding a workout partner can be helpful for support and encouragement, and your workout partner can help with the last repetition of an exercise, which can help improve your strength.

A balanced exercise program is best. Starting with an aerobic exercise is a good warmup to a resistance training session. Remember that learning the correct form in a weight training program will lessen the chance of injury. Go at your own pace. You are not competing with anyone. Listen to your body. If it hurts, stop.

Cautions

After an exercise session, you should feel a little tired. A little while later, however, you should have some energy.

- **Water:** Drink it before, during, and after you exercise. When you feel thirsty you have already lost important fluids and electrolytes and may be dehydrated.

- **Eat well:** Exercising tears down muscle in order to build it up stronger. You need nutrition to provide the raw materials to rebuild your muscles.

- **Sleep:** While you sleep, your body is rebuilding.

- **Listen to your body:** It will tell you to slow down or speed up.

If you are sick or have a cold, take a break. Your body will thank you.

Chapter 58

Sex and Sexuality If You Have HIV/AIDS

If you just tested positive for HIV, you may not want to think about having sex. Some people who get HIV feel guilty or embarrassed. These are common reactions, especially if you got HIV through sex. Chances are, however, that you will want to have sex again. The good news is that there is no reason why you can't. People with HIV enjoy sex and fall in love, just like other people.

If you are having a hard time dealing with negative feelings like anger or fear, you can get help. Talk to your doctor about support groups or counseling. Sex is a very tough topic for many people with HIV—you are not alone.

By reading this information, you are already taking a good first step toward a healthy sex life. Having good information will help you make good decisions.

Talking to Your Doctor

Your doctor or other members of your health care team may ask you about your sexual practices each time you go in for a checkup. It may feel embarrassing at first to be honest and open with your doctor. But he or she is trying to help you stay healthy.

Your doctor and staff will still give you care if you have had sex with someone of the same sex or someone other than your spouse. The

"Sex and Sexuality," U.S. Department of Veterans Affairs, National HIV/AIDS Program (http://www.hiv.va.gov), updated May 2, 2007.

doctor is not there to judge you. It's okay to tell your doctor the truth. It will not affect your medical benefits. It will help your health care team take better care of you.

Make sure you set aside time to ask your doctor questions about safer sex, sexually transmitted diseases (STDs), re-infection, or any other questions you might have. If you feel that you need help dealing with your feelings, ask about support groups or counseling.

Many people with HIV ask their doctor or nurse to talk with them and their partners about HIV and how it is transmitted. They can answer technical questions and address the specifics of your situation. If you live with someone, he or she may have questions about everyday contact as well as sexual contact.

Telling Your Sexual Partners

This may be one of the hardest things you have to do. But you need to tell your sexual partner that you are HIV positive, whether you have a primary partner such as a spouse or girlfriend or boyfriend, have more than one partner, or are single or casually dating.

What follows are tips for talking to your main partner, other partners, and former partners.

Talking to Your Main Partner

If you are in a relationship, one of the first things you will probably think about after learning that you have HIV is telling your partner or partners. For some couples, a positive HIV test may have been expected. For others, the news will be a surprise that can bring up difficult issues.

Your partner may not be prepared to offer you support during a time when you need it. Your partner may be worrying about his or her own HIV status. On the other hand, if you think you may have contracted HIV from your partner, you are probably dealing with your own feelings.

If your partner is not already HIV positive, he or she should get an HIV test right away. Don't assume that the results will come back positive, even if you have been having unsafe sex or sharing needles. Until he or she has been tested, your partner may assume the worst and may blame you for possibly spreading the disease. It is important that you discuss these feelings with each other in an open and honest way, perhaps with a licensed counselor.

Before telling your partner that you have HIV, take some time alone to think about how you want to bring up the subject.

If you or your partner is uncomfortable with sex after learning that you have HIV, keep in mind that you can both enjoy hugging, kissing, and touching. These actions carry no risk for HIV infection, and will definitely make you both feel better. Your partner's feelings may change with time and as he or she learns more about HIV and sex. Some people find it helpful to talk things over with a professional or in a support group.

Talking to New Partners

Talking with someone you are dating casually or someone you met recently about HIV may be difficult. You might not know this person very well or know what kind of reaction to expect. When telling a casual partner or someone you are dating, each situation is different and you might use a different approach each time. Sometimes you may feel comfortable being direct and saying, "Before we have sex, I want you to know that I have HIV."

Another time, you may want to bring it up by saying something like, "Let's talk about safer sex." Whichever approach you choose, you probably want to tell the person that you have HIV before you have sex the first time. Otherwise, there may be hurt feelings or mistrust later. Also be sure to practice safer sex. Whatever way you decide to tell, these tips might help.

Before telling your partner that you have HIV, take some time alone to think about how you want to bring it up.

Also, don't assume that your partner is negative. He or she also may be wondering, "Is this the right time to say that I have HIV?"

Talking to Former Partners

With people you have had sex with in the past or people you have shared needles with, it can be very difficult to explain that you have HIV. However, it is important that they know so that they can decide whether to get tested.

If you need help telling people that you may have been exposed to HIV, most city or county health departments will tell them for you, without using your name. Ask your doctor about this service.

What Is "Safer Sex"?

We know a lot about how HIV is transmitted from person to person. Having safer sex means you take this into account and avoid risky practices.

There are two reasons to practice safer sex: to protect yourself and to protect others.

Protecting Yourself

If you have HIV, you need to protect your health. When it comes to sex, this means practicing safer sex to avoid sexually transmitted diseases like herpes, hepatitis, and even HIV. HIV makes it harder for your body to fight off diseases. What might be a small health problem for someone without HIV could be big health problem for you.

Practicing safer sex can protect you from getting re-infected or "superinfected" with a different strain of HIV. Some strains are resistant to certain drugs, so getting a new strain of HIV could make the disease harder to treat. Experts believe that re-infection is possible although not very likely, but researchers are continuing to study the issue.

Protecting Your Partner

Taking care of others means making sure that you do not pass along HIV to them. If your sex partners already have HIV, you should still avoid infecting them with a different strain of HIV or with another sexually transmitted disease you may be carrying.

Most people would agree that you owe it to your sexual partners to tell them that you have HIV. This is being honest with them. Even though it can be very hard to do, in the long run you will probably feel much better about yourself.

Some people with HIV have found that people who love them think that unsafe sex is a sign of greater love or trust. If someone offers to have unsafe sex with you, it is still up to you to protect them by being safe.

To protect yourself and others, the rules are pretty simple, but you might need to make some changes. Because anal and vaginal sex have the highest risk of transmitting HIV, it is important that you use a condom every time you have anal or vaginal sex.

What Is Risky Sex?

HIV is passed through body fluids such as semen, vaginal fluid, or blood. The less contact you have with these, the lower the risk. The most sensitive areas where these fluids are risky are in the vagina or anus (ass). The skin there is thin, and is easily torn, which makes it easier for the virus to enter your body.

In general, vaginal or anal sex without a condom is the most risky. Kissing, touching, hugging, and mutual masturbation are very low risk. Saliva (spit) and tears aren't risky.

Here is a list of sexual activities organized by level of risk to help you and your partner make decisions:

High Risk

- anal sex without a condom (penis in the anus)
- vaginal sex without a condom (penis in the vagina)

Low Risk

- sex with a condom when you use it right
- oral sex, but don't swallow semen (cum)
- deep kissing (French kissing or tongue kissing)
- sharing sex toys that have been cleaned or covered with a new condom between uses

No Risk

- hugging, massage
- masturbation
- fantasizing
- dry kissing
- phone sex
- cyber sex
- sex toys you don't share

Talking about Safer Sex

You and your partners will have to decide what you are comfortable doing sexually. If you aren't used to talking openly about sex, this could be hard to get used to. Here are some tips:

- Find a time and place outside the bedroom to talk.
- Decide what are your boundaries, concerns, and desires before you start to talk.

- Make sure you clearly state what you want. Use only "I" statements, for example: "I want to use a condom when we have sex."

- Make sure you don't do, or agree to do, anything that you're not 100 percent comfortable with.

- Listen to what your partner is saying. Acknowledge your partner's feelings and opinions. You will need to come up with solutions that work for both of you.

- Be positive. Use reasons for safer sex that are about you, not your partner.

Of course, only you and your partner can decide what level of risk you are willing to take.

Birth Control and HIV

The only forms of birth control that will protect against HIV are abstinence, or using condoms while having sex. Other methods of birth control offer protection against unplanned pregnancy, but do not protect against HIV or other sexually transmitted diseases.

The following birth control options do protect against HIV:

- abstinence (not having sex)

- male condom

- female condom

Birth control options that do not protect against HIV are as follows:

- oral contraceptive ("the pill")

- Depo-Provera (shot)

- emergency contraception ("morning-after pill")

- Norplant

- IUD (intrauterine device)

- diaphragm, cap, and shield

- vasectomy (getting your tubes tied if you are a man)

- tubal ligation (getting your tubes tied if you are a woman)

- withdrawal

Considerations for HIV-Positive Women

If you are in a monogamous relationship and your partner also is HIV positive, you may decide to use a birth control method other than condoms. (These methods won't protect against other STDs or re-infection.)

Safe methods of birth control for HIV-positive women with an HIV-positive partner include the following:

- using a diaphragm
- tubal ligation (getting your tubes tied)

Use the following only after checking with your provider (these may interact with your anti-HIV medications):

- birth control pills
- Depo-Provera
- Norplant

IUD (intrauterine device) is not recommended (may cause irritation and infection, something you want to avoid).

Tips for Using Condoms and Dental Dams

Some people think that using a condom makes sex less fun. Other people have become creative and find condoms sexy. Not having to worry about infecting someone will definitely make sex much more enjoyable.

If you are not used to using condoms: practice, practice, practice.

Condom Dos and Don'ts

Shop around: Use lubricated latex condoms. Always use latex, because lambskin condoms don't block HIV and STDs, and polyurethane condoms break more often than latex. Shop around and find your favorite brand. Try different sizes and shapes. (Yes, they come in different sizes and shapes.) There are a lot of choices—one will work for you.

Keep it fresh: Store condoms loosely in a cool, dry place (not your wallet). Make sure your condoms are fresh—check the expiration date. Throw away condoms that have expired, been very hot, or been washed in the washer. If you think the condom might not be good, get a new one. You and your partner are worth it.

Take it easy: Open the package carefully, so that you don't rip the condom. Be careful if you use your teeth. Make sure that the condom package has not been punctured (there should be a pocket of air). Check the condom for damaged packaging and signs of aging such as brittleness, stickiness, and discoloration.

Keep it hard: Put on the condom after the penis is erect and before it touches any part of a partner's body. If a penis is uncircumcised (uncut), the foreskin must be pulled back before putting on the condom.

Heads up: Make sure the condom is right-side out. It's like a sock—there's a right side and a wrong side. Before you put it on the penis, unroll the condom about half an inch to see which direction it is unrolling. Then put it on the head of the penis and hold the tip of the condom between your fingers as you roll it all the way down the shaft of the penis from head to base. This keeps out air bubbles that can cause the condom to break. It also leaves a space for semen to collect after ejaculation.

Slippery when wet: Put lubricant on after you put on the condom, not before—it could slip off. Add more lube often. Dry condoms break more easily. If you use a lubricant (lube), it should be a water-soluble lubricant (for example, ID Glide, K-Y Jelly, Slippery Stuff, Foreplay, Wet, Astroglide) in order to prevent breakdown of the condom. Products such as petroleum jelly, massage oils, butter, Crisco, Vaseline, and hand creams are not considered water-soluble lubricants and should not be used.

Come and go: Withdraw the penis immediately after ejaculation, while the penis is still erect; grasp the rim of the condom between your fingers and slowly withdraw the penis (with the condom still on) so that no semen is spilled.

Clean up: Throw out the used condom right away. Tie it off to prevent spillage or wrap it in bathroom tissue and put it in the garbage. Condoms can clog toilets. Use a condom only once. Never use the same condom for vaginal and anal intercourse. Never use a condom that has been used by someone else.

Do You Have to Use a Condom for Oral Sex?

It is possible for oral sex to transmit HIV, whether the infected partner is performing or receiving oral sex. But the risk is low compared with unprotected vaginal or anal sex.

If you choose to perform oral sex, and your partner is male, use a latex condom on the penis; or if you or your partner is allergic to latex, plastic (polyurethane) condoms can be used.

If you choose to have oral sex, and your partner is female, use a latex barrier (such as a natural rubber latex sheet, a dental dam, or a cut-open condom that makes a square) between your mouth and the vagina. A latex barrier such as a dental dam reduces the risk of blood or vaginal fluids entering your mouth. Plastic food wrap also can be used as a barrier. If you choose to perform oral sex with either a male or female partner and this sex includes oral contact with your partner's anus (anilingus or rimming), use a latex barrier (such as a natural rubber latex sheet, a dental dam, or a cut-open condom that makes a square) between your mouth and the anus. Plastic food wrap also can be used as a barrier. This barrier is to prevent getting another sexually transmitted disease or parasites, not HIV.

If you choose to share sex toys, such as dildos or vibrators, with your partner, each partner should use a new condom on the sex toy; and be sure to clean sex toys between each use.

Female Condom

Most people have never heard of these, but they may be helpful for you. The female condom is a large condom made of polyurethane fitted with larger and smaller rings at each end that help keep it inside the vagina. They may seem a little awkward at first, but can be an alternative to the male condom. They are made of polyurethane, so any lubricant can be used without damaging them. Female condoms generally cost more than male condoms, and if you aren't used to them, you'll definitely need to practice.

- Store the condom in a cool dry place, not in direct heat or sunlight.

- Throw away any condoms that have expired—the date is printed on individual condom wrappers.

- Check the package for damage and check the condom for signs of aging such as brittleness, stickiness, and discoloration. The female condom is lubricated, so it will be somewhat wet.

- Before inserting the condom, you can squeeze lubricant into the condom pouch and rub the sides together to spread it around.

- Put the condom in before sex play because pre-ejaculatory fluid, which comes from the penis, may contain HIV. The condom can be inserted up to eight hours before sex.

- The female condom has a firm ring at each end of it. To insert the condom, squeeze the ring at the closed end between the fingers (like a diaphragm), and push it up into the back of the vagina. The open ring must stay outside the vagina at all times, and it will partly cover the lip area.

- Do not use a male condom with the female condom.

- Do not use a female condom with a diaphragm.

- If the penis is inserted outside the condom pouch or if the outer ring (open ring) slips into the vagina, stop and take the condom out. Use a new condom before you start sex again.

- Don't tear the condom with fingernails or jewelry.

- Use a female condom only once and properly dispose of it in the trash (not the toilet).

Dental Dams and Plastic Wrap

Even though oral sex is a low-risk sexual practice, you may want to use protection when performing oral sex on someone who has HIV.

Dental dams are small squares of latex that were made originally for use in dental procedures. They are now commonly used as barriers when performing oral sex on women, to keep in vaginal fluids or menstrual blood that could transmit HIV or other STDs.

Some people use plastic wrap instead of a dental dam. It's thinner. Here are some things to remember:

- Before using a dental dam, first check it visually for any holes.

- If the dental dam has cornstarch on it, rinse that off with water (starch in the vagina can cause an infection).

- Cover the woman's genital area with the dental dam.

- For oral-anal sex, cover the opening of the anus with a new dental dam.

- A new dental dam should be used for each act of oral sex; it should never be reused.

Chapter 59

Coping with Your Emotions If You Have HIV/AIDS

Chapter Contents

Section 59.1

Psychiatric Dimensions
of HIV/AIDS

"Let's Talk Facts about Coping with HIV and AIDS." Reprinted with
permission from www.healthyminds.org and the American Psychiatric
Association, © 2005.

What Is AIDS?

Acquired immunodeficiency syndrome (AIDS) is a disease that
compromises the body's immune system, causing it to break down
and rendering it unable to fight off infection. AIDS is caused by the
human immunodeficiency virus (HIV). When a person is infected
with HIV, the virus enters the body and lives and multiplies in the
white blood cells—cells that normally protect us from disease. The
HIV virus weakens the immune system, leaving the body vulnerable to infections and other illnesses, ranging from pneumonia to
cancer.

There are four primary means of becoming infected with HIV:
through sexual intercourse (anal or vaginal); through contact with
contaminated blood and blood products, tissues, and organs; through
use of contaminated needles, syringes, and other piercing instruments;
and, from mother to child during pregnancy or delivery. Some people
fear that HIV might be transmitted in other ways such as through
air, water, or insects; however, no scientific evidence to support any
of these fears has been found.

HIV-Related Mental Health Problems

Mental health problems can strike anybody, but people with HIV
are more likely to experience a range of mental health issues. More
common are feelings of acute emotional distress, depression, and
anxiety, which can often accompany adverse life-events. HIV also
can directly infect the brain, causing impairment to memory and
thinking. In addition, some anti-HIV drugs can have mental health
side effects.

Emotional Distress

Receiving an HIV diagnosis can produce strong emotional reactions. Initial feelings of shock and denial can turn to fear, guilt, anger, sadness, and a sense of hopelessness. Some people even have suicidal thoughts. It is understandable that one might feel helpless and fear illness, disability, and even death.

Support from family and friends can be very helpful at these times, as can professional help. If you are feeling emotionally distressed, it is important that you talk about your feelings. Your physician as well as knowledgeable and supportive friends and loved ones can help. Remember that any strong and lasting emotional reaction to an HIV diagnosis calls for some kind of assistance, and that there is always help through counseling.

Depression

Depression is a serious medical condition that can be paralyzing to sufferers. It is twice as common in people with HIV as in the general population. Depression is characterized by the presence of most or all of the following symptoms:

- low mood
- apathy
- fatigue
- inability to concentrate
- loss of pleasure in activities
- changes in appetite and weight
- trouble sleeping
- low self-worth, and, possibly, thoughts of suicide

There are many different types of treatments for depression, including antidepressants and specific types of psychotherapy, or "talk" therapy. Treatment, however, must be carefully chosen by a physician or a mental health professional based on the patient's physical and mental condition.

Anxiety

Anxiety is a feeling of panic or apprehension, which is often accompanied by the physical symptoms of sweating, shortness of breath, rapid heart beat, agitation, nervousness, headaches, and panic. Anxiety can accompany depression or be seen as a disorder by itself, often caused by circumstances that result in fear, uncertainty, or insecurity.

Each HIV patient and each experience of anxiety is unique and must be treated as such. Many drugs offer effective treatment, and many alternative remedies have proven useful, either alone or in combination with medication. Among them: muscle relaxation, acupuncture, meditation, cognitive behavioral therapy, aerobic exercise, and supportive group therapy.

Substance Use

Substance use is very common among those with HIV infection. Unfortunately, substance use can trigger and often complicate mental health problems. For many, mental health problems predate substance use activity. Substance use can increase levels of distress, interfere with treatment adherence, and lead to impairment in thinking and memory. Diagnosis and treatment by a psychiatrist or other qualified physician is critical as symptoms can mimic psychiatric disorders and other mental health problems.

Cognitive Disorders

Direct or indirect effects of the HIV virus can affect brain functioning. Some medications used to treat HIV infection also can cause similar complications. In people with HIV infection or AIDS, these complications can have significant impact on daily functioning and greatly diminish quality of life.

Among the most common disorders are the following:

- HIV-associated minor cognitive motor disorder

- HIV-1-associated dementia complex

- delirium

- psychosis

Signs of trouble may include forgetfulness, confusion, attention deficits, slurred or changed speech, sudden changes in mood or behavior, difficulty walking, muscle weakness, slowed thinking, and difficulty finding words.

Signs of any of these problems should be discussed with a physician immediately. New anti-HIV therapies in combination with psychiatric medication can reverse delirium and dementia and markedly improve cognition; however, special care must be taken to ensure that the drugs do not interact with HIV medications. Psychotherapy also can help patients understand their condition and adapt to their diminished level of functioning.

Conclusion

HIV infection and AIDS affect all aspects of a person's life. Those with HIV/AIDS must adapt to a chronic, life-threatening illness and corresponding physical and mental challenges. They often face a myriad of emotional demands such as stress, anger, grief, helplessness, depression, and cognitive disorders.

If you have concerns about your or a loved one's reaction to an HIV diagnosis or if you have questions about the mental problems associated with HIV/AIDS, discuss them with a doctor or counselor. Treatments are available and can greatly improve quality of life.

Because HIV infection and AIDS are associated with a number of physical, psychiatric, and psychological issues, this topic cannot be sufficiently reviewed in a brief summary. Readers are encouraged to consult a physician for further information. This summary is not intended to stand on its own as a comprehensive evaluation of HIV and AIDS.

Section 59.2

Depression and HIV/AIDS

"Depression and HIV/AIDS," National Institute of Mental Health
(http://www.nimh.nih.gov), National Institutes of Health (NIH),
NIH Publication No. 02-5005, May 2002.

Symptoms of Depression

If five or more of the following symptoms are present every day
for at least two weeks and interfere with routine daily activities such
as work, self-care, and childcare or social life, seek an evaluation for
depression.

- persistent sad, anxious, or "empty" mood

- feelings of hopelessness, pessimism

- feelings of guilt, worthlessness, helplessness

- loss of interest or pleasure in hobbies and activities that were
  once enjoyed, including sex

- decreased energy, fatigue, being "slowed down"

- difficulty concentrating, remembering, making decisions

- insomnia, early-morning awakening, or oversleeping

- appetite and/or weight changes

- thoughts of death or suicide or suicide attempts

- restlessness, irritability

Research has enabled many men and women, and young people
living with human immunodeficiency virus (HIV), the virus that
causes acquired immunodeficiency syndrome (AIDS), to lead fuller,
more productive lives. As with other serious illnesses such as cancer,
heart disease, or stroke, however, HIV often can be accompanied by
depression, an illness that can affect mind, mood, body, and behavior.
Treatment for depression helps people manage both diseases, thus
enhancing survival and quality of life.

Despite the enormous advances in brain research in the past 20 years, depression often goes undiagnosed and untreated. Although as many as one in three persons with HIV may suffer from depression, the warning signs of depression are often misinterpreted. People with HIV, their families and friends, and even their physicians may assume that depressive symptoms are an inevitable reaction to being diagnosed with HIV. But depression is a separate illness that can and should be treated, even when a person is undergoing treatment for HIV or AIDS. Some of the symptoms of depression could be related to HIV, specific HIV-related disorders, or medication side effects. However, a skilled health professional will recognize the symptoms of depression and inquire about their duration and severity, diagnose the disorder, and suggest appropriate treatment.

Depression Facts

Depression is a serious medical condition that affects thoughts, feelings, and the ability to function in everyday life. Depression can occur at any age. The National Institute of Mental Health (NIMH)-sponsored studies estimate that 6 percent of nine- to seventeen-year-olds in the U.S. and almost 10 percent of American adults, or about 19 million people age 18 and older, experience some form of depression every year. Although available therapies alleviate symptoms in over 80 percent of those treated, less than half of people with depression get the help they need.

Depression results from abnormal functioning of the brain. The causes of depression are currently a matter of intense research. An interaction between genetic predisposition and life history appear to determine a person's level of risk. Episodes of depression may then be triggered by stress, difficult life events, side effects of medications, or the effects of HIV on the brain. Whatever its origins, depression can limit the energy needed to keep focused on staying healthy, and research shows that it may accelerate HIV's progression to AIDS.

HIV/AIDS Facts

Many people do not develop any symptoms when they first become infected with HIV. Some people, however, have a flu-like illness within a month or two after exposure to the virus. More persistent or severe symptoms may not surface for a decade or more after HIV first enters the body in adults, or within two years in children born with HIV infection. This period of "asymptomatic"(without symptoms) infection is highly individual. During the asymptomatic period, however, the virus is actively multiplying, infecting, and killing cells of the immune system, and people are highly infectious.

As the immune system deteriorates, a variety of complications start to take over. For many people, their first sign of infection is large lymph nodes or "swollen glands" that may be enlarged for more than three months. Other symptoms often experienced months to years before the onset of AIDS include the following:

- lack of energy

- weight loss

- frequent fevers and sweats

- persistent or frequent yeast infections (oral or vaginal)

- persistent skin rashes or flaky skin

- pelvic inflammatory disease in women that does not respond to treatment

- short-term memory loss

Many people are so debilitated by the symptoms of AIDS that they cannot hold steady employment or do household chores. Other people with AIDS may experience phases of intense life-threatening illness followed by phases in which they function normally.

Because early HIV infection often causes no symptoms, a doctor or other health care worker usually can diagnose it by testing a person's blood for the presence of antibodies (disease-fighting proteins) to HIV. HIV antibodies generally do not reach levels in the blood which the doctor can see until one to three months following infection, and it may take the antibodies as long as six months to be produced in quantities large enough to show up in standard blood tests. Therefore, people exposed to the virus should get an HIV test within this time period.

Researchers have developed antiretroviral drugs to fight both HIV infection and its associated infections and cancers. Currently available drugs do not cure people of HIV infection or AIDS, however, and they all have side effects that can be severe. Because no vaccine for HIV is available, the only way to prevent infection by the virus is to avoid behaviors that put a person at risk of infection, such as sharing needles and having unprotected sex.

Get Treatment for Depression

While there are many different treatments for depression, they must be carefully chosen by a trained professional based on the circumstances of the person and family. Prescription antidepressant medications are generally well-tolerated and safe for people with HIV. There are, however, possible interactions among some of the medications and side effects that require careful monitoring. Specific types of psychotherapy, or "talk" therapy, also can relieve depression.

Some individuals with HIV attempt to treat their depression with herbal remedies. However, use of herbal supplements of any kind should be discussed with a physician before they are tried. Scientists have discovered that St. John's wort, an herbal remedy sold over-the-counter and promoted as a treatment for mild depression, can have harmful interactions with other medications, including those prescribed for HIV. In particular, St. John's wort reduces blood levels of the protease inhibitor indinavir (Crixivan) and probably the other protease inhibitor drugs as well. If taken together, the combination could allow the AIDS virus to rebound, perhaps in a drug-resistant form. [See chapter 35, "Alternative and Complementary Therapies."]

Treatment for depression in the context of HIV or AIDS should be managed by a mental health professional—for example, a psychiatrist, psychologist, or clinical social worker—who is in close communication with the physician providing the HIV/AIDS treatment. This is especially important when antidepressant medication is prescribed, so that potentially harmful drug interactions can be avoided. In some cases, a mental health professional that specializes in treating individuals with depression and co-occurring physical illnesses such as HIV/AIDS may be available. People with HIV/AIDS who develop depression, as well as people in treatment for depression who subsequently contract HIV, should make sure to tell any physician they visit about the full range of medications they are taking.

Recovery from depression takes time. Medications for depression can take several weeks to work and may need to be combined with ongoing psychotherapy. Not everyone responds to treatment in the same way. Prescriptions and dosing may need to be adjusted. No matter how advanced the HIV, however, the person does not have to suffer from depression. Treatment can be effective.

It takes more than access to good medical care for persons living with HIV to stay healthy. A positive outlook, determination, and discipline are also required to deal with the stresses of avoiding high-risk behaviors, keeping up with the latest scientific advances, adhering to complicated medication regimens, reshuffling schedules for doctor visits, and grieving over the death of loved ones.

Other mental disorders, such as bipolar disorder (manic-depressive illness) and anxiety disorders, may occur in people with HIV or AIDS, and they too can be effectively treated. For more information about these and other mental illnesses, contact NIMH.

Remember, depression is a treatable disorder of the brain. Depression can be treated in addition to whatever other illnesses a person might have, including HIV. If you think you may be depressed or know someone who is, don't lose hope. Seek help for depression.

Chapter 60

Preventing Infections from Pets

Should I keep my pets?

Yes. Most people with human immunodeficiency virus (HIV) can and should keep their pets. Owning a pet can be rewarding. Pets can help you feel psychologically and even physically better. For many people, pets are more than just animals—they are like members of the family. However, you should know the health risks of owning a pet or caring for animals. Animals may carry infections that can be harmful to you. Your decision to own or care for pets should be based on knowing what you need to do to protect yourself from these infections.

What kinds of infections could I get from an animal?

Animals can have cryptosporidiosis (crypto), toxoplasmosis (toxo), *Mycobacterium avium* complex (MAC), and other diseases. These diseases can give you problems like severe diarrhea, brain infections, and skin lesions.

What can I do to protect myself from infections spread by animals?

- Always wash your hands well with soap and water after playing with or caring for animals. This is especially important before eating or handling food.

Centers for Disease Control and Prevention (http://www.cdc.gov), National Center for HIV, STD, and TB Prevention, updated April 2003.

- Be careful about what your pet eats and drinks. Feed your pet only pet food or cook all meat thoroughly before giving it to your pet. Don't give your pet raw or undercooked meat. Don't let your pets drink from toilet bowls or get into garbage. Don't let your pets hunt or eat another animal's stool (droppings).

- Don't handle animals that have diarrhea. If the pet's diarrhea lasts for more than one or two days, have a friend or relative who does not have HIV take your pet to your veterinarian. Ask the veterinarian to check the pet for infections that may be the cause of diarrhea.

- Don't bring home an unhealthy pet. Don't get a pet that is younger than six months old—especially if it has diarrhea. If you are getting a pet from a pet store, animal breeder, or animal shelter (pound), check the sanitary conditions and license of these sources. If you are not sure about the animal's health, have it checked out by your veterinarian.

- Don't touch stray animals because you could get scratched or bitten. Stray animals can carry many infections.

- Don't ever touch the stool of any animal.

- Ask someone who is not infected with HIV and is not pregnant to change your cat's litter box daily. If you must clean the box yourself, wear vinyl or household cleaning gloves and immediately wash your hands well with soap and water right after changing the litter.

- Have your cat's nails clipped so it can't scratch you. Discuss other ways to prevent scratching with your veterinarian. If you do get scratched or bitten, immediately wash the wounds well with soap and water. (If you are bitten, you may need to seek medical advice.)

- Don't let your pet lick your mouth or any open cuts or wounds you may have.

- Don't kiss your pet.

- Keep fleas off your pet.

- Avoid reptiles such as snakes, lizards, and turtles. If you touch any reptile, immediately wash your hands well with soap and water.

- Wear vinyl or household cleaning gloves when you clean aquariums or animal cages and wash your hands well right after you finish.

- Avoid exotic pets such as monkeys and ferrets, or wild animals such as raccoons, lions, bats, and skunks.

I have a job that involves working with animals. Should I quit?

Jobs working with animals (such as jobs in pet stores, animal clinics, farms, and slaughterhouses) carry a risk for infections. Talk with your doctor about whether you should work with animals. People who work with animals should take these extra precautions:

- Follow your worksite's rules to stay safe and reduce any risk of infection. Use or wear personal protective gear, such as coveralls, boots, and gloves.

- Don't clean chicken coops or dig in areas where birds roost if histoplasmosis [his-to-plaz-MO-sis] is found in the area.

- Don't touch young farm animals, especially if they have diarrhea.

Can someone with HIV give it to their pets?

No. HIV can not be spread to, from, or by cats, dogs, birds, or other pets. Many viruses cause diseases that are like AIDS, such as feline leukemia virus, or FeLV, in cats. These viruses cause illness only in a certain animal and cannot infect other animals or humans. For example, FeLV infects only cats. It does not infect humans or dogs.

Are there any tests a pet should have before I bring it home?

A pet should be in overall good health. You don't need special tests unless the animal has diarrhea or looks sick. If your pet looks sick, your veterinarian can help you choose the tests it needs.

What should I do when I visit friends or relatives who have animals?

When you visit anyone with pets, take the same precautions you would in your own home. Don't touch animals that may not be healthy. You may want to tell your friends and family about the need for these precautions before you plan any visits.

Should children with HIV handle pets?

The same precautions apply for children as for adults. However, children may want to snuggle more with their pets. Some pets, like cats, may bite or scratch to get away from children. Adults should be extra watchful and supervise an HIV-infected child's handwashing to prevent infections.

Chapter 61

Tips and Strategies to Improve Medication Adherence

Staying on a treatment regimen is difficult under the best of conditions. Even doctors can find it difficult to take a simple course of antibiotics as directed. Regimens for HIV disease sometimes require a person to take a dozen or more pills a day, with specific timing and diet restrictions. When a person also uses drugs for other infections, the total daily pill count soars. Keeping up with your meds alone becomes a major activity. So it's little wonder that people have trouble keeping up with the program.

Things to Consider before You Start Therapy

Taking on complex, long-term treatment doesn't feel natural to most people. However, this challenge is not unique to people with HIV. Millions have learned to cope with diseases that require long-term management, including diabetes, mental illness, and heart disease, among others.

Whether or not you feel you're able to adhere to a new regimen may be one thing to consider—along with your lab results and overall general health—in deciding the right time to begin anti-HIV therapy. Your readiness, or ability to commit to the demands of therapy, is an important consideration to discuss with your doctor.

"Adherence: Keeping Up with Your Meds," From Project Inform, © 2007. For more information, contact the National HIV/AIDS Treatment Infoline, 1-800-822-7422, or visit our website at www.projectinform.org.

Giving careful thought to what benefits you hope to get from treatment, how you'll evaluate the benefit, and how you might manage side effects will be helpful. Some people try a "dry run" before beginning therapy, like taking empty gel caps, or candies like M&Ms, on the prescribed schedule while sticking to any diet requirements. While this doesn't prepare one for potential side effects, it can help you identify times when remembering to take therapy might be more of a challenge.

Perhaps the first and most important aspect of adherence lies in choosing the right therapy for you in the first place. Drugs can differ in many ways including:

- whether or not they can be taken with food;
- whether they are taken by mouth or injection;
- how many times a day they must be taken;
- how many pills per day are needed;
- what other drugs or complementary therapies they can and cannot be used with;
- their side effects and how they make a person feel; and
- some require refrigeration or other special handling.

Similarly, people differ widely in their habits and needs. A few examples:

- Some people are bound to rigid work schedules, such as hourly workers.
- Some have constantly changing schedules, or they routinely move in and out of different time zones, such as airline workers.
- Some people are unable to work and their schedules are dictated by a seemingly endless string of medical appointments.
- Some also have children, parents or partners to care for.
- Some have people around to help remind them of their drug schedules, while others are alone and must rely on timers, pill boxes or other devices.
- Some people have wasting syndrome or infections that might make eating difficult; others have no dietary problems but don't eat regularly.
- Finally, some people have to deal with other challenges like substance abuse or homelessness.

To find a treatment regimen you can live with, it's necessary to settle two sets of requirements: yours and the drug's. People who lead busy but largely unstructured lives might prefer drugs that can be taken easily with or without food. This may make it easier to fit therapy into changing routines. Others whose time is tightly structured by work might find it easier to go on more demanding regimens. These people can select a regimen purely on the basis of its potency.

People who have trouble eating or who struggle with weight loss may wish to avoid drugs that can't be taken with foods or even conversely, those requiring that they be taken with food. Others who take many other drugs for opportunistic infections or other health conditions might avoid anti-HIV drugs that have many drug interactions. They might even avoid creating regimens that require taking many more pills. Also, the more anti-HIV drugs you've already used, often the fewer choices you have about what to use next. Thus, often in more advanced disease, prior drug history tends to dictate what can and can't be done.

There may not be any perfect regimen for you, but there are options that are more and less easy to adapt to your life. The goal is to select a regimen you can live with—one that fits with who you are and how you live. Once you select a regimen, sticking to it requires planning, support, and commitment.

One study suggests that about 12 percent of people miss one dose in the past day, and 11 percent the day before that. Other studies report that nearly all who failed to achieve and sustain a viral load below the limit of detection had greatly deviated from their prescribed regimens for a month or more.

There are many reasons for failing to stay on your treatment regimen. One study showed that of those people who missed one or more doses:

- 40 percent simply forgot.
- 37 percent slept through a dose.
- 34 percent were away from home.
- 27 percent changed their therapy routine.
- 22 percent were busy.
- 13 percent were sick.
- 10 percent experienced side effects.
- 9 percent were depressed.

Planning

Stable access to drugs is critical for their effective use. People cannot stay on a regimen if they don't have constant access to their drugs. While it may sound obvious, many people taking HIV meds sometimes find themselves running short of one or another drug for a variety of reasons. This is often because of poor planning. Skipping doses because you've run out of a drug is still skipping doses.

Some drugs have different storage requirements than others, so your planning must also address these storage needs. This is primarily true of ritonavir and lopinavir, which for storage over one or two months respectively, need refrigeration. Once storage is addressed, it's helpful to put aside a full week's supply, in an accessible place, right after getting your drugs, and then start using the rest of that supply. This creates an emergency stash should unforeseen circumstances cause your basic supply to run short. Your stash should be rotated or replaced once a month to keep it fresh.

Keeping a steady supply of meds requires you to work closely with your doctor and pharmacist. And, when using AIDS Drug Assistance Programs or pharmaceutical company patient assistance programs, even more of the burden falls on you to make sure you order supplies as the program requires and still have a safety net for unforeseen situations. The main point is to always stay at least a week ahead of your needs.

People differ in their abilities to adhere to their regimens and this is influenced by lifestyle and other factors. People dealing with major life problems like active drug use or homelessness face difficult challenges with adherence. But that doesn't mean adherence is impossible. People with depression are also more likely to have difficulty with adherence. If you suffer from depression or mental illness and are considering treatment, consult a mental health expert as well as your regular doctor.

In reality, only you can decide whether you're ready and committed enough to maintain a steady course of treatment. If you are not ready or not in a position to make a serious effort at adherence, you might be better off to delay treatment. This doesn't jeopardize your ability to use effective treatment later. In contrast, misusing your drugs can jeopardize your future options by encouraging drug resistance. This can affect entire classes of anti-HIV therapy.

Building a Support Network for Yourself

Setting up a good relationship with your doctor is critical for maintaining your adherence. Your doctor should know the current standards of care for treating HIV. He or she should spend time with you to fully explain the benefits and challenges of treatment.

If you decide to start treatment, it's important to clarify your regimen with your doctor. Knowing what drugs you're taking and why will help you better understand the importance of adherence. One survey showed that the vast majority of people were unclear of their regimens only ten minutes after talking with their doctors. Some understood the dose but were confused about diet restrictions. Others were unclear on the correct doses or the timing of them.

Since adjusting your diet can be difficult at first, it's important to know what and when you can and cannot eat. Just as important, try to understand exactly what is meant by the drug's diet requirements. For example, many people interpret them for indinavir to mean that it should not be taken with food, which can be difficult for many people. The actual requirement is that it shouldn't be taken with fatty foods. Light snacks and non-fat foods can be taken with the drug without concern.

Similarly, the requirements for nelfinavir are often thought to mean that it must be taken with food. In fact, the label says only that it should be taken with food. In some cases, there's a genuine medical need to take a drug with or without food. In other cases, like for ddI, taking it with food is recommended only to lessen its side effects or unpleasant aftertaste.

A useful way to understand your treatment regimen is writing down instructions and repeating them back to your doctor. You can check them again with your pharmacist when you pick up or order the drugs. Use the team approach. Your doctor, nurse, pharmacist, and other providers can help you start and maintain effective therapy.

Some researchers note that people who foster friendly and supportive relationships with medical office staff get better service from them. Bringing another person—a family member, friend, or advocate—to appointments ensures that two people can ask questions and get information.

Ask your doctor to be clear about side effects and their management. Being mentally prepared for side effects can make them easier to manage if they occur. Make a plan with your doctor around what to do if you experience a difficult side effect. Knowing that you will have timely contact with a doctor may reassure you that side effects will be managed well.

It is also important to find out what to do if you miss a dose. If you do miss one, ask your doctor how you should handle it—if you should make it up or just take the next scheduled one at the usual time. Also, note the missed dose and the reason for missing. There may be a strategy you can use to avoid missing future doses.

If you are not able to take all the drugs in your regimen, don't take a partial dose. Contact your doctor immediately if you can't take your full dose for whatever reason. In this situation it might be necessary for you to stop all of your anti-HIV drugs until you're able to take a complete dose of all the medications in the regimen again.

Committing to Staying on Your Therapy

Resistance is another reason to adhere to your regimen. Today's potent combination therapy has brought new hope and new challenges to people living with HIV. However, if therapy is not used properly (like skipping doses, taking lower than prescribed doses, or not taking them on time), drug resistance will probably develop faster. In this case, the potential benefits of therapy can be lost.

In order to prevent drug resistance, it's important to keep enough drug in your bloodstream 24 hours a day. Each time you miss a dose, the drug blood level falls below the minimum necessary level for several hours. This creates an opportunity for HIV to develop resistance to the drug(s).

Moreover, resistance to one drug may result in resistance to other drugs of the same class, called cross-resistance. This is particularly true about non-nucleoside reverse transcriptase inhibitors (NNRTIs). High level resistance to any one of these drugs almost certainly passes on some degree of resistance to all the other NNRTIs.

There's little debate about it being difficult to always adhere to today's complex regimens. It is somewhat less clear how much non-adherence is tolerable before resistance becomes a threat. There are no data telling us exactly when resistance begins. There is, however, plenty of evidence that people who are adherent have better and more sustained anti-HIV responses. While no single episode of a skipped or late dose is likely—by itself—to trigger resistance, the more often they occur, the more likely it is to develop drug resistance.

A Final Thought

Perhaps the greatest way that adherence to HIV treatments differs from adherence in other chronic illnesses is the lack of immediate symptoms or consequences when adherence fails. This lack of a rapid response places more of the burden for adherence on the mind and less on the immediate reaction of the body. A person living with HIV must take a long-term view in order to have a long-term future.

Adherence also challenges many of the support systems for people living with HIV. Some doctors have less time to spend educating their patients. As well, most doctors have little or no training in the tools that might help people stay on their treatment regimens. Sometimes, in order to be fully supported, people may need to seek help from others, like treatment support groups, case managers or treatment buddies.

The best long-term solutions for treating HIV—outside of a cure—must focus on making better and longer-lasting therapies. These include ones that are easier to use, more easily absorbed, have fewer side effects and drug interactions, and maintain more consistent drug levels in blood. This work is underway for some treatments that may require only once-a-day dosing. [See chapter 34, "Once-a-Day Medications for HIV Treatment."]

In the meantime, there are many ideas for what you can do to make the most out of your treatment regimen. Consider the ones presented here or come up with your own solutions that make the most sense for your life.

Strategies for Adherence

Adherence strategies may not work for everyone. Because of cultural, gender, and socioeconomic differences, these suggestions are more appropriate for some people than others. Different issues are more important in some settings than others.

For example, some people have a great need for privacy around their HIV status and taking medications. This places greater emphasis on planning ahead for moments of privacy each day. For people struggling with lack of housing, active drug use, or untreated mental health conditions, adherence strategies will often go beyond what we cover here. Still, even in the most challenging situations, people have daily routines that can be used as triggers for taking meds.

Adherence strategies can and must vary from person to person. The best way to ensure success is your motivation and commitment to your regimen. It may help to know that many people have accommodated long-term treatment in their lives. People with chronic illnesses have long shown that it can be done. It may take a few tries before you find the approach that works best for you.

Some of the following strategies and tools have worked for many people taking combination therapy:

- Integrate your regimen into your daily routines. Most people find it easier to fit medications into their lives, rather than scheduling their lives around their medication. Use a daily activity, one that you do every day without fail, to prompt you to take your meds. Take them before the activity; it's easier to remember.

- Count out all your meds in daily doses for a week at a time. Use a pillbox or a nail organizer from a hardware store to hold each dose. Setting up a weekly pillbox needs to become routine each weekend. Drugs can also be divided daily by dose and put in separate canisters marked with the dosage times—some use film canisters. Some people put each canister near the place they'll take a dose. For example, put the morning dose by the coffee pot, evening dose by the TV.

- Keep a checklist for doses taken with a space to note how you're feeling.

- Use an electronic pillbox or beeping alarm to remind you when to take your meds. The downside of these mechanisms is that the electronic pillboxes are too small and the alarms may be very obvious.

- Use a daily planner, especially at the start of a new regimen. Inserting medication requirements in a planner, as if they were appointments, can be a useful reminder for many people. Others use hand-held computers or electronic organizers to remind them of daily doses. These kinds of devices can be purchased for under $50.

- Evaluate your regimen about two weeks after you start it. It may take a few weeks of experimenting to figure out how to best schedule your meds with other events in your life. For this reason it may be useful to start a dry run of therapy, allowing time to adjust your routines before actually taking the drugs.

- Plan ahead for weekends and vacations. People often miss doses when they're away from home. For most, weekends are different from normal weekday routines, so it's important to plan ahead. Take into account the changed environment. Will you feel comfortable with your normal routine or will you need other strategies?

- Keep all your meds with you when you travel. Baggage can be lost or delayed.

- Plan ahead for privacy if you need to hide the fact that you're taking medication. In this situation, try to find at least one person with a similar problem with whom you can discuss strategy. You could adjust your lunch or break schedule to ensure privacy or keep water in your bedroom at all times.

- Keep a diary. Include whatever is important to you: when you took treatment, reason for missed doses, how you feel, etc. Keeping a record like this reminds you how well, or poorly, you are doing with adherence.

- Use your support network to remind you of your medication needs. Some people have a treatment buddy who can make daily reminder phone calls.

- Set up a support network for your emotional needs. It's hard to take treatment and also deal with daily stress, whether it's taking care of children, working or dealing with illness.

Chapter 62

Caring for Someone with AIDS at Home

How to Get Ready to Take Care of Someone at Home

Every situation is different, but here are some tips to get you started.

First, read this chapter. Have the person living with HIV or AIDS read it. Have other people living in the same house as the person with AIDS read it. The information in this chapter is for both people with diagnosed AIDS and people with HIV infection who are sick and need care. If you have trouble understanding any of the words, see the glossary chapter.

Take a home care course, if possible. Learn the skills you need to take care of someone at home and how to manage special situations. Your local Red Cross chapter, Visiting Nurses Association, state health department, or HIV/AIDS service organization can help you find a home care course. See chapter 74, "Directory of Organizations and Hotlines," for more information.

Talk with the person you will be caring for. Ask them what they need. If you are nervous about caring for them, say so. Ask if it

Centers for Disease Control and Prevention (http://www.cdc.gov); National Center for HIV, STD, and TB Prevention; revised June 2001. This revision is the most recent available from CDC; despite the older date, the information is still helpful to those providing home care for somcone with HIV/AIDS.

is okay for you to talk to their doctor, nurse, social worker, case manager, other health care professional, or lawyer when you need to. Together you can work out what is best for both of you.

Talk with the doctor, nurse, social worker, case manager, and other health care workers who are also providing care. They may need the patient's permission, sometimes in writing, to talk to you, but you need to talk to these people to find out how you can help. Work with them and the person you are caring for to develop a plan for who does what.

- Get clear, written information about medicines and other care you'll give. Ask what each drug does and what side effects to look out for.

- Ask the doctor or nurse what changes in the person's health or behavior to watch for. For example, a cough, fever, diarrhea, or confusion may mean an infection or problem that needs a new medicine or even putting the person in the hospital.

- You also need to know whom to call for help or information and when to call them. Make a list of doctors, nurses, and other people you might need to talk to quickly, their phone numbers, and when they are available. Keep this list by the phone.

Talk to a lawyer or AIDS support organization. For some medical care or life support decisions, you may need to be legally named as the care coordinator. If you are going to help file insurance claims, apply for government aid, pay bills, or handle other business for the person with AIDS, you may also need a power of attorney. There are many sources of help for people with AIDS, and you can help the person with AIDS get what they are entitled to.

Think about joining a support group or talking to a counselor. Taking care of someone who is sick can be hard emotionally as well as physically. Talking about it with people with the same kind of worries helps sometimes. You can learn how other people cope and realize that you are not alone.

Take care of yourself. You can't take care of someone else if you are sick or upset. Get the rest and exercise you need to keep going. You also need to do some things you enjoy, such as visit your friends and relatives. Many AIDS service organizations can help with "respite care" and send someone to be with the person you're caring for while you get out of the house for awhile.

Giving Care

People living with AIDS should take care of themselves as much as they can for as long as they can. They need to be and feel as independent as possible. They need to control their own schedules, make their own decisions, and do what they want to do as much as they are able. They should develop their own exercise program and eating plan. In addition to regular visits to the doctor, many people with AIDS work at staying healthy by eating properly, sleeping regularly, doing physical exercises, praying or meditating, or other things. If the person you are caring for finds something that helps them, encourage them to keep it up. An exercise program can help maintain weight and muscle tone and can make a person feel better if it is tailored to what the person can do. Well-balanced, good-tasting meals help people feel good, give them energy, and help their body fight illness. People with HIV infection are better off if they don't drink alcoholic drinks, smoke, or use illegal drugs. Keeping up-to-date on new treatments and understanding what to expect from treatments the person is taking are also important.

There are some simple things you can do to help someone with AIDS feel comfortable at home.

- Respect their independence and privacy.

- Give them control as much as possible. Ask to enter their room, ask permission to sit with them, etc., saying, "Can I help you with that?" lets them keep control.

- Ask them what you can do to make them comfortable. Many people feel shy about asking for help, especially help with things like using the toilet, bathing, shaving, eating, and dressing.

- Keep the home clean and looking bright and cheerful.

- Let the person with AIDS stay in a room that is near a bathroom.

- Leave tissues, towels, a trash basket, extra blankets, and other things the person might need close by so these things can be reached from the bed or chair.

If the person you care caring for has to spend most of their time in bed, be sure to help them change position often. If possible, a person with AIDS should get out of bed as often as they can. A nurse can show you how to help someone move from a bed to a chair without hurting yourself or them. This helps prevent stiff joints, bedsores, and some kinds of pneumonia. They may also need your help to turn over or to adjust the pillows or blankets. A medical "trapeze" over the bed can help the person shift position by themselves if they are strong enough. If they are so weak they can't turn over, have a nurse show you how to use a sheet to help roll the person in bed from side to side. Usually a person in bed needs to change position at least every four hours.

Bedsores

Bedsores or other broken skin can be serious problems for someone with AIDS. In addition to changing position in bed often, to help keep skin healthy, put extra-soft material (sheepskin, "egg crate" foam, or water mattresses) under the person, keep the sheets dry and free from wrinkles, and massage the back and other parts of the body (like hips, elbows, and ankles) that press down on the bed. Report any red or broken areas on the skin to the doctor or nurse right away.

Exercises

Even in bed, a person can do simple arm, hand, leg, and foot exercises. These are usually called "range of motion" exercises. These exercises help prevent stiff, sore points and help keep the blood moving. A doctor, nurse, or physical therapist can show you how to help.

Breathing

If someone is having trouble breathing, sitting them up may help. Raise the head of a hospital-type bed or use extra pillows or some other soft back support. If they have severe trouble breathing, they need to see a doctor.

Comfort

A good back rub can help a person relax as well as help their circulation. A nurse, physical therapist, or book on massage can give you some tips on how to give a good back rub. Put books, remote controls, water, tissues, and a bell to call for help within easy reach. If the person can't get up, put a urinal or bedpan within easy reach.

Providing Emotional Support

You are caring for a person, not just a body; their feelings are important too. Since every person is different, there are no rules about what to do or say, but here are some ideas that may help.

- Keep them involved in their care. Don't do everything for them or make all their decisions. Nobody likes feeling helpless.

- Have them help out around the house if they can. Everybody likes to feel useful. They want to be part of the group, contributing what they can.

- Include them in the household. Make them part of normal talk about books, TV shows, music, what is going on in the world, and so on. Many people will want to feel involved in the things that are happening around them. But you don't always have to talk; just being there is sometimes enough. Just watching TV together or sitting and reading in the same room is often comforting.

- Talk about things. Sometime they may need to talk about AIDS or talk through their own situation as a way to think out loud. Having AIDS can make a person angry, frustrated, depressed, scared, and lonely, just like any other serious illness. Listening, trying to understand, showing you care, and helping them work through their emotions is a big part of home care. A support group of other people with AIDS can also be a good place for them to talk things out. Contact the National Association of People with AIDS for information about support groups in your area. [See chapter 74, "Directory of Organizations," for contact information.] If they want professional counseling, help them get it.

- Invite their friends over to visit. A little socializing can be good for everyone.

- Touch them. Hug them; kiss them; pat them; hold their hands to show that you care. Some people may not want physical closeness, but if they do, touch is a powerful way of saying you care.

- Get out together. If they are able, go to social events, shopping, riding around, walking around the block, or just into the park, yard, or porch to sit in the sun and breathe fresh air.

Guarding against Infections

People living with AIDS can get very sick from common germs and infections. Hugging, holding hands, giving massages, and many other types of touching are safe for you, and needed by the person with AIDS. But you have to be careful not to spread germs that can hurt the person you are caring for.

Wash Your Hands

Washing your hands is the single best way to kill germs. Do it often. Wash your hands after you go to the bathroom and before you fix food. Wash your hands again before and after feeding them, bathing them, helping them go to the bathroom, or giving other care. Wash your hands if you sneeze or cough; touch your nose, mouth, or genitals; handle garbage or animal litter; or clean the house. If you touch anybody's blood, semen, urine, vaginal fluid, or feces, wash your hands immediately. If you are caring for more than one person, wash your hands after helping one person and before helping the next person. Wash your hands with warm, soapy water for at least 15 seconds. Clean under your finger nails and between your fingers. If your hands get dry or sore, put on hand cream or lotion, but keep washing your hands frequently.

Cover Your Sores

If you have any cuts or sores, especially on your hands, you must take extra care not to infect the person with AIDS or yourself. If you have cold sores, fever blisters, or any other skin infection, don't touch the person or their things. You could pass your infection to them. If you have to give care, cover your sores with bandages, and wash your hands before touching the person. If the rash or sores are on your hands, wear disposable gloves. Do not use gloves more than one time; throw them away and get a new pair. If you have boils, impetigo, or shingles, if at all possible, stay away from the person with AIDS until you are well.

Keep Sick People Away

If you or anybody else is sick, stay away from the person with AIDS until you're well. A person with AIDS often can't fight off colds, flu, or other common illnesses. If you are sick and nobody else can do what needs to be done for the person with AIDS, wear a well-fitting, surgical-type mask that covers your mouth and nose and wash your hands before coming near the person with AIDS.

Watch Out for Chickenpox

Chickenpox can kill a person with AIDS. If the person you are caring for has already had the chickenpox, they probably won't get it again. But, just to be on the safe side, see the following list:

- Never let anybody with chickenpox in the same room as a person with AIDS, at least not until all the chickenpox sores have completely crusted over.

- Don't let anybody who recently has been near somebody with chickenpox in the same room as a person who has AIDS. After three weeks, the person who was exposed to the chickenpox can visit, if they aren't sick. Most adults have had chickenpox, but you have to be very careful about children visiting or living in the house if they have not yet had chickenpox. If you are the person who was near somebody with chickenpox and you have to help the person with AIDS, wear a well-fitting, surgical-type mask, wash your hands before doing what you have to do for the person with AIDS, and stay in the room as short a time as you can. Tell the person with AIDS why you are staying away from them.

- Don't let anybody with shingles (herpes zoster) near a person with AIDS until all the shingles have healed over. The germ that causes shingles can also cause chickenpox. If you have shingles and have to help the person with AIDS, cover all the sores completely and wash your hands carefully before helping the person with AIDS.

- Call the doctor as soon as possible if the person with AIDS does get near somebody with chickenpox or shingles. There is a medicine that can make the chickenpox less dangerous, but it must be given very soon after the person has been around someone with the germ.

Get Your Shots

Everybody living with or helping take care of a person with AIDS should make sure they took all their "childhood" shots (immunizations). This is not only to keep you from getting sick, but also to keep you from getting sick and accidentally spreading the illness to the person with AIDS. Just to be sure, ask your doctor if you need any shots or boosters for measles, mumps, or rubella since these shots may not have been available when you were a child. Discuss any vaccinations with your doctor and the doctor of the person with AIDS before you get the shot. If the person with AIDS is near a person with measles, call the doctor that day. There is a medicine that can make the measles less dangerous, but it has to be given very soon after the person is around the germ.

Children or adults who live with someone with AIDS and who need to get vaccinated against polio should get an injection with "inactivated virus" vaccine. The regular oral polio vaccine has weakened polio virus that can spread from the person who got the vaccine to the person with AIDS and give them polio.

Everyone living with a person with AIDS should get a flu shot every year to reduce the chances of spreading the flu to the person with AIDS. Everyone living with a person with AIDS should be checked for tuberculosis (TB) every year.

Be Careful with Pets and Gardening

Pets can give love and companionship. Having a pet around can make a person with AIDS feel better and enjoy life more. However, people with HIV or AIDS should not touch pet litter boxes, feces, bird droppings, or water in fish tanks. Many pet animals carry germs that don't make healthy people sick, but can make the person with AIDS very sick. A person with AIDS can have pets, but must wash their hands with soap and water after handling the pet. Someone who does not have HIV infection must clean the litter boxes, cages, fish tanks, pet beds, and other things. Wear rubber gloves when you clean up after pets and wash your hands before and after cleaning. Empty litter boxes every day, don't just sift. Just like the people living with AIDS, pets need yearly checkups and current vaccinations. If the pet gets sick, take it to the veterinarian right away. Someone with AIDS should not touch a sick animal.

Gardening can also be a problem. Germs live in garden or potting soil. A person with AIDS can garden, but they must wear work gloves while handling dirt and must wash their hands before and after handling dirt. You should do the same.

Personal Items

A person with HIV infection should not share razors, toothbrushes, tweezers, nail or cuticle scissors, pierced earrings or other "pierced" jewelry, or any other item that might have their blood on it.

Laundry

Clothes and bed sheets used by someone with AIDS can be washed the same way as other laundry. If you use a washing machine, either hot or cold water can be used, with regular laundry detergent. If clothes or sheets have blood, vomit, semen, vaginal fluids, urine, or feces on them, use disposable gloves and handle the clothes or sheets as little as possible. Put them in plastic bags until you can wash them. You can but you don't need to add bleach to kill HIV; a normal wash cycle will kill the virus. Clothes may also be dry cleaned or hand-washed. If stains from blood, semen, or vaginal fluids are on the clothes, soaking them in cold water before washing will help remove the stains. Fabrics and furniture can be cleaned with soap and water or cleansers you can buy in a store; just follow the directions on the box. Wear gloves while cleaning. See the section on gloves, under "Protect Yourself" heading, for more information on types of gloves.

Cleaning House

Cleaning kills germs that may be dangerous to the person with AIDS. You may want to clean and dust the house every week. Clean tubs, showers, and sinks often; use household cleaners, then rinse with fresh water. You may want to mop floors at least once a week. Clean the toilet often; use bleach mixed with water or a commercial toilet bowl cleaner. You may clean urinals and bedpans with bleach after each use. Replace plastic urinals and bedpans every month or so. About one-fourth cup of bleach mixed with one gallon of water makes a good disinfectant for floors, showers, tubs, sinks, mops, sponges, etc. (Or one tablespoon for bleach in one quart of water for small jobs). Make a new batch each time because it stops working after about 24 hours. Be sure to keep the bleach and the bleach and water mix, like other dangerous chemicals, away from children.

Protect Yourself

A person who has AIDS may sometimes have infections that can make you sick. You can protect yourself, however. Talk to the doctor or nurse to find out what germs can infect you and other people in the house. This is very important if you have HIV infection yourself.

For example, diarrhea can be caused by several different germs. Wear disposable gloves if you have to clean up after or help a person with diarrhea and wash your hands carefully after you take the gloves off. Do not use disposable gloves more than one time.

Another cause of diarrhea is the cryptosporidiosis parasite. It is spread from the feces of one person or animal to another person or animal, often by contaminated water, raw food, or food that isn't cooked well enough. Again, wash your hands after using the bathroom and before fixing food. You can check with your local health department to see if cryptosporidiosis is in the water. If you hear that the water in your community may have cryptosporidiosis parasites, boil your drinking water for at least one minute to kill the parasite, then let the water cool before drinking. You may want to buy bottled (distilled) water for cooking and drinking if the cryptosporidiosis parasite or other organisms that might make a person with HIV infection sick could be in the tap water.

If the person with AIDS has a cough that lasts longer than a week, the doctor should check them for TB. If they do have TB, then you and everybody else living in the house should be checked for TB infection, even if you aren't coughing. If you are infected with TB germs, you can take medicine that will prevent you from developing TB.

If the person with AIDS gets yellow jaundice (a sign of acute hepatitis) or has chronic hepatitis B infection, you and everybody else living in the house and any people the person with AIDS has had sex with should talk to their doctor to see if anyone needs to take medicine to prevent hepatitis. All children should get hepatitis B vaccine whether or not they are around a person with AIDS.

If the person with AIDS has fever blisters or cold sores (herpes simplex) around the mouth or nose, don't kiss or touch the sores. If you have to touch the sores to help the person, wear gloves and wash your hands carefully as soon as you take the gloves off. This is especially important if you have eczema (allergic skin) since the herpes simplex virus can cause severe skin disease in people with eczema. Throw the used gloves away; never use disposable gloves more than once.

Many persons with or without AIDS are infected with a virus called Cytomegalovirus (CMV), which can be spread in urine or saliva. Wash your hands after touching urine or saliva from a person with AIDS. This is especially important for someone who may be pregnant because a pregnant woman infected with CMV can also infect her unborn child. CMV causes birth defects such as deafness.

Remember, to protect yourself and the person with AIDS from these diseases and others, be sure to wash your hands with soap and water before and after giving care, when handling food, after taking gloves of, and after going to the bathroom.

Gloves

Because the virus that causes AIDS is in the blood of infected persons, blood or other body fluids (such as bloody feces) that have blood in them could infect you. You can protect yourself by following some simple steps. Wear gloves if you have to touch semen, vaginal fluid, cuts, or sores on the person with AIDS, or blood or body fluids that may have blood in them. Wear gloves to give care to the mouth, rectum, or genitals of the person with AIDS. Wear gloves to change diapers or sanitary pads or to empty bedpans or urinals. If you have any cuts, sores, rashes, or breaks in your skin, cover them with a bandage. If the cuts or sores are on your hands, use bandages and gloves. Wear gloves to clean up urine, feces, or vomit to avoid all the germs (HIV and other kinds) that might be there.

There are two types of gloves you can use. Use disposable, hospital-type latex or vinyl gloves to take care of the person with AIDS if there is any blood you might touch. Use these gloves one time, then throw them away. Do not use latex gloves more than one time even if they are marked "reusable." You can buy hospital-type gloves by the box at most drug stores, along with urinals, bedpans, and many other medical supplies. Many insurance companies and Medicaid will pay for these gloves if the doctor writes a prescription for them. For cleaning blood or bloody fluids from floors, bed, etc., you can use household rubber gloves, which are sold at any drug or grocery store. These gloves can be cleaned and reused. Clean them with hot, soapy water and with a mixture of bleach and water (about one-fourth cup bleach to one gallon of water). Be sure not to use gloves that are peeling, cracked, or have holes in them. Don't use the rubber gloves to take care of a person with AIDS; they are too thick and bulky.

To take gloves off, peel them down by turning them inside out. This will keep the wet side on the inside, away from your skin and other people. When you take the gloves off, wash your hands with soap and water right away. If there is a lot of blood, you can wear an apron or smock to keep your clothes from getting bloody. (If the person with AIDS is bleeding a lot or very often, call the doctor or nurse.) Clean up spilled blood as soon as you can. Put on gloves, wipe up the blood with paper towels or rags, put the used paper towels or rags in plastic bags to get rid of later, then wash the area where the blood was with a mix of bleach and water.

Since HIV can be in semen, vaginal fluid, or breast milk just as it can be in blood, you should be as careful with these fluids as you are with blood.

If you get blood, semen, vaginal fluid, breast milk, or other body fluid that might have blood in it in your eyes, nose, or mouth, immediately pour as much water as possible over where you got splashed, then call the doctor, explain what happened, and ask what else you should do.

Needles and Syringes

A person with AIDS may need needles and syringes to take medicine for diseases caused by AIDS or for diabetes, hemophilia, or other illnesses. If you have to handle these needles and syringes, you must be careful not to stick yourself. That is one way you could get infected with HIV.

Use a needle and syringe only one time. Do not put caps back on needles. Do not take needles off syringes. Do not break or bend needles. If a needle falls off a syringe, use something like tweezers or pliers to pick it up; do not use your fingers. Touch needles and syringes only by the barrel of the syringe. Hold the sharp end away from yourself.

Put the used needle and syringe in a puncture-proof container. The doctor, nurse, or an AIDS service organization can give you a special container. If you don't have one, use a puncture-proof container with a plastic top, such as a coffee can. Keep a container in any room where needles and syringes are used. Put it well out of the reach of children or visitors, but in a place you can easily and quickly put the needle and syringe after they are used. When the container gets nearly full, seal it and get a new container. Ask the doctor or nurse how to get rid of the container with the used needles and syringes.

If you get stuck with a needle used on the person with AIDS, don't panic. The chances are very good (better than 99 percent) that you will not be infected. However, you need to act quickly to get medical care. Put the needle in the used needle container, then wash where you stuck yourself as soon as you can, using warm, soapy water. Right after washing, call the doctor or the emergency room of a hospital, no matter what time it is, explain what happened, and ask what else you should do. Your doctor may want you to take medicine, such as AZT. If you are going to take AZT, you should begin taking it as soon as possible, certainly within a few hours of the needlestick.

Wastes

Flush all liquid waste (urine, vomit, etc.) that has blood in it down the toilet. Be careful not to splash anything when you are pouring liquids into the toilet. Toilet paper and tissues with blood, semen, vaginal fluid, or breast milk may also be flushed down the toilet.

Paper towels, sanitary pads and tampons, wound dressings and bandages, diapers, and other items with blood, semen, or vaginal fluid on them that cannot be flushed should be put in plastic bags. Put the items in the bag, then close and seal the bag. Ask the doctor, nurse, or local health department about how to get rid of things with blood, urine, vomit, semen, vaginal fluid, or breast milk on them. If you can't have plastic bags handy, wrap the materials in enough newspaper to stop any leaks. Wear gloves when handling anything with blood, semen, vaginal fluids, or breast milk on it.

Sex

If you used to or still do have sex with a person with HIV infection, and you didn't use latex condoms the right way every time you had sex, you could have HIV infection, too. You can talk to your doctor or a counselor about taking an HIV antibody test. Call CDC-INFO 24 hours/day at 800-CDC-INFO (232-4636), 888-232-6348 (TTY) for information about HIV antibody testing and referrals to places in your area that you can get confidential or anonymous HIV testing. The idea of being tested for HIV may be scary. But, if you are infected, the sooner you find out and start getting medical care, the better off you will be. Talk to your sex partner about what will need to change. It is very important that you protect yourself and your partner from transmitting HIV infection and other sexually transmitted diseases. Talk about types of sex that don't risk HIV infection. If you decide to have sexual intercourse (vaginal, anal, or oral), use condoms. Latex condoms can protect you from HIV infection if they are used the right way every time you have sex. Ask your doctor, counselor, or call CDC-INFO 24 hours/day at 800-CDC-INFO (232-4636), 888-232-6348 (TTY) for more information about safer sex. [See chapter 24, "HIV Prevention through Changing Behavior."]

Other Help You Can Give

Dealing with hospitals or insurance companies, filling out forms, and looking up records can be difficult even if you are well. Many people with AIDS need help with these tasks.

- Getting a ride to the doctor's office, clinic, drug store, or other places can be a problem. Don't wait to be asked, offer to help.

- Keeping a diary of medical events and other information for the person you are taking care of can help them and any other people who are helping. Be sure the person you are caring for knows what you are writing and helps keep the diary if they can.

- Keeping a record of medicine and other care for the doctor or the other people providing care can help a lot. Make sure you know what drugs the person is taking, how often they should take them, and what side effects to watch out for. The doctor, nurse, or pharmacist can tell you what to do. People who are sick sometimes forget to take medicine or take too much or too little. Divided pill boxes or a chart showing what medicines to take, when to take them, and how much of each to take can help.

- If the person you are caring for has to go into the hospital, you can still help. Take a special picture or other favorite things to the hospital. Tell the hospital staff of any special needs or habits the person has or if you see any problems. Most of all, visit often.

Children with AIDS

Infants and children with HIV infection or AIDS need the same things as other children—lots of love and affection. Small children need to be held, played with, kissed, hugged, fed, and rocked to sleep. As they grow, they need to play, have friends, and go to school, just like other kids. Kids with HIV are still kids, and need to be treated like any other kids in the family.

Kids with AIDS need much of the same care that grown-ups with AIDS need, but there are a few extra things to look out for such as the following:

- Watch for any changes in health or the way the child acts. If you notice anything unusual for that child, let the doctor know. For a child with AIDS, little problems can become big problems very quickly. Watch for breathing problems, fever, unusual sleepiness, diarrhea, or changes in how much they eat. Talk to the child's doctor about what else to look for and when to report it.

- Talk to the doctor before the child gets any immunizations (including oral polio vaccine) or booster shots. Some vaccines could make the child sick. No child with HIV or anyone in the household should ever take oral polio vaccine.

- Stuffed and furry toys can hold dirt and might hide germs that can make the child sick. Plastic and washable toys are better. If the child has any stuffed toys, wash them in a washing machine often and keep them as clean as possible.

- Keep the child away from litter boxes and sandboxes that a pet or other animal might have been in.

- Ask the child's doctor what to do about pets that might be in the house.

- Try to keep the child from getting infectious diseases, especially chickenpox. If the child with HIV infection gets near somebody with chickenpox, tell the child's doctor right away. Chickenpox can kill a child with AIDS.

- Bandage any cuts or scrapes quickly and completely after washing with soap and warm water. Use gloves if the child is bleeding.

Taking care of a child who is sick is very hard for people who love that child. You will need help and emotional support. You are not alone. There are people who can help you get through this. [See chapter 74, "Directory of Organizations and Hotlines," for contact information.]

Changing Symptoms

People with AIDS seem to get very sick, then get better, then get very sick, then better, and so on. Sometimes they get sicker and sicker. You can't always tell if they are going to live through a particular illness or not. These times are very rough on everyone involved. If you know what to expect, you can deal with these rough times better.

Dementia

Dementia (having trouble thinking) can be a problem for a person with AIDS. AIDS can affect the brain and cause poor memory; short attention span; trouble moving, speaking, or thinking; less alertness; loss of interest in things; and wide mood swings. These problems can upset the person with AIDS as well as the people around them. Mental problems can make it hard to follow the planned routines for care and make it difficult to protect the person with AIDS from infections. Be prepared to recognize these problems; understand what is happening; and talk to the doctor, nurse, social worker, or mental health worker about what to do.

549

If the person you are caring for does develop mental problems, you can help:

- Keep important things in the same place all the time, a place that is easy to reach and easy to see.

- If you need to, remind the person you are caring for where they are and who you are.

- Put a clock and a calendar where the person you are caring for can see them. Mark off the days on the calendar. Write in what will happen each day.

- Put up pictures of people who might be in the house with their names on the pictures where the person with AIDS can see them.

- Speak in short, simple sentences.

- Don't be afraid to be firm. Remove things like dangerous objects from reach.

- Keep the sound from TVs, radios, and other noises down so the person doesn't get confused by unexpected sounds.

- Talk to a health care worker who deals with people with dementia about how to handle problems.

As AIDS Progresses

Here are some of the things to expect as AIDS enters its final stages and ways to try to cope. Like other people nearing death, the following apply to a person with AIDS who is near death:

- He/she sleeps more and more and is hard to wake up. Try to talk to them and do things during those times when they do seem alert.

- He/she becomes confused about where they are, the time or date, or who people are. Tell them where they are, what time and day it is, and who people are. Don't scold them for forgetting, just tell them.

- He/she begins to wet their pants or lose bowel control. Clean them, using gloves, and use powder or lotion to prevent rashes. A catheter for passing urine may become necessary.

- He/she has skin that feels cool to the touch and may turn darker on the side of their body touching the bed as the circulation slows down. Keep them covered with warm blankets, but don't use electric blankets because they can burn a person with poor circulation.

- He/she may have trouble seeing or hearing. Even so, never talk to other people as if the person with AIDS can't hear you. Always talk to the person with AIDS or anyone else in the room as if the person with AIDS hears you.

- He/she may seem restless, pulling at the sheets on the bed or acting as if they see things that you don't. Stay calm, speak slowly, and reassure the person. Comfort them with gentle reminders about who you are and where they are.

- He/she may stop eating and drinking. Wipe their mouth often with a wet cloth. Keep their lips wet with lip moisturizer.

- He/she may almost stop urinating. If there is a catheter, it may need to be rinsed or flushed to keep it from getting blocked. A nurse can show you how to do this.

- He/she has noisy breathing because they can't cough up the fluids that collect in the back of their throat. Talk to their doctor; the doctor may suggest raising the head of the bed or putting extra pillows under their head. Turning them on their side may also help. If they can swallow, feed them some ice chips. If they have trouble swallowing, a cool, wet washcloth on the lips can keep their mouth and lips moist and may satisfy their thirst. If they begin to have irregular breathing or seem to stop breathing for a minute, call the doctor.

Hospice Care

Many people have found hospice care (programs for people who are dying and their caregivers) for adults and children a big help. Others feel that hospice care isn't right for them. Hospice services can help caregivers, family, and other loved ones, as well as help the dying person deal with the concerns and fears that may come near the end of their life. You should be able to find hospice organizations listed in your local phone book.

Final Arrangements

A person with AIDS, like every other adult, should have a will. This can be a difficult subject to discuss, but a will may need to be written before there is any question of the mental competence of the person with AIDS. You may want to be sure the person you are caring for has a will and that you know where it is.

Living wills, which specify what medical care the person with AIDS wants or does not want, also have to be written before their mental competence could be questioned. You, as the caregiver, may be the person asked to see that the doctors follow the wishes of the person with AIDS. This can be a very hard experience to deal with, but is another way of showing respect for a dying person. You may want to be sure the person you are caring for knows that they can control their medical care through living wills.

Often, people who know that they will die soon choose to make their own funeral or memorial arrangements. This helps make sure that the funeral will be done the way they want it done. It also makes things easier for those left behind. They no longer have to guess what their friend or loved one would have wanted. You may be asked to help the person with AIDS plan the funeral, make arrangements with the funeral home, and select a cemetery plot or mausoleum. You may be able to help the person with AIDS decide how they wish to be buried or if they want to be cremated.

After the death, there will still be things to do. Programs that have been providing help, such as Supplemental Security Income, will have to be officially informed of the death. Some money already sent or received may have to be returned. The will may name you, a relative, or another person as the one to handle these tasks.

Dying at Home

Whether or not to die at home is a big decision, but it may not have to be made right away. As the health of the person with AIDS changes, you and they may change your minds several times. However, it is something you should talk about with the person with AIDS ahead of time. Plans should be made; legal papers may need to be signed. What the dying person wants and needs, the needs and abilities of the caregivers and other loved ones, the advice of the doctors and other medical professionals, the advice of clergy or other spiritual leaders, may all need to be considered in deciding what is best. Consideration must be given to everyone living in the home. Small children and others may not be ready to cope with death in their home. Others in the home may prefer to face the final moments of the person with AIDS in familiar surroundings. Just be sure the person with AIDS knows that they will not die alone, that the people they love will try to be with them, wherever they choose to die. You also should get help to deal with your own grief after the death.

Help for You

Taking care of someone who is very sick is hard. It wears you down physically and emotionally and creates stress. You can get very angry watching a person you love get sicker and sicker no matter how hard you work or how much you care. You have to do something with this anger. Many people can talk out their anger with other people who have the same problems or with counselors, ministers, rabbis, friends, family, or health workers. Many AIDS service organizations can help you find people to talk to.

You should not try to be the only person taking care of someone with AIDS. You need some time for yourself. The sicker the person you are taking care of becomes, the more important this is. If you try to do everything yourself, you will wear yourself out and not be able to go on. You are not alone. Other people have done this before. Learn from them. Call the places listed in chapter 74, "Directory of Organizations and Hotlines," for help.

Chapter 63

Your Rights as a Person with HIV Infection or AIDS

The Office for Civil Rights (OCR) of the U.S. Department of Health and Human Services (HHS) enforces federal laws that prohibit discrimination by health care and human service providers. Two of these laws are Section 504 of the Rehabilitation Act of 1973 (Section 504), and Title II of the Americans with Disabilities Act of 1990 (ADA).

Section 504 and the ADA protect individuals with human immunodeficiency virus (HIV) or acquired immunodeficiency syndrome (AIDS) from discrimination on the basis of their disability. The information in this chapter applies to persons who have tested positive for HIV, persons who have AIDS, and persons regarded as having HIV or AIDS.

Protections against Discrimination

Both Section 504 and the ADA prohibit discrimination against qualified persons with HIV and other disabilities. Section 504 prohibits discrimination by health care and human service providers (called "entities") that receive federal funds or some other types of federal assistance. Title II of the ADA prohibits discrimination by state and local government entities even if they do not receive federal financial assistance. Examples of entities that may be covered by Section 504 and the ADA include hospitals, clinics, social services agencies, drug treatment centers, and nursing homes.

U.S. Department of Health and Human Services, Office for Civil Rights (http://www.hhs.gov/ocr), revised January 31, 2007.

Discrimination may occur if the entity excludes a person with HIV from participating in a service, or denies them a benefit. The person living with HIV must meet the essential eligibility requirements for the benefit or service he or she is seeking. The entity may be required to make a reasonable accommodation to enable the person with HIV to participate. The ADA also protects other persons, such as family and friends, who are discriminated against because of their association with someone who has HIV.

Types of Discrimination against Persons with HIV/AIDS

Persons with HIV infection have been denied access to social services, or denied medical treatment, or had treatment or services delayed, solely because they have HIV or AIDS. Such actions by an agency, organization, hospital, nursing home, drug treatment center, clinic, medical or dental office, or other entity, may be unlawful discrimination under either Section 504 or the ADA, or both.

The following are examples of practices which may be illegal discrimination:

- A nursing home that has space available denies admission to a person with HIV, because their staff is not trained to care for HIV-related conditions, even though the home could easily provide the necessary training.

- A social services agency removes a foster child from his foster home because the agency learns that one of the foster parents is a person with HIV.

How to File a Complaint

If you believe that you have been discriminated against because of your HIV infection, you or your representative may file a complaint with OCR. The deadline for filing a complaint is 180 days from the date the discrimination occurred, unless there is good reason for delay. You may request a complaint form from OCR [see contact information at the end of this chapter].

If you do not use OCR's complaint form, please write down the following information and send it to OCR:

1. Your name, address, and telephone number; please sign your name (You may send a complaint for another person, providing their contact information and stating your relationship to that person, such as spouse or friend.)

2. Name and address of the entity you believe discriminated against you

3. How, why, and when you believe you were discriminated against, and

4. Any other important information

Send the complaint to the nearest OCR regional office; please see contact information which follows. OCR staff will review the complaint to decide if Section 504 or the ADA may cover it.

- If OCR does not have authority to investigate your complaint, we will refer it to the correct agency, if possible.

- If OCR does have authority to investigate the complaint and finds that there is discrimination, OCR will work with the entity to correct the action.

- Once you file a complaint with OCR, it is against the law for the entity to take any action against you, or any other person who provides information about the complaint to OCR. If this happens, tell OCR about it immediately.

Under Section 504 and ADA, you may also file a private lawsuit. A private attorney or your local legal aid office can tell you what the court deadlines are for filing a lawsuit.

For further information, contact the U.S. Department of Health and Human Services, Office for Civil Rights:

Director—Office for Civil Rights
U. S. Department of Health and Human Services
200 Independence Avenue, SW
Room 509-F, HHH Building
Washington, DC 20201
Toll-Free: 800-368-1019
TDD: 800-537-7697
Website: http://www.hhs.gov/ocr
E-mail: ocrmail@hhs.gov

Part Eight

Research Initiatives and Clinical Trials

Chapter 64

The Future of AIDS Research

Mario Stevenson, PhD, is the newly appointed chairman of amfAR's Research and Scientific Advisory Committees. A native Scot, Dr. Stevenson received his PhD from the University of Strathclyde, Glasgow. In 1984, he moved to the United States to pursue his scientific interest in viruses and has since become a leader in AIDS research. Now director of the Center for AIDS Research and professor of molecular medicine at the University of Massachusetts Medical School, Dr. Stevenson's primary area of research involves studying how viruses such as HIV cause disease. In his challenging new volunteer role at amfAR, Dr. Stevenson will help shape the Foundation's research priorities in the years to come. amfAR's Dr. Rowena Johnston, director of research, spoke with him about what those priorities are most likely to be.

amfAR: One of your first tasks as chairman of amfAR's Research Committee was to convene a think tank. What was its purpose?

Stevenson: The think tanks are designed to bring together a group of individuals to come up with a strategy to support a particular problem in the field. The problem that we're facing right now is: why do the available drugs not cure AIDS? Now it's a simple question, but the answer is anything but simple. We have antiretroviral agents that are incredibly effective at suppressing HIV. Unfortunately, the drugs are failing in many individuals because they're toxic, and the virus becomes resistant to the drugs in some individuals, meaning that they are no longer effective. So about 25 percent of patients who are on these drugs eventually fail therapy. The drugs are a stopgap measure. They're not a long-term solution.

amfAR: So if the drugs are so capable of suppressing the virus, why don't they eradicate it completely?

Stevenson: One possibility is that the virus has either found a niche—a compartment—in the body where it's protected from the drug, or that the virus has somehow become dormant so that the drugs don't do anything. When the drugs are removed, the virus comes back again.

Despite all the research that's been done in the past, we still don't know the answer to those questions. The think tank participants identified the ways this question could be addressed by amfAR's research program, and then those discussions became the basis for our latest research request for proposals.

amfAR: The request for proposals (RFP) is called "Exploring the Potential for HIV Eradication." Do you think this reflects a new optimism that eradication may be possible?

Stevenson: I think the issue of eradication has been played with by a number of individuals, and people feel very strongly one way or the other. What a burgeoning body of literature is supporting is that perhaps the reason HIV is resisting therapy is because it's actually found a niche; it's found a way to protect itself. But there is no really definitive evidence for that. So the first thing you have to do, if you want to eradicate the virus, is identify how it's able to survive in the face of comprehensive therapy. Once you know the answer to that question, then you can come up with better strategies to achieve eradication.

This will lay the groundwork for more ambitious studies that may lead to therapeutic strategies that actually do achieve eradication. Now if you want to believe in eradication, you have to be a little bit of an optimist. Obviously, I'm one of the optimists.

amfAR: What other areas of research do you think are important or hold a lot of promise right now?

Stevenson: I think one of the subjects of a recent amfAR RFP was particularly important: the area of cellular defenses.

Humans, it turns out, are a very hostile environment for viruses like HIV. Our cells have proteins that carry out natural functions in the cell. Some of these proteins have a very toxic effect on HIV.

amfAR: So if our bodies carry these natural defenses that protect us against HIV, why do we get infected?

Stevenson: The virus has evolved a strategy to protect itself. So if we can find a way to foil the virus's defense mechanisms, then we would render it sensitive to the human body's natural defenses and hopefully make us resistant to HIV. If we can mobilize our natural defenses, I think we'd have a very powerful protection against HIV. And if I were betting the mortgage, I'd put my money on the natural cellular defenses rather than a vaccine strategy.

amfAR: Do you see that in the form of a therapeutic strategy?

Stevenson: Right. If we could come up with small molecules that prevent the ability of the virus to counteract these cellular defenses, then the virus would be rendered susceptible to our body's natural defenses. We would be able to protect ourselves from HIV. I should emphasize that these cellular defenses are incredibly potent.

amfAR: They're more potent than any vaccine currently used to prevent other diseases?

Stevenson: Right. The main weakness in a vaccine strategy is that the virus is incredibly variable. Because HIV is continually changing its structure, the immune system can't get a fix on it. The virus is continually evolving to avoid recognition by the immune system.

In contrast, these natural defenses are oblivious to the variability of the virus. They attack the virus regardless of what type of HIV it is. So this sort of strategy would work against all HIV variants.

amfAR: Last September [2005] you agreed to chair amfAR's Research Committee and the Scientific Advisory Committee. What made you decide you wanted to accept?

Stevenson: I'm probably one of amfAR's biggest fans. I got my first grant through amfAR in 1987. At the time I was trying to transition to being an independent investigator. It's a stage where you're trying to establish your laboratory, teach, write grants, and it's also the most difficult time in terms of finding funding for your research. So I applied to amfAR and got funded, and that really set me off on an independent career in HIV. Two years later, I was able to apply for funding from the National Institutes of Health (NIH). I owe amfAR a lot for that, and I feel that I have a commitment to help amfAR support other young investigators and to fill a void that's been left by federal agencies in terms of supporting young investigators.

amfAR: Do you think it's equally difficult now for young investigators to get funding? Have things changed?

Stevenson: Right now it's incredibly difficult for young investigators to find funding. When I was establishing my career as a young investigator, the NIH had a mechanism to support young investigators. It was called a First Investigator Award and it was specifically for those who were applying for their first NIH grant. Because of this, those investigators didn't have to compete with established investigators.

A number of years ago, the NIH phased that program out and young investigators had to compete with established investigators. As a result, it's not a level playing field.

At the NIH now, one in every eight grants gets funded, meaning that young investigators really have very little chance of getting funded, because the established investigators are competing hard for the little money that's there. Rather than thinking of the science and doing the science, young investigators are spending all their time chasing up ways to raise money. And it's not unusual for people to have to wait a year or more before they actually receive funding they've applied for.

amfAR: How does amfAR help fill that need now?

Stevenson: amfAR supports young investigators through its research fellowship program. Plus, amfAR has a quick turnaround time. If an investigator needs to have their research funded, they can't wait a year, a year and a half. By then, the field has moved on and the research is out of date.

What amfAR is doing is trying to prioritize the most important issues. And that can be a tall order, because the field is changing so rapidly. What is hot today will be history in six months. amfAR is well placed because it's so mobile, because it's able to respond and grant funding quickly. It can really keep zeroing in on the most important issues as they evolve.

amfAR: Are there other ways in which amfAR supports young researchers?

Stevenson: Yes. It's not enough just to give an investigator money, particularly a young investigator, because at some point in time that investigator has to be presenting results to an audience of peers. And ultimately the investigator gets a wake-up call when they find that their research is not well received, or they submit an application for a more ambitious grant and they find that the reviewers don't like the direction they are taking.

In other words, there is no mentoring of young investigators to help them identify the most important issues in the field, and to show them how to go for more ambitious federal funding. By requesting that grantees go to meetings and participate in some of the workshops at these meetings, amfAR is helping to start them off on the right foot. You're preparing them for a tough career as an independent scientist.

amfAR: In a recent article calling for more spending on research, someone made the point that people who suffer from various diseases are concerned mostly with "the fix." I like to think that amfAR is also concerned largely with the fix—the solution. We understand that we need to know details in order to get there, but the fix is clearly our goal. Would you agree?

Stevenson: In theory I agree with that, but in reality you have to have research in a wider theater. We need to have the serendipity element. Scientists have to be allowed free rein to also create conditions for accidental breakthroughs. They don't happen by design. They happen because a lot of good scientists are pursuing different ideas and those findings come together to form a new solution.

Chapter 65

Research on HIV Infection and AIDS in Minority Populations

National Institute of Allergy and Infectious Diseases (NIAID) Research on HIV Infection and AIDS

NIAID is the lead institute for HIV/AIDS research at the National Institutes of Health (NIH) and is at the forefront of the war against this continuing health crisis.

NIAID supports scientific research at universities, medical schools, hospitals, and research institutions, both in the United States and internationally. This research is aimed at preventing, diagnosing, and treating HIV/AIDS and other infectious diseases as well as allergic and other immune system disorders.

NIAID's HIV/AIDS research agenda includes conducting clinical trials that address the specific needs and concerns of minority populations, ensuring that all populations have access to clinical trials and the latest information on HIV/AIDS treatment and prevention. In addition, NIAID's Office of Special Populations Research and Training encourages research aimed at improving the health of minority populations and also works to increase the effectiveness of outreach and education programs.

NIAID works with community-based organizations to disseminate information about HIV infection, AIDS, and NIAID research activities, especially HIV vaccine development, to minority communities. NIAID is currently implementing an HIV Vaccine Communications Campaign

"HIV Infection in Minority Populations," National Institute of Allergy and Infectious Diseases (http://www.niaid.nih.gov), a component of the National Institutes of Health (NIH), April 22, 2005.

(HVCC), which is aimed at increasing awareness of and support for HIV vaccine research, especially in at-risk populations. NIAID receives input and guidance for developing appropriate and culturally sensitive messages from its HIV Vaccine Communications Steering Group, which consists of representatives from community groups, other government agencies, pharmaceutical companies, and HIV vaccine advocacy groups. In addition, HVCC supports the Community Education and Outreach Partnership Program, which is designed to create local and national partnerships. The goal of these partnerships is to enhance NIAID's ability to provide messages on HIV vaccine, treatment, and prevention research to African Americans, Hispanic, and men who have sex with men (MSM) populations.

Clinical Research

NIAID supports a comprehensive clinical research agenda to evaluate treatment and prevention strategies for HIV/AIDS and its associated complications and co-infections. NIAID supports the following clinical trial networks:

- Adult AIDS Clinical Trials Group (AACTG)
- Pediatric AIDS Clinical Trials Group (PACTG)
- Terry Beirn Community Programs for Clinical Research on AIDS (CPCRA)
- HIV Prevention Trials Network (HPTN)
- HIV Vaccine Trials Network (HVTN)
- Acute Infection and Early Disease Research Program (AIEDRP)

NIAID's Vaccine Research Center (VRC) also conducts Phase I trials of HIV vaccines at the VRC Clinic housed in the NIH Clinical Center in Bethesda, Maryland.

Together, these programs represent the largest HIV/AIDS treatment and prevention initiative in the world. Recruiting minorities into clinical trials is a priority for NIAID to ensure that research results will apply to all populations affected by HIV. With the epidemic disproportionately affecting minority communities, inclusion of these populations is particularly urgent.

AACTG investigates therapeutic interventions for HIV infection, AIDS, complications of HIV-associated immunodeficiency, and associated co-infections in adults. AACTG sites receive additional funding from the National Institute on Drug Abuse (NIDA) to increase participation of injection drug users, who are also disproportionally affected by the AIDS epidemic.

PACTG evaluates clinical interventions for treating HIV infection and HIV-associated illnesses in neonates, infants, children, and adolescents. Both PACTG and HPTN are researching approaches to interrupt mother-to-child transmission (MTCT) of HIV. In 2004, 6,367 and 2,815 participants were enrolled in AACTG and PACTG studies respectively. In AACTG, 30 percent were African American, 19 percent Hispanic, 2 percent Asian/Pacific Islander, and less than 1 percent American Indian/Alaska Native. In PACTG, 58 percent were African American, 27 percent Hispanic, 1 percent Asian/Pacific Islander, and less than 1 percent American Indian/Alaska Native.

CPCRA is a network of community-based health centers and clinics that support clinical research in community settings. CPCRA conducts large comparative studies that examine how to use available therapies more effectively as well as the long term consequences of different treatments. Currently, CPCRA trials are under way in 17 cities at 18 units. In 2004, 4,869 people participated in CPCRA studies. Of those, 45 percent were African American, 13 percent Hispanic, 1 percent American Indian/Alaska Native, and 1 percent Asian/Pacific Islander.

NIAID also supports clinical research on vaccine and non-vaccine strategies to prevent HIV infection. Vaccine studies are carried out through HVTN, and non-vaccine prevention studies are conducted by HPTN. HVTN is a global network of clinical sites that evaluate preventive HIV vaccine in all phases of clinical trials. They allow for studies that examine differences in HIV diversity and genetic background, all of which may prove crucial to developing an effective vaccine for use around the world.

HPTN is a global multicenter network dedicated to non-vaccine biomedical and behavioral interventions. The primary areas of research of HPTN include topical microbicides, sexually transmitted infection prevention and treatment, behavioral and barrier interventions, antiretroviral drugs, interventions related to drug abuse, and modalities to decrease MTCT. HPTN is also funded by the National Institute of Child Health and Human Development (NICHD), NIDA, and the National Institute of Mental Health.

Through close collaborations and education outreach programs with communities where vaccines will be tested, HVTN and HPTN hope to enroll a diversified population in their clinical trials, ensuring access and representation of populations most affected by and vulnerable to HIV spread.

HVTN and HPTN opened in 2000 and have since enrolled thousands of study participants. In FY 2004, 1,348 and 11,091 people participated in HVTN and HPTN, respectively. Of those in the HVTN, 29 percent were African American, 44 percent Hispanic, 1 percent Asian/Pacific Islander, and less than 1 percent American Indian/Alaska Native. In HPTN, 64 percent of participants were African American, 8 percent Hispanic, 15 percent Asian/Pacific Islander, and less than 1 percent American Indian/Alaska Native.

AIEDRP is a multi-site network that studies how HIV causes disease in adults. Each AIEDRP site works with universities or hospitals that conduct research with people who have been recently infected with HIV. In FY 2004, AIEDRP enrolled 726 patients. Of those patients enrolled, 5 percent were black, 12 percent Hispanic, 4 percent Asian, and less than 1 percent American Indian/Alaska Native.

Epidemiologic Research

NIAID conducts and supports research on HIV infection in a variety of population groups. These studies are conducted through the Women and Infants Transmission Study (WITS), the Women's Interagency HIV Study (WIHS), and the Multicenter AIDS Cohort Study (MACS). Inner-city women, children, and injection drug users are the focus of the WITS. Ninety percent of the women in this study are from minority populations.

Similar populations of women are the focus of WIHS. NIAID awarded funds to six U.S. sites in 1993 to investigate primarily the impact of HIV infection on women. Several other NIH institutes also collaborate on WIHS and provide funds for various components. They include NIDA, the National Cancer Institute, NICHD, and the National Institute of Dental and Craniofacial Research.

Active community involvement through WIHS sites and the WIHS National Community Advisory Board helps encourage minority women to participate in the studies. More than 80 percent of the women currently enrolled in WIHS are from minority populations.

In the United States, MACS and WIHS are the two largest observational studies of HIV/AIDS in homosexual or bisexual men and in women, respectively. These studies have made major contributions to understanding how HIV is spread, how the disease progresses, and how it can best be treated. These studies expanded their enrollment to increase the size of the study groups by 60 percent and increase the number of minority participants in 2004. The enlarged groups will focus on contemporary questions regarding HIV infection and treatment.

Chapter 66

Hope for AIDS Cure Remains Alive

In the hide-and-seek game played out between scientists and HIV over the last 25 years, the virus has so far been winning.

"All of the drugs that we have now are specific antiretroviral agents that inhibit some step in the virus' life cycle, so they hit HIV only when it is replicating," explained researcher Paul Bieniasz, an associate professor at the Aaron Diamond AIDS Research Center in New York City.

That strategy has brought many infected patients long-term health.

"But there's always a small but significant population of virus present in infected individuals that is not replicating," Bieniasz said.

For patients on effective drug therapy, that means HIV remains dormant in tissues at levels that are undetectable by standard tests.

These tiny reservoirs of "latent" HIV lie curled up as bits of foreign DNA buried deep within the nucleus of cells. Like a tiny time bomb, this dormant virus may stay sleeping for years. On the other hand, it may also switch over to replicating status and re-start the deadly progression to AIDS.

"It's a tricky virus, and latency is an excellent strategy for HIV," said Dr. Rowena Johnston, director of basic research at the Foundation for AIDS Research (amfAR). "If the virus is latent, not only is antiretroviral therapy not going to get at it, but it's also impossible for the immune system to target it, too."

Latent virus is the major reason why scientists have failed to find a cure for HIV/AIDS. According to Bieniasz, latent virus has no real "hook" for drugs to latch onto. And because latent HIV lies deep within the nucleus, any drug that could attack it might prove far too toxic to healthy cells.

But that isn't stopping researchers from pursuing a solution to the problem.

"At amfAR, we like to think that if we haven't proven that it's impossible, then we're not doing our job if we don't go after it," Johnston said.

In fact, amfAR is funding the work of Bieniasz' lab, where researchers are creating artificial pools of latent virus in cell cultures. They are using these cultures to test the effects of thousands of compounds—watching to see if any particular molecule pushes latent HIV into an active, replicating state.

"It's thought that one strategy to eradicate HIV and effectively cure people is to make these latent viruses replicate," Bieniasz said. "Because once they replicate, you can then hit them with existing antiretroviral drugs."

The cell cultures in the Aaron Diamond lab are engineered to switch on a fluorescent biochemical tag, if and when a candidate molecule flips the virus from latency to replication.

Bieniasz said a cure for AIDS isn't around the corner, but these experiments are a vital first step. "What we are looking for here is essentially proof-of-principal that you can do this without having wide-ranging effects on cells," he said.

Other research is also yielding valuable clues to latency.

Dr. Stephen Deeks is an associate professor of medicine at the University of California, San Francisco's General Clinical Research Center. His work, also funded by amfAR, focuses on that tiny minority of HIV-infected individuals—less than 1 percent—who have remained healthy for more than 20 years without the need for drug therapy.

These so-called "elite controllers" typically carry virus that stays at low or undetectable levels. "So, the question remains, what makes these individuals different?" said Deeks.

"One model is that they have an immune system that allows them to control the virus very effectively," he said. In fact, some—but not all—of these people have immune cells that are especially rich in human leukocyte antigen (HLA) receptors. "These receptors allow immune cells to recognize very specific parts of an infection, such as a virus," he said.

That could be part of the story. Or, these individuals might have been lucky enough to contract what researchers call a "replication-impaired" form of HIV—a kind of weakling strain that is easy to keep at bay.

"That remains a theory," Deeks said, "mainly because the virus is actually very hard to find in these individuals. But we are aggressively trying to find that out."

The answers his team comes up with could help the 99 percent of infected patients with no such defenses against HIV.

"If it's the immune response that's key, and if we can figure out what those responses are, then we can develop vaccines that focus in those areas," Deeks said. Vaccine research could also receive a boost if it's a particular strain of virus that causes long-term control, he said.

Cutting-edge drug therapies have already beaten HIV down to infinitesimally low levels. In 2005, a team led by Dr. David Margolis of the University of North Carolina made a big splash by announcing in the *Lancet* that it had significantly depleted levels of latent virus in four patients.

In the study, Margolis' team added a common epilepsy drug, valproic acid, to the patients' standard mix of antiretroviral drugs. All of the patients had already exhibited very low viral loads for years.

Valproic acid is known to inhibit an enzyme called histone deacetylase 1 (HDAC1), which HIV needs to stay hidden in cells.

By the end of the four-month trial, reservoirs of latent HIV in immune CD4 cells had been depleted by 75 percent, the researchers reported. "This new approach, in the future, may allow us to make progress in eradication of infection in an HIV-infected person," Margolis told HealthDay at the time.

Still, experts say the bulk of latent HIV hides out in a wide variety of tissues, including the gut, lymph nodes, and drug-impermeable areas such as the brain or testes. So, this line of research still has a very long way to go, according to amfAR's Johnston.

"I don't want anyone to come away with the impression that amfAR thinks that we're close to a cure—we're absolutely not," she said. "We need to work at understanding what the barriers are, let alone work out how to overcome them."

Deeks agreed. But he also agreed that the search for a cure must go on.

"All of this has to be put into the context of the fact that antiretroviral treatment, although it works great, has its limitations," he said. "Many people can't adhere to these drugs for a lifetime, they are complicated, and all these toxicities keep piling up."

"A drug-free way to manage patients is a highly desirable thing," Deeks said. "I'd call that a cure. And that's what we should be reaching for."

Chapter 67

Why Develop an AIDS Vaccine?

Why an AIDS Vaccine?

Background

Since the U.S. Centers for Disease Control reported the first cases of a novel immunodeficiency disease a quarter of a century ago, the need for a vaccine to prevent HIV/AIDS has never been clearer. Out of an estimated 38.6 million people living with HIV worldwide by the end of 2005, 4.1 million were newly infected last year alone, 95 percent of them in developing countries.[1]

With dramatic increases in funding and technical assistance from the Global Fund to fight AIDS, Tuberculosis, and Malaria, the U.S. President's Emergency Plan for AIDS Relief (PEPFAR), and the World Health Organization (WHO)'s '3 by 5' program, antiretroviral drugs (ARVs) now reach 20 percent of those who need them in low- and middle-income countries, and coverage continues to expand.[2] But drug treatment is expensive, difficult to manage on a large scale, and becomes ineffective over time as the ever-evolving virus becomes resistant. Unless new infections are reduced drastically through expansion and strengthening of existing HIV prevention initiatives, underpinned

This chapter includes text from "Why an AIDS Vaccine?" © 2006 International AIDS Vaccine Initiative (www.iavi.org), reprinted with permission; and "Scientists Unveil Piece of HIV Protein that May Be Key to AIDS Vaccine Development," National Institutes of Health (NIH), February 14, 2007.

by new tools like AIDS vaccines, the financial burden of AIDS treatment will continue to escalate, pushing adequate supplies of medicines increasingly out of reach for poor nations.

The Challenges of Developing an AIDS Vaccine

The science of designing AIDS vaccines remains complex. The traditional vaccine development approach—utilizing a weakened version of a virus to prompt a protective immune response against the real disease—has not been feasible with HIV. Unlike many other epidemics for which successful vaccines have been developed, there are no known cases of infected individuals recovering from the virus and gaining protective immunity. Scientists are thus attempting to develop a vaccine without a definitive roadmap.

The biology of HIV infection presents other obstacles. Like other retroviruses, HIV inserts copies of its genetic material into human cells to create a persistent, yet immunologically invisible, reservoir of infection. Most importantly, HIV is also a moving target: the ability of the virus to evolve and mutate rapidly to escape immune responses and the enormous diversity worldwide of HIV pose monumental challenges to the development of an effective vaccine.

Progress Towards an AIDS Vaccine

Nevertheless, scientists believe that an AIDS vaccine is possible. Virtually all persons' immune systems are able to keep the virus in check for a number of years, some for over two decades. There is also good evidence that some rare individuals have a natural ability to avoid HIV infection despite repeated exposure to the virus. Furthermore, experimental vaccines have successfully protected monkeys from simian immunodeficiency virus (SIV), a virus that causes a disease in monkeys that is much like AIDS.

Thanks to increased political and financial commitment over the past few years—from $160 million spent annually in 1993 to $759 million last year [2005][3]—new scientific consortia comprising leading HIV researchers are tackling crucial scientific questions in vaccine development.

A wide range of major players are coming together under the umbrella of the Global HIV Vaccine Enterprise to further enhance scientific coordination and information sharing and to identify new strategies and mechanisms to accelerate the global vaccine development effort. The Bill and Melinda Gates Foundation, for example, established the Collaboration for AIDS Vaccine Discovery (CAVD), a network of laboratories focused on designing AIDS vaccines. The U.S. government, through its National Institute of Allergy and Infectious Diseases (NIAID), is focusing consortia work on examining virologic, genetic, and immunologic responses to HIV infection. For its own part, the International AIDS Vaccine Initiative (IAVI)'s Neutralizing Antibody Consortium is analyzing how antibodies work to neutralize different HIV subtypes. Bringing together five leading scientific laboratories, researchers in IAVI's Live Attenuated Consortium (LAC) also are studying successful immunization and antiretroviral strategies against SIV in the non-human primate model.

As of June 2006, there are close to 30 ongoing trials with preventive AIDS vaccine candidates in approximately two dozen countries,[4] with advanced testing now taking place or planned for several candidates. Much of this cutting-edge research is being conducted in Africa and Asia, where most new HIV infections are occurring. Over the past couple of years for example, clinical teams from several countries— India, China, Rwanda, and Zambia among them—have launched the first AIDS vaccine trials in their respective countries, and in doing so increased global site preparations for future AIDS vaccine efficacy trials. Other Phase I and II studies of preventive AIDS vaccines currently under way also stand to significantly inform the field in coming years.

The Way Forward

IAVI estimates that even a modestly effective AIDS vaccine could slash the number of new infections over a decade by one-third, saving tens of millions of lives.[5] But in addition to scientific roadblocks, economic and political barriers impede vaccine development progress. In the past 30 years, the scientific community has not been able to develop and license a vaccine against any disease without industry involvement. Yet today, only a handful of private companies are engaged in AIDS vaccine research and development, with less than 10 percent of vaccine research and development spending coming from the private sector.[6] New government incentives, including advance market commitments and tax credits, are urgently needed to spur private-sector involvement in new vaccine discovery.

Global spending on AIDS vaccine development, although growing, is still falling short of what is needed. Recent figures on the overall funding gap for AIDS vaccine research and development estimate the deficit to be between $340 and $400 million annually.[7] Expanded research and development capacity in developing countries where AIDS is taking its greatest toll, investments in scientific teams and clinical trial site infrastructure, and stronger ethical and regulatory agencies would also speed research and development and help prepare communities for the distribution of a safe and effective preventive AIDS vaccine.

With 14,000 persons becoming newly infected with HIV each day, accelerating the timetable towards a vaccine is a global health and development priority. A comprehensive approach to HIV/AIDS that includes adequate and sustained attention to the development of new AIDS prevention technologies is the best path to eventually reversing the 25-year-old pandemic.

The International AIDS Vaccine Initiative (IAVI) is a global not-for-profit organization whose mission is to ensure the development of safe, effective, accessible, preventive HIV vaccines for use throughout the world. Founded in 1996 and operational in 23 countries, IAVI and its network of collaborators research and develop vaccine candidates. For more information, see http://www.iavi.org.

References

1. UNAIDS, 2006 Report on the Global AIDS Epidemic, May 2006, available from http://www.unaids.org/en/HIV_data/ 2006GlobalReport/default.asp.

2. WHO, Progress on Global Access to HIV Antiretroviral Therapy—A Report on "3 x 5" and Beyond, March 2006, available from http://www.who.int/hiv/fullreport_en_highres.pdf.

3. HIV Vaccines and Microbicides Resource Tracking Working Group, Adding It All Up: Funding for HIV Vaccine and Microbicide Development, 2000–2006 (New York: IAVI, August 2006).

4. International AIDS Vaccine Initiative, IAVI Database of AIDS Vaccines in Human Trials, February 2006, available from http://www.iavireport.org/trialsdb.

5. Stover J, Estimating the Global Impact of an AIDS Vaccine (New York: International AIDS Vaccine Initiative, October 2005).

6. HIV Vaccines and Microbicides Resource Tracking Working Group (2005).

7. International AIDS Vaccine Initiative, Investing in AIDS Vaccines: Estimated Resources Required to Accelerate R&D (New York: International AIDS Vaccine Initiative, June 2005).

Scientists Unveil Piece of HIV Protein that May Be Key to AIDS Vaccine Development

In a finding that could have profound implications for AIDS vaccine design, researchers led by a team at the National Institute of Allergy and Infectious Diseases (NIAID), part of the National Institutes of Health (NIH), have generated an atomic-level picture of a key portion of an HIV surface protein as it looks when bound to an infection-fighting antibody. Unlike much of the constantly mutating virus, this protein component is stable and—more importantly, say the researchers—appears vulnerable to attack from this specific antibody, known as b12, that can broadly neutralize HIV.

"Creating an HIV vaccine is one of the great scientific challenges of our time," says NIH Director Elias A. Zerhouni, MD. "NIH researchers and their colleagues have revealed a gap in HIV's armor and have thereby opened a new avenue to meeting that challenge."

The research team was led by Peter Kwong, PhD, of NIAID's Vaccine Research Center (VRC). His collaborators included other scientists from NIAID and the National Cancer Institute, NIH, as well as investigators from the Dana-Farber Cancer Institute, Boston, and The Scripps Research Institute in La Jolla, CA. Their paper appears in the February 15, [2007], issue of *Nature* and is now available online.

"This elegant work by Dr. Kwong and his colleagues provides us with a long-sought picture of the precise interaction between the HIV gp120 surface protein and this neutralizing antibody," says NIAID Director Anthony S. Fauci, MD. "This finding could help in the development of an HIV vaccine capable of eliciting a robust antibody response."

For years, AIDS vaccine developers have been stymied by the seemingly unlimited ways HIV eludes natural and vaccine-induced immune defenses. Notes Dr. Kwong, "The more we learned about HIV, the more we realized just how many levels of defense the virus has against attacks by the immune system." For example, not only does HIV mutate rapidly and continuously—defeating attempts by the immune system to identify and destroy it—the virus is also swathed by sugary molecules. This nearly impenetrable sugar cloak prevents antibodies from slipping in and blocking the proteins the virus uses to latch onto a cell and infect it.

In 1998, Dr. Kwong and colleagues published the first x-ray snapshot of the core of HIV gp120 as it attaches to a cellular receptor known as CD4. That image gave researchers a glimpse of some sites on the virus that could be targets of drugs or vaccines, but it also revealed the extent of HIV's overlapping defenses. For example, scientists subsequently learned that CD4-gp120 contact causes gp120 to change shape, a viral feint known as conformational masking, which acts to further shield HIV from immune system attack.

While the earlier study provided a picture of the CD4-gp120 complex, the new finding delineates the precise stepwise engagement between gp120 and CD4. The researchers found that the gp120-CD4 encounter starts with a highly focused contact and then expands to a broader surface that stabilizes the interaction.

"The first contact is like a cautious handshake, which then becomes a hearty bear hug," says Gary Nabel, MD, PhD, director of NIAID's VRC and co-author of the new paper.

An effective HIV vaccine likely needs to induce antibodies that can sense and destroy multiple HIV strains. Scientists have sought such broadly neutralizing antibodies by studying the blood of people whose immune systems appear to hold the virus at bay for long periods of time—b12 is one of these rare, broadly neutralizing antibodies.

Until now, no one had succeeded in determining the detailed structure of b12 in complex with gp120. It was extremely difficult to crystallize b12 bound to gp120, says Dr. Kwong, in part due to the inherently flexible nature of the chemical bonds in gp120. To overcome the problem, the investigators created a variety of gp120s and eventually made the protein stiff enough to capture a picture of it in complex with b12. They saw that b12 binds gp120 at the same point where gp120 initially attaches to CD4. Unlike the gp120-CD4 interactions, however, b12 can latch onto the site of CD4's first contact without requiring a shape change in gp120 to create a stable bond between the two molecules. Essentially, the scientists found that the initial point of CD4 contact is a site of gp120 weakness because it is the site of recognition—called an epitope—for b12.

"One of our primary goals is to develop HIV vaccines that can stimulate broadly neutralizing antibodies," says Dr. Nabel. "The structure of this gp120 epitope, and its susceptibility to attack by a broadly neutralizing antibody, shows us a critical area of vulnerability on the virus that we may be able to target with vaccines. This is certainly one of the best leads to come along in recent years."

References

Zhou T, et al. Structural definition of a conserved neutralization epitope on HIV-1 gp120. *Nature* DOI: 10.1038/Nature05580 (2007).

Kwong PD, et al. Structure of an HIV gp120 envelope glycoprotein in complex with CD4 receptor and a neutralizing human antibody. *Nature* 393:648–59 (1998).

Vaccine Research Center Structural Biology Laboratory online at http://www.niaid.nih.gov/vrc/labs_kwong.htm

Chapter 68

Clinical Trials

Chapter Contents

Section 68.1

What Is an AIDS Clinical Trial?

From AIDSinfo (http://www.aidsinfo.nih.gov), a service of the U.S. Department of Health and Human Services, September 2005.

HIV/AIDS clinical trials are research studies in which new therapies and prevention strategies for HIV infection and AIDS are tested in humans. These studies are conducted by physicians and other health care professionals and can help determine the usefulness of experimental drugs and vaccines in treating or preventing HIV infection. Carefully conducted clinical trials are the fastest and safest way to help find treatments and prevention strategies that work.

New therapies are tested in humans only after laboratory and animal studies show promising results. In Phase I clinical trials, the experimental therapies are given to small numbers of people to help determine safe doses. Larger groups of patients may then receive the therapies in Phase II trials to help measure side effects and preliminary effectiveness. The treatments may then be used in even larger Phase III studies to compare the new treatment to ones already in use or to help estimate other effects of the drug.

What is a clinical trial protocol?

A clinical trial protocol is a detailed plan of how the trial will be conducted. Potential clinical trial participants learn details about the clinical trial protocol in a process called informed consent. Informed consent is the process of learning key facts about a clinical trial before deciding whether or not to participate. To help someone decide whether or not to participate, study staff explain the details of the trial. Then the research team provides an informed consent document that includes details about the study, such as its purpose, duration, required procedures, and key contacts. Risks and potential benefits are also explained in the document. The participant then decides whether or not to sign the document. Informed consent is an ongoing process and the participant may withdraw from the trial at any time.

What are the benefits of participating in an HIV/AIDS clinical trial?

- Participants may gain access to new treatments not yet available to the public.
- Participants may receive expert medical care at leading health care facilities.
- Participants have a chance to help others by contributing to medical research.
- Experimental drugs are often provided free of charge.

What are the risks of participating in an HIV/AIDS clinical trial?

- Experimental drugs may not have any benefits or may even be harmful.
- New drugs may have unanticipated side effects.
- Protocols may require a lot of the participant's time and frequent trips to the study site.

What questions should I ask?

If you are interested in participating in a clinical trial, you may want to ask the following questions:

- What is the purpose of the study?
- What are the drug's side effects?
- What other treatment options do I have?
- Will I have to be in the hospital?
- How often will I have study visits?
- How long will the study last?
- Who will provide my medical care after the study is completed?
- What other drugs can I take if I participate in the study?
- What treatments must I avoid while participating in the study?
- Who will pay the costs of the study?
- How will my confidentiality be protected?

Section 68.2

Federally Funded Clinical Research Trials

"HIV/AIDS Therapeutics: Clinical Trials," National Institute of
Allergies and Infectious Diseases (NIAID), a component of the National
Institutes of Health (NIH), July 15, 2006.

National Institute of Allergies and Infectious Diseases (NIAID)-
Funded Clinical Research: NIAID pursues HIV/AIDS therapeutics
clinical research through its Division of Intramural Research, individual investigator-initiated grants, and clinical trial networks administered by its Division of AIDS.

- **NIAID Division of Intramural Research (DIR):** This Division conducts all of NIAID's in-house research. DIR scientists
carry out basic and clinical research in immunologic, allergic,
and infectious diseases. Patients are frequently admitted to the
clinical service to participate in new and promising treatment
or diagnostic procedures derived from basic research that was
conducted in DIR laboratories.

- **Adult AIDS Clinical Trials Group (AACTG):** A network of
academic research institutions performing all phases of clinical
trials to investigate therapeutic interventions to manage HIV
infection, and its complications including co-infections and
disorders of advancing disease and its therapy.

- **Pediatric AIDS Clinical Trials Group (PACTG):** A network
of academic research institutions performing all phases of clinical
trials to evaluate clinical interventions for treating HIV infection
and HIV-associated illnesses in neonates, infants, children, adolescents, and pregnant women, and new approaches to prevent
mother-to-infant transmission.

- **Terry Beirn Community Programs for Clinical Research
on AIDS (CPCRA):** A network of community-based primary care
units performing large scale, comparative trials to evaluate questions related to optimal clinical management of HIV infection,
including when to start, change, or sequence therapy.

- **Acute Infection and Early Disease Research Program (AIEDRP):** A program of investigator-initiated research focused on innovative ways to study how HIV-1 causes disease in adults.

- **Evaluation of Subcutaneous Proleukin in a Randomized International Trial (ESPRIT):** A randomized, international, five-year, 4000-person study of interleukin-2 (IL-2) in people with HIV infection and a CD4+ (also called T4) cell count of at least 300/mm^3. The goal of the study is to evaluate and compare the effectiveness of IL-2 plus anti-HIV therapy versus anti-HIV therapy alone on numbers and severity of AIDS-related illnesses and deaths

Other NIH-Funded Clinical Trials Networks: Other networks working in collaboration with the Division of Acquired Immunodeficiency Syndrome (DAIDS) on clinical research pertaining to adolescents and co-infections and complications of HIV respectively, include:

- **AIDS Malignancy Consortium (AMC)** conducts clinical trials of therapies for AIDS malignancies, including non-Hodgkin lymphoma, primary central nervous system lymphoma, Kaposi sarcoma, and cervical cancer.

- **Adolescent Trials Network (ATN)** is the only national study of HIV/AIDS in teens infected through sex or injecting-drug behaviors. Funded by the National Institute of Child Health and Human Development (NICHD), ATN research will be able to inform the nation's adolescent-specific HIV/AIDS scientific agenda to improve the prevention of HIV infection and the medical treatment of HIV-positive teens.

- **Bacteriology and Mycology Study Group (BAMSG)** directs trials for antimicrobial therapies of systemic fungal infections.

- **Collaborative Antiviral Study Group (CASG)** conducts studies to evaluate experimental therapies for severe herpes, congenital CMV, human papillomavirus, respiratory viruses, enteroviruses, and hepatitis viruses.

- **Neurology AIDS Research Consortium (NARC)** conducts studies on HIV-associated neurological complications.

- **Studies of Ocular Complications of AIDS (SOCA)** conducts clinical trials and epidemiological research on ocular complications of AIDS, primarily CMV retinitis.

AIDSinfo: The Department of Health and Human Services supports a comprehensive website with a database of all federally-funded and privately-sponsored HIV/AIDS clinical trials, as well as information on HIV/AIDS treatment and prevention guidelines, therapeutic and preventive drugs and vaccines, and other HIV/AIDS related health topics can be found on their website at http://aidsinfo.nih.gov. [Information on clinical trials may also be found online at the National Institutes of Health website at http://www.clinicaltrials.gov/ct/info/resources.]

Section 68.3

Clinical Trial of Experimental Gene Therapy to Treat HIV Shows Encouraging Results

"Fighting HIV with HIV: New Gene Therapy Vector Shows Promise in Penn HIV Study," University of Pennsylvania Health System, November 6, 2006, © 2006 Trustees of the University of Pennsylvania. Available online at http://www.uphs.upenn.edu/news/News_Releases/nov06/HIV genether_print.htm.

Researchers at the University of Pennsylvania School of Medicine (Penn) report the first clinical test of a new gene therapy based on a disabled AIDS virus carrying genetic material that inhibits HIV replication. For the first application of the new vector five subjects with chronic HIV infection who had failed to respond to at least two antiretroviral regimens were given a single infusion of their own immune cells that had been genetically modified for HIV resistance.

The researchers, led by Carl June, MD, and Bruce Levine, PhD, of the Abramson Family Cancer Research Institute and the Department of Pathology and Laboratory Medicine, along with Rob Roy MacGregor, MD, Professor of Medicine, report their findings in the online edition of the *Proceedings of the National Academy of Sciences*. Viral loads of the patients remained stable or decreased during the study, and one subject showed a sustained decrease in viral load. T-cell counts remained steady or increased in four patients during the nine-month trial. Additionally, in four patients, immune function specific to HIV improved.

Overall, the study results are significant, say the researchers, because it is the first demonstration of safety in humans for a lentiviral vector (of which HIV is an example) for any disease. Additionally, the vector, called VRX496, produced encouraging results in some patients where other treatments have failed.

"The goal of this Phase I trial was safety and feasibility and the results established that," says June. "But the results also hint at something much more."

Each patient received one infusion of his or her own gene-modified T cells. The target dose was 10 billion cells, which is about 2 to 10 percent of the number of T cells in an average person. The T-cell count was unchanged early after the infusions. "We were able to detect the gene-modified cells for months, and in one or two patients, a year or more later," says Levine. "That's significant—showing that these cells just don't die inside the patient. The really interesting part of the study came when we saw a significant decrease in viral load in two patients, and in one patient, a very dramatic decrease.

But, cautions Levine, "just because this has produced encouraging results in one or two patients doesn't mean it will work for everyone. We have much more work to do." In the current study, each patient will be followed for 15 years.

Trojan horses: "The new vector is a lab-modified HIV that has been disabled to allow it to function as a Trojan horse, carrying a gene that prevents new infectious HIV from being produced," says Levine. "Essentially, the vector puts a wrench in the HIV replication process." Instead of chemical- or protein-based HIV replication blockers, this approach is genetic and uses a disabled AIDS virus to carry an anti-HIV genetic payload. The modified AIDS virus is added to immune cells that have been removed from the patients' blood by apheresis, purified, genetically modified, and expanded by a process June and Levine developed. The modified immune cells are then returned to the patients' body by simple intravenous infusion.

This approach enables patients' own T cells, which are targets for HIV, to inhibit HIV replication—via the HIV vector and its anti-viral cargo. The HIV vector delivers an antisense RNA molecule that is the mirror image of an HIV gene called envelope to the T cells. When the modified T cells are given back to the patient, the antisense gene is permanently integrated into the cellular DNA. When the virus starts to replicate inside the host cell, the antisense gene prevents translation of the full-length HIV envelope gene, thereby shutting down HIV replication by preventing it from making essential building blocks for progeny virus. VRX496 was designed and produced by the Gaithersburg, MD, biotech company VIRxSYS Corp.

A new field: The new vector is based on a lentivirus, a subgroup of the well-known retroviruses. The study and its safety profile to date have now opened up the field of lentiviral vectors, which have potential advantages over other viral vectors currently being studied because they infect T cells better than adenoviruses, a commonly used viral vector. Lentiviruses also infect non-dividing or slowly dividing cells, which improves delivery to cells such as neurons or stem cells, thus enabling the evaluation of gene therapy in an even wider array of diseases than before. Furthermore, lentiviral vectors insert into cellular DNA in such a way that may be safer than other gene therapy vectors. This is because lentiviruses appear to insert differently from other retroviruses that have caused side effects in other trials involving stem-cell therapy. In addition, gene insertion by lentiviral vectors is attractive for potential therapeutics since it enables long-term gene expression, unlike other viral vectors where expression is lost over time.

Penn researchers are now recruiting for a second trial using the VRX496 vector with HIV patients whose virus is well controlled by existing antiretroviral drugs, a group of patients who are generally healthier and have more treatment options available. This trial will use six infusions rather than one and is designed to evaluate the safety of multiple infusions and to test the effect of infusions on the patients' ability to control HIV after removal of their antiretroviral drugs. The hope is that this treatment approach may ultimately allow patients to stay off antiretroviral drugs for an extensive period, which are known to have significant toxicity, especially after long-term use.

The research was supported by the National Institute of Allergy and Infectious Disease; the Abramson Family Cancer Research Institute; and VIRxSYS Corp. In addition to June, Levine, and MacGregor, co-authors on the paper are: Jean Boyer and Frederic Bushman from Penn; Laurent M. Humeau, Tessio Rebello, Xiaobin Lu (now with U.S. Pharmacopeia), Gwendolyn K. Binder (now with Penn), Vladimir Slepushkin, Frank Lemiale, and Boro Dropulic (now with Lentigen Corp, Baltimore) from VIRxSYS; and John R. Mascola from the National Institutes of Health.

Part Nine

Additional Help and Information

Chapter 69

Glossary of AIDS- and HIV-Related Terms

acquired immunodeficiency syndrome (AIDS): A deficiency of cellular immunity induced by infection with the human immunodeficiency virus (HIV-1) and characterized by opportunistic diseases, including *Pneumocystis carinii/jiroveci* pneumonia, Kaposi sarcoma, oral hairy leukoplakia, cytomegalovirus disease, tuberculosis, *Mycobacterium avium* complex (MAC) disease, candidal esophagitis, cryptosporidiosis, isosporiasis, cryptococcosis, non-Hodgkin lymphoma, progressive multifocal leukoencephalopathy (PML), herpes zoster, and lymphoma. HIV is transmitted from person to person in cell-rich body fluids (notably blood and semen) through sexual contact, sharing of contaminated needles (as by IV drug abusers), or other contact with contaminated blood (as in accidental needlesticks among health care workers).[1]

adherence: The extent to which a patient continues an agreed-upon mode of treatment without close supervision.[1]

The terms in this glossary marked "1" are excerpted from *Stedman's Electronic Medical Dictionary* v. 5.0, Copyright © 2000 Lippincott Williams and Wilkins. All rights reserved. Terms marked "2" are from documents produced by AIDSinfo, a service of the U.S. Department of Health and Human Services, and the National Institute of Allergy and Infectious Diseases (NIAID), a component of the U.S. National Institutes of Health (NIH). "List of Acronyms" is excerpted from "How to Find Reliable HIV/AIDS Treatment Information on the Internet," National Library of Medicine, prepared by the Medical Education and Outreach Group, Oak Ridge Institute for Science and Education, April 2005.

afebrile: Without fever, denoting apyrexia; having a normal body temperature.[1]

AIDS dementia complex (ADC): A subacute or chronic HIV-1 encephalitis, the most common neurologic complication in the later stages of HIV infection; manifested clinically as a progressive dementia, accompanied by motor abnormalities. Syn: AIDS dementia, HIV encephalopathy.[1]

AIDS-defining condition: Any of a list of illnesses that, when occurring in an HIV-infected person, leads to a diagnosis of AIDS. The Centers for Disease Control and Prevention (CDC) published a list of AIDS-defining conditions in 1993. The 26 conditions include candidiasis, cytomegalovirus disease, Kaposi sarcoma, *Mycobacterium avium* complex, *Pneumocystis carinii/jiroveci* pneumonia, recurrent pneumonia, progressive multifocal leukoencephalopathy, pulmonary tuberculosis, invasive cervical cancer, and wasting syndrome.[1]

AIDS-related complex (ARC): Manifestations of AIDS in persons who have not yet developed major deficient immune function, characterized by fever with generalized lymphadenopathy, diarrhea, weight loss, minor opportunistic infections, cytopenias.[1]

antibody: A protein produced by the body's immune system that recognizes and fights infectious organisms and other foreign substances that enter the body. Each antibody is specific to a particular piece of an infectious organism or other foreign substance.[2]

antiviral: Opposing a virus; interfering with its replication; weakening or abolishing its action (e.g., zidovudine, acyclovir).[1]

apoptosis: Cellular suicide, also known as programmed cell death. HIV may induce apoptosis in both infected and uninfected immune system cells.[2]

asymptomatic: Without symptoms, or producing no symptoms.[1]

AZT (azidothymidine): A thymidine analog that is an inhibitor of in vitro replication of HIV virus, the causative agent of AIDS and ARC, and is used in the management of these diseases. Syn: zidovudine.[1]

B cells: White blood cells of the immune system that produce infection-fighting proteins called antibodies.[2]

cachexia: A general weight loss and wasting occurring in the course of a chronic disease or emotional disturbance.[1]

CD4 receptor: A protein present on the outside of infection-fighting white blood cells. CD4 receptors allows HIV to bind to and enter cells.[2]

CD4: A type I transmembrane protein found on helper/inducer T cells, monocytes, macrophages, and dendritic cells that is involved in T-cell recognition of antigens; expressed in T-cell lymphomas.[1]

CD4+ T cells: White blood cells that orchestrate the immune response, signaling other cells in the immune system to perform their special functions. Also known as T helper cells, these cells are killed or disabled during HIV infection.[2]

colposcopy: Examination of vagina and cervix by means of an endoscope. Colposcopy is used chiefly to identify areas of cervical dysplasia in women with abnormal Pap smears.[1]

co-infection: Infection with more than one virus, bacterium, or other micro-organism at a given time. For example, an HIV-infected individual may be co-infected with hepatitis C virus (HCV) or tuberculosis (TB).[2]

co-receptor: In addition to binding a CD4 receptor, HIV must also bind either a CCR5 or CXCR4 co-receptor protein to get into a cell.[2]

cytokines: Proteins used for communication by cells of the immune system. Central to the normal regulation of the immune response.[2]

dendritic cells: A type of antigen-presenting cell that picks up foreign substances from the bloodstream and "presents" them to other parts of the immune system, activating an immune response against the foreign invader.[2]

drug resistance: The capacity of disease-causing microorganisms to withstand drugs previously toxic to them; achieved by spontaneous mutation or through selective pressure after exposure to the drug in question. Usually an organism that has acquired resistance to a given antibiotic is resistant to others in the same chemical class. Drug resistance is a growing problem worldwide.[1]

emerging viruses: In epidemiology, a class of viruses that have long infected humans or animals but now have the opportunity to attain epidemic proportions. A number of viruses have been termed emergent. Virologists speculate that the strain of HIV that causes AIDS may also fall into this category, having entered humans through contact with monkeys in central Africa, possibly having existed among monkey populations for some 50,000 years.[1]

epitope: The simplest form of an antigenic determinant, on a complex antigenic molecule, which can combine with antibody or T cell receptor.[1]

gene: A short segment of DNA or RNA that acts as a blueprint for building a specific protein.[2]

genetic engineering: A laboratory technique that can produce custommade proteins for use as drugs and vaccines.[2]

hairy leukoplakia: A white lesion appearing on the tongue, occasionally on the buccal mucosa, of patients with AIDS; a manifestation of Epstein-Barr virus infection in an immunocompromised host; the lesion appears raised, with a corrugated, shaggy, or "hairy" surface due to keratin projections. Oral hairy leukoplakia was first recognized in 1981 as a marker of immunosuppression in patients with AIDS.[1]

highly active antiretroviral therapy (HAART): The name given to treatment regimens that aggressively suppress HIV replication and progression of HIV disease. The usual HAART regimen combines three or more anti-HIV drugs.[2]

immunodeficiency/immune deficiency: The inability of the immune system to work properly, resulting in susceptibility to disease.[2]

human immunodeficiency virus (HIV): The virus that causes acquired immunodeficiency syndrome (AIDS). HIV is in the retrovirus family, and two types have been identified: HIV-1 and HIV-2. HIV-1 is responsible for most HIV infections throughout the world, while HIV-2 is found primarily in West Africa.[2]

immunocompetent: Possessing the ability to mount a normal immune response.[1]

immunocompromised: Denoting an individual whose immunologic mechanism is deficient either because of an immunodeficiency disorder or because it has been rendered so by immunosuppressive agents.[1]

immunosuppression: Immune system response to foreign invaders such as HIV is reduced.[2]

integrase: An HIV enzyme used by the virus to integrate its genetic material into the host cell's DNA.[2]

lentivirus: "Slow" virus characterized by a long interval between infection and the onset of symptoms. HIV is a lentivirus as is the simian immunodeficiency virus (SIV), which infects nonhuman primates.[2]

lipodystrophy: Defective metabolism of fat. Syn: lipodystrophia.[1]

log: This mathematical term represents a change in value of what is being measured by a factor of 10. Changes in viral load (the amount of HIV in the blood) are often reported as logarithmic or "log" changes.[1]

macrophage: A large immune system cell that devours invading pathogens and other intruders. Stimulates other immune system cells by presenting them with small pieces of the invaders.[2]

microbes: Microscopic living organisms, including viruses, bacteria, fungi, and protozoa.[1]

microbicide: An agent destructive to microbes; a germicide; an antiseptic. Syn: microbicidal.[1]

microorganisms: Small life forms that can be seen only through a microscope, including bacteria, protozoa, viruses, and fungi.[2]

monocyte: A circulating white blood cell that develops into a macrophage when it enters tissues.[2]

mother-to-child transmission (MTCT): The passage of HIV from an HIV-infected mother to her infant. The infant may become infected while in the womb, during labor and delivery, or through breast-feeding.[2]

***Mycobacterium avium-intracellulare* complex (MAC):** An opportunistic agent of infection, particularly in people with AIDS. Difficult to treat because *Mycobacterium avium-intracellulare* is resistant to many antibiotics.[1]

opportunistic infection: An illness caused by an organism that usually does not cause disease in a person with a normal immune system. People with advanced HIV infection suffer opportunistic infections of the lungs, brain, eyes, and other organs.[2]

p24: An HIV protein that makes up the virus core that surrounds HIV's genetic material.[2]

palliative: Reducing the severity of; denoting the alleviation of symptoms without curing the underlying disease.[1]

pandemic: Denoting a disease affecting or attacking the population of an extensive region, country, continent, global; extensively epidemic.[1]

Pap test: Microscopic examination of cells exfoliated or scraped from a mucosal surface after staining with Papanicolaou stain; used especially for detection of cancer of the uterine cervix. Syn: Papanicolaou smear test.[1]

pathogens: Disease-causing organisms.[2]

perinatal: Occurring during, or pertaining to, the periods before, during, or after the time of birth.[1]

***Pneumocystis carinii* pneumonia (PCP):** Pneumonia resulting from infection with *Pneumocystis carinii / jiroveci,* frequently seen in the immunologically compromised, such as persons with AIDS. In AIDS patients the tissue damage is usually restricted to the pulmonary parenchyma. Patients may be only slightly febrile [feverish] (or even afebrile), but are likely to be extremely weak, dyspneic [out of breath], and cyanotic. This is a major cause of morbidity among patients with AIDS. Syn: pneumocystosis, interstitial plasma cell pneumonia.[1]

post-exposure prophylaxis (PEP): Administration of anti-HIV drugs within 72 hours of a high-risk exposure, including unprotected sex, needle sharing, or occupational needlestick injury, to help prevent development of HIV infection.[2]

progressive multifocal leukoencephalopathy (PML): A rare, subacute, afebrile disease characterized by areas of demyelinization surrounded by markedly altered neuroglia; it occurs usually in individuals with AIDS, leukemia, lymphoma, or other debilitating diseases. Caused by JC virus, a human polyoma virus. Syn: progressive subcortical encephalopathy.[1]

prophylaxis: Prevention of disease or of a process that can lead to disease.[1]

provirus: DNA of a virus, such as HIV, that has been integrated into the genes of a host cell.[2]

regimen: A program, including drugs, which regulates aspects of one's lifestyle for a hygienic or therapeutic purpose; a program of treatment; sometimes mistakenly called regime.[1]

resistance: The natural or acquired ability of an organism to maintain its immunity to or to resist the effects of an antagonistic agent, e.g., pathogenic microorganism, toxin, drug.[1]

retrovirus: HIV and other viruses that carry their genetic material in the form of RNA and that have the enzyme reverse transcriptase.[2]

reverse transcriptase: The enzyme produced by HIV and other retroviruses that allows them to synthesize DNA from their RNA.[2]

safe sex: Sexual practices that limit the risk of transmitting or acquiring an infectious disease via exchanges of semen, blood, and other bodily fluids, e.g., use of a condom, mutual masturbation, and avoidance of anal intercourse.[1]

seroconversion: Development of detectable specific antibodies in the serum as a result of infection or immunization.[1]

sexually transmitted disease (STD): Any contagious disease acquired during sexual contact; e.g., syphilis, gonorrhea, chancroid. Syn: venereal disease.[1]

superinfection: A new infection in addition to one already present.[1]

T lymphocyte: A type of white blood cell that detects and fights foreign invaders of the body.[2]

titer: The standard of strength of a volumetric test solution; the assay value of an unknown measure by volumetric means.[1]

vector: A harmless virus or bacteria used as a vaccine carrier to deliver pieces of a disease-causing organism (such as HIV) into the body's cells.[2]

viral load: The plasma level of viral RNA, as determined by various techniques including target amplification assay by reverse transcriptase polymerase chain reaction and branched DNA technology with signal amplification. Reported as the number of copies of viral RNA per mL of plasma, assessment of viral load provides important information about the number of lymphoid cells actively infected with HIV. This laboratory procedure has supplanted the CD4 count as an indicator of prognosis of persons infected with HIV, in determining when to start antiretroviral therapy, and in measuring the response to therapy. Because the CD4 count is regarded as superior in determining the level of immune compromise and the risk of opportunistic infection, both tests are currently used.[1]

virion: The complete virus particle that is structurally intact and infectious.[1]

wasting: Becoming abnormally thin from extreme loss of flesh. Syn: emaciation.[1]

wild-type virus: A term to describe virus strains (including strains of HIV) that have not acquired any genetic mutations that create special characteristics, such as resistance to particular drugs.[2]

List of Acronyms

ACTIS: AIDS Clinical Trials Information Service

ADAP: AIDS Drug Assistance Program

AEGIS: AIDS Education Global Information System

AETC: AIDS Education and Training Centers

AACTG: Adult AIDS Clinical Trials Group

APC: antigen-presenting cells

ARI: AIDS Research Institute

ARIC: AIDS Research Information Center

ASO: AIDS Service Organization

ATIS: HIV/AIDS Treatment Information Service

AVN: avascular necrosis

BETA: Bulletin of Experimental Treatments for AIDS

BFR: Body Fat Redistribution Syndrome

BUARC: Bastyr University AIDS Research Center

CARE Act: Ryan White Comprehensive AIDS Resources Emergency Act of 1990 (Public Law 101-381)

CBCT: Community-Based Clinical Trials

CBO: Community-Based Organization

CMHRA: Center for Mental Health Research on AIDS

CMV: Cytomegalovirus

CPAT: Community Provider AIDS Training Project

CPCRA: Community Programs for Clinical Research on AIDS

CRIA: Community Research Initiative on AIDS

DAAIR: Direct AIDS Alternative Information Resources

DAIDS: Division of Acquired Immunodeficiency Syndrome

DIRLINE: Directory of Information Resources Online

FY: fiscal year

G.A.R.D.: Global AIDS Resource Directory

GMHC: Gay Men's Health Crisis

HIVCIN: HIV Clinical Information Network

HRSA: Health Resources and Services Administration

IAPAC: International Association of Physicians in AIDS Care

IAS: International AIDS Society

IAS-USA: International AIDS Society, United States of America

ICAAC: Interscience Conference on Antimicrobial Agents and Chemotherapy

ICAR: International Conference on Antiviral Research

IDSA: Infectious Disease Society of America

IND: investigational new drug

JAMA: *Journal of the American Medical Association*

KS: Kaposi sarcoma

MATEP: Midwest AIDS Training Center Partners

MMWR: *Morbidity and Mortality Weekly Report*

NATAP: National AIDS Treatment Advocacy Project

NLM: National Library of Medicine

NMAC: National Minority AIDS Council

OAM: Office of Alternative Medicine

OHL: oral hairy leukoplakia

OI: opportunistic infections

PAETC: Pacific AIDS Education and Training Center

PCP: *Pneumocystis carinii/jiroveci* pneumonia

PDQ: Physician Data Query

PEP: post-exposure prophylaxis

PHS: Public Health Service

PI: Project Inform

PIV: Partnership in Vision

PWA: Persons with AIDS

RITA!: Research Initiative/Treatment Action!

STD: sexually transmitted disease

SIT: Structured Intermittent Therapy

STI: Structured Treatment Interruption

T cells: T lymphocytes

T4 cell: T-helper cell

TAG: Treatment Action Group

TB: tuberculosis

TST: tuberculin skin test

TPAN: Test Positive Aware Network

UCSF: University of California, San Francisco

UN: United Nations

USPHS: U.S. Public Health Service

Chapter 70

Medical and Support Services for People Living with HIV/AIDS

Chapter Contents

Section 70.1

The Basics: The Ryan White CARE Act

"The Basics: The Ryan White CARE Act," September 14, 2005.
© National Health Policy Forum. Reprinted with permission.

In the early 1980s, the United States was confronted by an epidemic of the human immunodeficiency virus (HIV). This virus, left untreated, progresses to a disease called the acquired immunodeficiency syndrome (AIDS) that severely hampers the body's ability to ward off illness and infection. As of 2003, between 1,039,000 and 1,185,000 people are estimated to be living with HIV/AIDS in the United States, and one-quarter of them do not know they are infected.

The Centers for Disease Control and Prevention (CDC) believes that 40 to 60 percent of the infected population does not receive regular treatment. Of those that receive treatment, one study estimated that 20 percent were uninsured, 29 percent were covered by Medicaid only, 6 percent were covered by Medicare only, 13 percent were dually eligible for Medicaid and Medicare, and 31 percent had private insurance. Many of those who are uninsured or underinsured turn to the health care "safety net" for free or low-cost treatment. Medicaid and the Ryan White Comprehensive AIDS Resources Emergency (CARE) Act are two key federal funders of the HIV/AIDS safety net. A variety of private providers, free clinics, community health centers, hospital outpatient departments, and local health departments, among others, receive these funds in return for providing treatment to this population.

Congress created the Ryan White CARE Act in 1990 in response to calls for assistance from a number of urban public hospitals that were struggling financially from uncompensated care provided to individuals dying of AIDS. The Act was named for Ryan White, a teenager who contracted HIV through a blood transfusion and died after an eight-year struggle with the disease.

The Ryan White CARE Act is a series of grant programs that fund treatment services for people with HIV/AIDS who are either uninsured or underinsured; it is not a health insurance program like Medicaid or

Medicare. Since its creation, the Act has been reauthorized twice, in 1996 and 2000. Its current authorization expires on September 30, 2005. [See the next section for information on the 2006 reauthorization.] The authorizing committees of jurisdiction are the Senate Committee on Health, Education, Labor, and Pensions and the House Committee on Energy and Commerce.

The Act funds medical and support services for approximately 533,000 individuals and families living with HIV/AIDS each year. In 2002, 46 percent of people who receive these services through Ryan White were African American, 20 percent were Hispanic, and about one-third were women. At least one of every two clients lived below the federal poverty level, about 25 percent were uninsured, less than 10 percent had any private health insurance, and about 28 percent were enrolled in Medicaid. The Health Resources and Services Administration within the Department of Health and Human Services administers the Act through the HIV/AIDS Bureau.

CARE Act Components

The Act is organized into four titles and one part. Each title directs funds to a different type of recipient. For example, Title I is geared to cities, Title II to states, and Titles III and IV to community-based providers. The funding distribution mechanisms vary among the titles. Title I funds formula grants, which are awarded noncompetitively based on statutorily established factors, as well as competitive grants; Title II funds only formula grants, and Titles III and IV fund only competitive grants. Eighty-five percent of Ryan White funds are distributed through Titles I and II of the Act.

Title I (Part A) of the CARE Act

The first title of the Act provides funds to eligible metropolitan areas (EMAs) that have a population of at least 500,000 and more than 2,000 estimated living AIDS cases (ELCs) within the past five years. Half of the funds are distributed through formula grants and the other half through competitive, supplemental grants based on the severity of the EMA's need. An EMA's formula grant is based on its proportion of ELCs compared to all ELCs across all EMAs. In FY 2005, 51 EMAs were funded.

Title I grant funds may be used for outpatient and ambulatory health services, including dental, substance abuse, and mental health services, and support services such as case management, transportation and housing assistance, nutrition services, day care, and respite care. They may also be used for outreach to people who know their HIV status but are not receiving treatment.

Funds are directed to the chief elected official of the public health agency within the EMA that serves the largest number of people with AIDS. That official appoints a local planning council that has broad responsibilities for targeting funds to the local population living with HIV/AIDS.

Title II (Part B) of the CARE Act

Title II funds three types of formula grants: base grants, AIDS Drug Assistance Program (ADAP) grants, and grants to emerging communities.

Base Grants

The Title II base grant is a formula grant that goes to all 50 states, the District of Columbia, Puerto Rico, Guam, the U.S. Virgin Islands, and five U.S. Pacific territories. It has two parts; 80 percent of the award is based on a state's proportion of all estimated living AIDS cases, and the other 20 percent comes from the state's proportion of AIDS cases within the state but outside its EMAs. For states with less than 90 AIDS cases, the minimum grant is $200,000; states with over 90 cases receive a minimum of $500,000 and territories receive at least $50,000. Most states provide some services directly but also award subgrants of these dollars to public or nonprofit providers.

AIDS Drug Assistance Program

About one-third of all Ryan White funding and the majority of Title II funds—$788 million in FY 2005—is earmarked by Congress for the AIDS Drug Assistance Program (ADAP). Federal ADAP funds are distributed by a formula based on each state's proportion of the nation's living AIDS cases. In addition to the federal grant, some ADAPs receive state general revenue funding, funds from other parts of the CARE Act, or funds from drug rebates negotiated with drug manufacturers.

ADAPs operate in 57 jurisdictions including all 50 states, Puerto Rico, the District of Columbia, the U.S. Virgin Islands, the Marshall Islands, Guam, American Samoa, and the Northern Mariana Islands. They primarily provide prescription drugs approved by the Food and Drug Administration to eligible individuals, but they may also use funds to pay to continue an eligible individual's private health insurance, if it has prescription drug coverage, or to fund treatment adherence programs for clients.

States must ensure that an individual has been medically diagnosed with HIV and that he or she qualifies as "low income," as defined by the state, to receive services from an ADAP. The statute gives states flexibility in designing their program including setting income and medical eligibility criteria and developing formularies.

The 2000 reauthorization added a supplemental ADAP grant program to help states expand access to treatment specifically for their HIV/AIDS population with income below 200 percent of the federal poverty level. States may only use these funds to purchase drugs, and they must match one dollar for every four federal dollars.

Emerging Communities Grants

In an attempt to respond to the growing epidemic in small urban centers, suburban, and rural areas, Congress added the emerging communities formula grant program to Title II in the 2000 reauthorization. Funds are distributed to communities with a population of at least 50,000 that have between 500 and 1,999 reported AIDS cases over the last five years. Funding is divided into two tiers, with 50 percent awarded to communities with 1,000 to 1,999 AIDS cases and 50 percent to communities with 500 to 999 AIDS cases. Within each tier, funds are distributed to communities based on their proportion of AIDS cases within the tier.

Title III (Part C) of the CARE Act

Whereas the first two titles of the Act provide funds to metropolitan areas and states, the third title funds community-based organizations through a competitive process. Funds are awarded to public and private, nonprofit, primary care providers such as federally qualified health centers (FQHCs), city and county health departments, hemophilia treatment centers, and outpatient facilities at academic medical centers that serve people living with HIV/AIDS. Ninety-eight percent of Title III funds are used to provide early intervention services for uninsured and underinsured individuals. Early intervention services include counseling, testing, primary care, drug therapy, case management, and mental health services, among others. The remaining 2 percent of funds is awarded for capacity building and planning at these same organizations.

Title IV (Part D) of the CARE Act

Title IV funds are targeted to women, infants, children, and youth with HIV/AIDS. Grants are awarded competitively to public and private non-profit organizations to provide primary and specialty care; substance abuse and mental health services; support services such as transportation, child care, and housing assistance; care coordination; access to clinical trials and clinical research; and supportive services to family members and others who care for this population. A special focus of Title IV is to identify HIV-positive pregnant women and ensure that they have access to prenatal care to prevent mother-to-child transmission of the virus.

Part E

Part E authorizes grants for emergency response employees and establishes notification procedures in case of exposure to infectious diseases; the corresponding funds have never been appropriated to implement this program.

Part F: Provider Training, Dental Reimbursement, and Special Projects

Part F of the Act includes three other competitive grant programs. The AIDS Education and Training Centers Program (AETC) is the clinical training component of the Act and funds a network of 11 regional centers with more than 130 sites that conduct multidisciplinary training and education programs for health care providers who treat patients with HIV/AIDS.

The Ryan White dental program was created to alleviate significant difficulties in access to dental care for people living with HIV/AIDS. The program reimburses dental schools, postdoctoral dental programs, and, since the 2000 reauthorization, dental hygiene programs, for the uncompensated services they provide to people living with HIV/AIDS.

The Special Projects of National Significance Program supports the development and replication of innovative models in HIV/AIDS care and service delivery. Grantee organizations include academic health center clinics, FQHCs, community-based organizations, and state and local health departments, among others.

Section 70.2

The Ryan White HIV/AIDS Treatment Modernization Act of 2006

"Fact Sheet: The Ryan White HIV/AIDS Treatment Modernization Act of 2006," Office of the Press Secretary, the White House, December 19, 2006.

President Bush signed The Ryan White HIV/AIDS Treatment Modernization Act of 2006 on December 19. This bill focuses on life-saving and life-extending services and increased accountability for funding. It will also provide more flexibility to the Secretary of Health and Human Services to direct funding to the areas of greatest need.

The President is committed to addressing the needs of the 1 million Americans living With HIV/AIDS and to preventing new HIV infections within the United States. Since 2001, the Administration has devoted more than $74 billion to HIV/AIDS treatment and care, increasing annual treatment funding by 37 percent. The Administration has also devoted more than $15 billion to HIV/AIDS research to help develop new methods of treatment and prevention, increasing annual research funding by 20 percent.

The Ryan White CARE Act is an important tool in turning the tide against HIV/AIDS in America. For 16 years, the Ryan White CARE Act has provided medical care, antiretroviral treatments, and counseling to people living with HIV who would otherwise have little or no access to care. It also supports HIV testing to prevent this disease from spreading further.

The Ryan White HIV/AIDS Treatment Modernization Act revises and extends services under the Ryan White Care Act (RWCA) Program. This Act will do the following:

- Provide more flexibility to direct funding to areas of greatest need. New supplemental grants will be provided to States with an increasing need for HIV/AIDS-related services due to limited access to health care, high prevalence of HIV/AIDS, and other relevant factors. The program's formula for awarding funds will also be updated to consider the number of HIV and AIDS cases—the previous formula considered only the number of AIDS cases.

- Target money to core life-saving medical services for those in need. Grantees under Titles I, II, and III of the program will use no less than 75 percent of funds to provide core medical services. In addition, the reauthorization calls for the Early Intervention Services grant program to provide core medical services for individuals with HIV/AIDS in underserved populations.

- Require more aggressive oversight of RWCA programs. For example, the Secretary of Health and Human Services will be required to submit biennial reports describing barriers to HIV program integration. In addition, the Government Accountability Office (GAO) will be required to conduct an evaluation concerning how funds are used to provide family-centered care involving outpatient or ambulatory care services under Title IV of the RWCA Program.

- Standardize minimum requirements for the AIDS Drug Assistance Program (ADAP). The Secretary of Health and Human Services will develop and maintain a list of core ADAP medications needed to manage symptoms associated with HIV infection. States will be required to ensure that their programs, at a minimum, provide these core medications.

The Ryan White HIV/AIDS Treatment Modernization Act authorizes programs to address HIV/AIDS in women, children, and minorities. This Act will do the following:

- Expand resources for women, infants, and children. The reauthorization provides for grants to States for the universal testing of newborns for HIV/AIDS. It also supports the provision of family-centered care for women and children with HIV/AIDS, including the provision of support services such as referrals for inpatient hospital services, treatment for substance abuse, mental health services, and other social services.

- Codify the Minority AIDS Initiative. HIV/AIDS has had a devastating impact on minorities in the United States—African Americans accounted for 49 percent of all HIV/AIDS cases diagnosed in 2005. The Minority AIDS Initiative provides funding for activities to evaluate and address the disproportionate impact of HIV/AIDS and disparities in access, treatment, care, and outcome on racial and ethnic minorities.

Chapter 71

Social Security for People Living with HIV/AIDS

If you have HIV/AIDS and cannot work, you may qualify for disability benefits from the Social Security Administration. Your disability must be expected to last at least a year or end in death, and must be serious enough to prevent you from doing substantial gainful work. The amount of earnings considered substantial and gainful changes each year. For the current figure, refer to the annual *Update* (Publication No. 05-10003).

If your child has HIV/AIDS, he or she may be able to get Supplemental Security Income (SSI) if your household income is low enough.

What two programs are benefits paid under?

Disability benefits are paid under two programs: the Social Security disability insurance program for people who paid Social Security taxes and the Supplemental Security Income program for people who have little income and few resources. If your Social Security benefits are very low and you have limited other income and resources, you may qualify for benefits from both programs.

How do I qualify for Social Security disability benefits?

When you work and pay Social Security taxes, you earn Social Security credits. (Most people earn the maximum of four credits a

Social Security Administration (http://www.socialsecurity.gov), SSA Publication No. 05-10019, February 2005.

year.) The number of years of work needed for disability benefits depends on how old you are when you become disabled. Generally, you need five years of work in the ten years before the year you become disabled. Younger workers need fewer years of work. If your application is approved, your first Social Security disability benefit will be paid for the sixth full month after the date your disability began.

What will I get from Social Security?

The amount of your monthly benefits depends on how much you earned while you were working. You also will qualify for Medicare after you have been getting disability benefits for 24 months. Medicare helps pay for hospital and hospice care, lab tests, home health care, and other medical services. For more information on Medicare, contact the SSA for the publication, *Medicare* (Publication No. 05-10043).

How do I qualify for SSI disability payments?

If you have not worked long enough to get Social Security or your Social Security benefits are low, you may qualify for SSI payments if your total income and resources are low enough.

If you get SSI, you most likely will be eligible for food stamps and Medicaid. Medicaid takes care of your medical bills while you are in the hospital or receiving outpatient care. In some states, Medicaid pays for hospice care, a private nurse, and prescription drugs used to fight HIV disease. For more information about Medicaid, contact your local social services office.

How do I file for benefits?

You can apply for Social Security disability benefits online at www.socialsecurity.gov, or you can call the toll-free number, 800-772-1213 (for the deaf or hard of hearing, call the TTY number, 800-325-0778), to ask for an appointment. The SSA can answer specific questions and provide information by automated phone service 24 hours a day.

All calls are treated confidentially. The SSA also wants to make sure you receive accurate and courteous service. That is why they have a second Social Security representative monitor some telephone calls.

How does the SSA decide my claim?

All applications received from people with HIV/AIDS are processed as quickly as possible. Social Security works with an agency in each state called the Disability Determination Services.

The state agency will look at the information you and your doctor give them and decide if you qualify for benefits.

SSI benefits can be paid right away for up to six months before a final decision on your claim is made if you meet the following conditions:

- you are not working

- you meet the SSI rules about income and resources

- your doctor or other medical source certifies that your HIV infection is severe enough to meet the medical eligibility rules

How can I help speed up my claim?

You can help speed up the processing of your claim by having certain information, including the following, when you apply.

- your Social Security number and birth certificate

- the Social Security numbers and birth certificates of any family members who may be applying for benefits

- a copy of your most recent W-2 form

- information about your income and resources (bank statements, unemployment records, rent receipts, and car registration), if applying for SSI

The SSA also needs information about the following:

- the names and addresses of any doctors, hospitals, or clinics you have been to for treatment

- how HIV/AIDS has affected your daily activities, such as cleaning, shopping, cooking, taking the bus, etc.

- the kinds of jobs you have had during the past 15 years

Additionally, your doctor will be asked to complete a form telling the SSA how your HIV infection has affected you. Call 800-772-1213 to ask for form "SSA-4814" for adults or "SSA-4815" for children.

You should take the form to your doctor to complete and bring or send the completed form to a Social Security office.

What happens if I go back to work?

If you return to work, there are special rules that let your benefits continue while you work. These rules are important for people with HIV/AIDS who may be able to go back to work when they are feeling better.

For more information on these rules, ask any Social Security office for a copy of the publication, *Working While Disabled—How We Can Help* (Publication No. 05-10095).

Chapter 72

The AIDS Drug Assistance Program (ADAP)

The AIDS Drug Assistance Program (ADAP) provides medications for the treatment of HIV disease. Program funds may also be used to purchase health insurance for eligible clients. Amendments to the Ryan White Comprehensive AIDS Resources Emergency (CARE) Act in October 2000 added language allowing ADAP funds to be used for services that enhance access to, adherence to, and monitoring of drug treatments. The program is funded through Title II of the CARE Act, which provides grants to states and territories.

CARE Act programs work with cities, states, and local community-based organizations to provide services to more than 500,000 individuals each year who do not have sufficient health care coverage or financial resources for coping with HIV disease. The majority of CARE Act funds support primary medical care and essential support services. A smaller but equally critical portion is used to fund technical assistance, clinical training, and research on innovative models of care. The CARE Act, which was first authorized in 1990, is currently funded at $2.06 billion.

Funding

- Grants are awarded to all 50 States, the District of Columbia, Puerto Rico, Guam, and the U.S. Virgin Islands. In FY 2002, two

"ADAP Fact Sheet," Department of Health and Human Services (HHS), Health Resources and Services Administration (HSRA), HIV/AIDS Bureau (http://hab.hrsa.gov), July 2006.

additional jurisdictions in the Pacific, the Marshall Islands and North Marianas, received funds.

- Congress "earmarks" funds that must be used for the ADAP, an important distinction since other Title II spending decisions are made locally. The ADAP earmark is by far the fastest growing component of CARE Act appropriations. It was $52 million in 1996 and $790 million in 2006. But total ADAP spending is even higher, because state ADAPs also receive money from their respective states, from other CARE Act programs, and through cost-savings strategies.

- A formula based on AIDS prevalence is used to award ADAP funds to states and territories. However, 3 percent of the total earmark is reserved for supplemental grants to states and territories with demonstrated severe need that prevents them from providing medications consistent with Public Health Service Guidelines.

Clients

- Approximately 142,653 people received medications through ADAP in FY 2004.

- None had adequate health insurance or the financial resources necessary to cover the cost of medications.

- Many clients are enrolled in ADAP only temporarily while they await acceptance into other insurance programs, such as Medicaid. On average, 73,000 clients are served each month.

Implementation

The ADAP in each state and territory is unique in that it decides which medications will be included in its formulary and how those medications will be distributed.

- Many states and territories provide medications through a pharmacy reimbursement model. Patients show enrollment cards at participating pharmacies to receive their medications, and the pharmacy invoices the ADAP for payment.

- Some ADAPs use pharmacies located within public health clinics to distribute drugs.

- A few ADAPs purchase drugs and mail them to clients directly.

Eligibility

Each state and territory establishes its own eligibility criteria. All require that program participants document their HIV status. Nine programs require a CD4 count of 500 or less. Fifteen states have established income eligibility at 200 percent or less of the Federal Poverty Level (FPL). Nationally, more than 80 percent of ADAP clients have incomes at 200 percent or less of the FPL.

Increasing Demand

Pressure on ADAP resources has increased substantially.

- Highly active antiretroviral therapy (HAART) is the standard of care for the majority of individuals living with HIV disease. Its cost may be $12,000 per year or more, in addition to the costs of addressing opportunistic infections, side affects, and other treatment issues.

- AIDS mortality has decreased dramatically in the United States since 1995, and HIV incidence remains constant at approximately 40,000 new infections annually. Therefore, the total number of people living with HIV disease continues to climb.

- The epidemic is growing rapidly among minorities, who have historically experienced higher risk for poverty, lack of health insurance, comorbidity, and disenfranchisement from the health care system. The result is a growing number of people living with HIV disease who require public support.

Additional Resources

Additional fact sheets on ADAP eligibility, formularies, and cost-saving mechanisms are available on the HIV/AIDS Bureau website at http://hab.hrsa.gov.

Chapter 73

Housing Options for Persons Living with HIV/AIDS

HIV/AIDS Housing

The Need for HIV/AIDS Housing Assistance

Throughout many communities, persons living with HIV or AIDS risk losing their housing due to compounding factors, such as increased medical costs or limited ability to keep work due to AIDS.

The lack of affordable and medically appropriate housing for persons living with HIV/AIDS and their families is an ongoing concern for AIDS housing providers, policy makers, and advocates across the country. Stable housing promotes improved health status, sobriety or decreased use of nonprescription drugs, and a return for some persons with AIDS to productive work and social activities. Stable housing is the cornerstone of HIV/AIDS treatment.

Recent studies confirm that persons living with HIV/AIDS must have stable housing to access comprehensive health care and adhere to complex HIV/AIDS drug therapies. Even though stable housing has been shown to be a necessary link to medical and supportive services, accessing housing is difficult as the wait for affordable housing increases in many communities across the country. Compounding the problem of waiting lists is access to housing with the services to care

This chapter includes text from "HIV/AIDS Housing" and "Housing Opportunities for Persons with AIDS (HOPWA) Program," U.S. Department of Housing and Urban Development (http://www.hud.gov), Office of HIV/AIDS Housing, Office of Community Planning and Development, updated May 8, 2007.

619

and treat the increasing number of persons living not only with HIV/AIDS but also with histories of homelessness, mental illness, and substance abuse.

Department of Housing and Urban Development (HUD)'s Response

In recognition of the unique effect HIV/AIDS has on housing for persons with HIV/AIDS and their families, HUD established the Office of HIV/AIDS Housing. The mission of the Office is to ensure that each HUD program and initiative is responsive to the needs of persons living with HIV/AIDS. The office performs policy, program, liaison, outreach, and program evaluation functions.

One of the primary functions of the Office of HIV/AIDS is to manage the Housing Opportunities for Persons with AIDS (HOPWA) program. The HOPWA program is the only federal program dedicated to the housing needs of persons living with HIV/AIDS and their families.

In addition to HOPWA, HUD has other programs designated to serve persons with a variety of needs that can be used to serve persons living with HIV/AIDS. HUD programs such as HUD's Homeless Assistance Programs, Programs for Persons with Disabilities, and HOME Initiatives can be directed to persons living with HIV/AIDS and their families.

Housing Options

Persons living with HIV/AIDS and their families may require housing that provides emergency, transitional, or long-term affordable solutions. A variety of HUD programs and projects provide such housing; however, this housing often is not the typical structure we think of as a "house." HIV/AIDS housing includes short- and long-term rental assistance, live-in medical facilities, and housing sites developed exclusively for people living with AIDS.

Community Planning Options

An additional resource for communities striving to meet the housing needs of persons living with HIV and AIDS is the HOPWA National Technical Assistance Program. The HOPWA National TA Program provides assistance to communities in developing strategies and plans to address the housing needs of persons living with HIV and AIDS. Through comprehensive needs analysis, HOPWA TA providers in partnership with community leaders, providers, and consumers develop needs assessments to determine existing projected housing needs for persons living with HIV/AIDS. Through these assessments, communities may address the housing needs of persons living with HIV and AIDS through a holistic approach, which maximizes resources and provides a continuum of housing options.

Housing Opportunities for Persons with AIDS (HOPWA) Program

About the HOPWA Program

HUD's Office of HIV/AIDS Housing manages the HOPWA program in collaboration with 44 state and area Community Planning and Development (CPD) offices in providing guidance and program oversight. The Office works with other HUD offices to ensure that all HUD programs and initiatives are responsive to the special needs of people with HIV/AIDS. One of the primary functions of the Office is to administer the Housing Opportunities for Persons with HIV/AIDS (HOPWA) program.

The HOPWA Program was established by HUD to address the specific needs of persons living with HIV/AIDS and their families. HOPWA makes grants to local communities, States, and nonprofit organizations for projects that benefit low income persons medically diagnosed with HIV/AIDS and their families.

HOPWA Programs

HOPWA funds are awarded as grants from one of three programs:

- The HOPWA Formula Program uses a statutory method to allocate HOPWA funds to eligible States and cities on behalf of their metropolitan areas.

- The HOPWA Competitive Program is a national competition to select model projects or programs.

- The HOPWA National Technical Assistance Funding awards are provided to strengthen the management, operation, and capacity of HOPWA grantees, project sponsors, and potential applicants of HOPWA funding.

HOPWA funding provides housing assistance and related supportive services as part of HUD's Consolidated Planning initiative that works in partnership with communities and neighborhoods in managing federal funds appropriated to HIV/AIDS programs. HOPWA grantees are encouraged to develop community-wide strategies and form partnerships with area non-profit organizations. HOPWA funds may be used for a wide range of housing, social services, program planning, and development costs. These include, but are not limited to, the acquisition, rehabilitation, or new construction of housing units; costs for facility operations; rental assistance; and short-term payments to prevent homelessness. HOPWA funds also may be used for health care and mental health services, chemical dependency treatment, nutritional services, case management, assistance with daily living, and other supportive services.

Many beneficiaries receive supportive services that are funded by HOPWA or other related public and private programs. In fact, states and cities leverage approximately two dollars for every one dollar provided by the HOPWA program.

The Background

Since the beginning of the HOPWA program in 1992, the federal government has made available over $2.3 billion in HOPWA funds to support community efforts to create and operate HIV/AIDS housing initiatives. HUD estimates that the FY 2004 HOPWA appropriation of $294.75 million provided housing assistance to about 73,700 households. This number included family members who reside with the persons living with HIV/AIDS. More than half of those units (approximately 45,000) involved clients who receive small, short-term payments to prevent homelessness. An additional 25,000 units involved ongoing rental assistance payments. Approximately 5,000 units in supportive housing facilities, single room occupancy (SRO) dwellings, or community residences also were developed or operated with HOPWA funds.

Chapter 74

Directory of Organizations and Hotlines Providing HIV/ AIDS Services and Information

Government Agencies and Organizations That Provide Information about HIV/AIDS

Agency for Healthcare Research and Quality (AHRQ)
HIV Research Program
540 Gaither Road, Suite 2000
Rockville, MD 20850
Phone: 301-427-1364
Fax: 301-427-1430
Website: http://www.ahrq.gov

Resources in this chapter were compiled from a variety of sources. Hotline information was taken from "U.S. National AIDS Hotlines and Resources," Body Health Resources Corporation (http://www.thebody.com), January 16, 2007. AIDSinfo Live Help information is from AIDSinfo (http://www.aidsinfo .nih.gov), a service of the U.S. Department of Health and Human Services, May 30, 2007. All contact information in this chapter was verified and updated in May 2007.

AIDSinfo
U.S. Department of Health and Human Services
P.O. Box 6303
Rockville, MD 20849-6303
Toll-Free: 800-HIV-0440 (800-448-0440) (M–F, 12–4 Eastern)
Phone: 301-519-0459
Fax: 301-519-6616
TTY/TDD: 888-480-3739
Website: http://www.aidsinfo .nih.gov; http://www.aidsinfo.nih .gov/LiveHelp/default.aspx
E-mail: ContactUs@aidsinfo.gov

Brain Resources and Information Network
P.O. Box 5801
Bethesda, MD 20824
Toll-Free: 800-352-9424
Website: http://www.ninds.nih.gov

Centers for Disease Control and Prevention (CDC)
1600 Clifton Road, NE
Atlanta, GA 30333
Toll-Free: 800-CDC-INFO
(232-4636), open 24 hours
TTY: 888-232-6348
Website: http://www.cdc.gov;
http://www.cdc.govhiv; http://
www.cdc.gov/omh/Partnerships/
resourcesSHD.htm (State
Health Departments)
E-mail: cdcinfo@cdc.gov

CDC National HIV Testing Resources
Website: http://www.hivtest.org

Child Health Insurance Program
Toll-Free: 877-543-7669

Health Resources and Services Administration (HRSA)
HIV/AIDS Bureau
5600 Fishers Lane, Suite 7-05
Rockville, MD 20857
Phone: 301-443-1993
Website: http://www.hab.hrsa.gov

National Institute of Allergy and Infectious Diseases (NIAID)
6610 Rockledge Drive, MSC 6612
Bethesda, MD 20892-6612
Toll-Free: 800-HIV-0440
Phone: 301-496-5717
Fax: 301-402-3573
Website: http://www.niaid.nih.gov

National Institute of Dental and Craniofacial Research (NIDCR)
Bethesda, MD 20892-2190
Phone: 301-496-4261
Website: http://
www.nidcr.nih.gov
E-mail: nidcrinfo@mail.nih.gov

National Institute of Mental Health (NIMH)
6001 Executive Blvd.
Room 8184, MSC 9663
Bethesda, MD 20892-9663
Toll-Free: 866-615-6464
Phone: 301-443-4513
Fax: 301-443:4279
Website: http://
www.nimh.nih.gov
E-mail: nimhinfo@nih.gov

National Institute of Neurological Disorders and Stroke (NINDS)
P.O. Box 5801
Bethesda, MD 20824
Toll-Free: 800-352-9424
Phone: 301-496-5751
Website: http://
www.ninds.nih.gov

National Institute on Aging Information Center (NIA)
P.O. Box 8057
Gaithersburg, MD 20898-8057
Toll-Free: 800-222-2225
TTY: 800-222-4225
Website: http://
www.niapublications.org

National Institute on Drug Abuse (NIDA)
Website: http://www.nida.nih.gov
E-mail: information@nida.nih.gov

National Women's Health Information Center (NWHIC)
200 Independence Avenue, SW
Room 712E
Washington, DC 20201
Toll-Free: 800-994-9662
Phone: 703-289-7923
Fax: 703-663-6942
Website: http://www.womenshealth.gov/hiv

Office of AIDS Research (OAR)
National Institutes of Health
5635 Fishers Lane, Suite 4000
Rockville, MD 20852
Phone: 301-496-0357
Fax: 301-496-2119
Website: http://www.oar.nih.gov

Office of Minority Health Resource Center (OMHRC)
P.O. Box 37337
Washington, DC 20013-7337
Toll-Free: 800-444-6472
Website: http://www.omhrc.gov
E-mail: info@omhrc.gov

Office of National AIDS Policy
Website: http://www.whitehouse.gov/onap/aids.html

Presidential Advisory Council on HIV/AIDS
200 Independence Avenue, SW
Washington, DC 20201
Phone: 202-690-7694
Website: http://www.pacha.gov

Social Security Administration (SSA)
Toll-Free: 800-772-1213
TTY: 800-325-0778
Website: http://www.ssa.gov

State Health Departments
http://www.cdc.gov/omh/Partnerships/resourcesSHD.htm

Substance Abuse and Mental Health Services Administration (SAMHSA)
Website: http://www.samhsa.gov

TARGET Center — Technical Assistance for Ryan White CARE Act
c/o WriteProcess, Inc.
1850 Newton Street, NW
Washington, DC 20010
Website: http://www.careacttarget.org
E-mail: TARGETteam@careacttarget.org

U.S. Department of Health and Human Services (DHHS)
Director—Office for Civil Rights
200 Independence Avenue, SW
Room 506-F
Washington, DC 20201
Toll-Free: 800-368-1019
TDD: 800-537-7697
Website: http://www.hhs.gov/ocr
E-mail: ocrmail@hhs.gov

U.S. Department of Veterans Affairs (VA)
National HIV/AIDS Program
810 Vermont Avenue, NW
Washington, DC 20420
Website: http://www.hiv.va.gov

Private, Nonprofit, and Faith-Based Organizations That Provide Information about HIV/AIDS

AIDS Community Research Consortium
1048 El Camino Real, Suite B
Redwood City, CA 94063
Phone: 650-364-6563
Fax: 650-364-9001
Website: http://www.acrc.org

AIDS Community Research Initiative of America
230 West 38th Street, 17th Floor
New York, NY 10018
Website: www.acria.org/
treatment/
treatment_edu_viral_hep.html

AIDS Vaccine Advocacy Coalition (AVAC)
101 West 23rd Street, #2227
New York, NY 10011
Website: http://www.avac.org
E-mail: avac@avac.org

American Foundation for AIDS Research (amfAR)
120 Wall Street, 13th Floor
New York, NY 10005-3908
Phone: 212-806-1600
Fax: 212-806-1601
Website: http://www.amfar.org

American Red Cross National Headquarters
HIV/AIDS Programs
2025 East Street, NW
Washington, DC 20006
Website: http://
www.redcross.org/services/hss/
hivaids

Body Health Resources Corporation
Website: http://www.thebody.com

Council of Religious AIDS Networks (C.R.A.N.)
c/o Dr. Jon A. Lacey
P.O. Box 4188
East Lansing, MI 48826-4188
Website: http://www.aidsfaith.com

Family Health International
P.O. Box 13950
Research Triangle Park, NC 27709
Phone: 919-544-7040
Fax: 919-544-7261
Website: http://www.fhi.org

Bill and Melinda Gates Foundation
P.O. Box 23350
Seattle, WA 98102
Phone: 206-709-3100
Website: http://www.gatesfoundation.org
E-mail: info@gatesfoundation.org

Elizabeth Glaser Pediatric AIDS Foundation
1140 Connecticut Avenue, NW
Suite 200
Washington, DC 20036
Toll-Free: 888-499-4673
Phone: 202-296-9165
Fax: 202-296-9185
Website: http://www.pedaids.org
E-mail: info@pedaids.org

International AIDS Vaccine Initiative (IAVI)
110 William Street, Floor 27
New York, NY 10038-3901
Website: http://www.iavi.org
E-mail: info@iavi.org

Elton John AIDS Foundation
P.O. Box 17139
Beverly Hills, CA 90209-3139
Website: http://www.ejaf.org

Henry J. Kaiser Family Foundation (KFF)
2400 Sand Hill Road
Menlo Park, CA 94025
Phone: 650-854-9400
Fax: 650-854-4800
Website: http://www.kff.org
E-mail: http://www.kff.org/about/contact.cfm

KNOWHIVAIDS.ORG
Toll-Free: 866-344-KNOW
Website: http://www.knowhivaids.org

National AIDS Treatment Advocacy Project (NATAP)
Website: http://www.natap.org

National Association of People with AIDS (NAPWA)
8401 Colesville Road, Suite 750
Silver Spring, MD 20910
Phone: 240-247-0880
Fax: 240-247-0574
Website: http://www.napwa.org
E-mail: info@napwa.org

National Association on HIV over Fifty
23 Miner Street
Boston, MA 02215-5318
Website: http://www.hivoverfifty.org

National Minority AIDS Council
1931 13th Street, NW
Washington, DC 20009
Website: http://www.nmac.org
E-mail: info@nmac.org

National NeuroAIDS Tissue Consortium
401 N. Washington St., Suite 700
Rockville, MD 20850
Toll-Free: 800-510-1678
Phone: 301-251-1161, ext. 186
Fax: 301-251-1355
Website: http://www.hivbrainbanks.org
E-mail: nntc@emmes.com

New York State Department of Health AIDS Institute
Corning Tower, Empire State Plaza
Albany, NY 12237
Website: http://www.nyhealth/diseases/aids/index.htm

Project Inform
205 13th Street, Suite 2001
San Francisco, CA 94103-2461
Toll-Free: 800-822-7422 (Infoline)
Phone: 415-558-9051
Fax: 415-558-0684
Website: http://www.projectinform.org

Service and Advocacy for GLBT Elders (SAGE)
305 Seventh Avenue, 16th Floor
New York, NY 10001
Phone: 212-741-2247
Website: http://www.sageusa.org

University, Academic, and Research Organizations

Center for AIDS Prevention Studies (CAPS)
University of California, San Francisco
50 Beale Street, Suite 1300
San Francisco, CA 94105
Toll-Free: 800-458-5231
Phone: 415-597-9100
Fax: 415-597-9213
Website: http://www.caps.ucsf.edu; http://www.hivinsite.ucsf.edu
E-mail: CAPS.web@ucsf.edu

Harvard School of Public Health AIDS Initiative
651 Huntington Avenue
Boston, MA 02115
Phone: 617-432-4400
Fax: 617-432-4545
Website: http://www.aids.harvard.edu
E-mail: hai@hsph.harvard.edu

New Mexico AIDS Education and Training Center
University of New Mexico
Health Sciences Center
P.O. Box 810
Arroyo Seco, NM 87514
Website: http://www.aidsinfonet.org
E-mail: hivcc@nmia.com

Rural Center for AIDS/STD Prevention
Indiana University
801 E. Seventh Street
Bloomington, IN 47405-3085
Website: http://www.indiana.edu/~aids
E-mail: aids@indiana.edu

UCSF Center for HIV Information, HIV InSite
University of California, San Francisco
4150 Clement Street, Box 111V
San Francisco, CA 94121
Fax: 415-379-5547
Website: http://chi.ucsf.edu

U.S. National AIDS Hotlines and Resources

AIDS Treatment Data Network
Toll-Free: 800-734-7104
Phone: 212-260-8868

Americans with Disabilities Act Information and Assistance Hotline
Toll-Free: 800-514-0301
TTY: 800-514-0383

CDC Business and Labor Resource Service
Toll-Free: 877-242-9760
Phone: 301-562-1098
Fax: 888-282-7681; 301-562-1050
TTY: 800-243-7012
E-mail: info@hivatwork.org

CDC National AIDS Clearinghouse
Toll-Free: 800-458-5231
Phone: 301-562-1098
TTY: 800-243-1098;
301-588-1586

Childhelp USA® National Child Abuse Hotline
Toll-Free: 800-4-A-CHILD
(800-422-4453)

Drug and Alcohol Treatment Hotline
Toll-Free: 800-662-HELP (4357)

Gay Men's Health Crisis Hotline
Toll-Free: 800-AIDS-NYC (243-7692)
Phone: 212-807-6655
TTY: 212-645-7470
E-mail: hotline@gmhc.org

Hemophilia AIDS Network/ National Hemophilia Foundation
Toll-Free: 800-424-2634
Phone: 212-328-3700

HIPS Hotline
Toll-Free: 800-676-HIPS (800-676-4477)

National AIDS Hotline
Toll-Free: 800-CDC-INFO (800-232-4636)
TTY: 888-232-6348
E-mail: cdcinfo@cdc.gov

National Domestic Violence Hotline
Toll-Free: 800-799-7233
TTY: 800-787-3224

National Herpes Hotline
Phone: 919-361-8488

National Native American AIDS Prevention Center
Phone: 720-382-2244
Fax: 720-382-2248
E-mail: information@nnaapc.org

National Prevention Information Network (NPIN)
Toll-Free: 800-458-5231 (English and Spanish)
Phone: 301-562-1098
TTY/TDD: 800-243-7012

National Runaway Switchboard
Toll-Free: 800-RUNAWAY (786-2929)
TDD: 800-621-0394

National Sexually Transmitted Diseases (STD) Hotline
Toll-Free: 800-227-8922 (English); 800-344-7432 (Spanish)
TTY/TDD: 800-243-7889

Rape Abuse and Incest National Network
Toll-Free: 800-656-Hope
TTY: 800-810-7440

Suicide Hotline
Toll-Free: 800-SUICIDE (800-784-2433)

Women Alive
Toll-Free: 800-554-4876
Phone: 323-965-1564 (Main Office)

Help for Addiction

AL ANON and ALATEEN
Toll-Free: 800-4AL-ANON (888-425-2666)

Cocaine Anonymous
Toll-Free: 800-347-8998
(National Referral Line)

Pride Institute
Toll-Free: 800-547-7433

Sex Addicts Anonymous
Website: http://www.sexaa.org

Sexual Compulsives Anonymous
Toll-Free: 800-977-HEAL

AIDSinfo Live Help

AIDSinfo Live Help, available Monday–Friday, 12:00 p.m.–4:00 p.m. Eastern Time, is designed to provide one-on-one assistance via the internet to help you navigate the AIDSinfo website and find answers to your questions about federally approved information on HIV/AIDS treatment and prevention research, HIV/AIDS clinical trials, and treatment and prevention guidelines.

Is it confidential?

Your privacy is important to us. All AIDSinfo Live Help users are anonymous. Though we have designed this service to keep all of your information private, we cannot guarantee the security of any information you send over the internet.

Is there really a person on the other end?

Yes. AIDSinfo health information specialists respond to questions via AIDSinfo Live Help. By typing your questions, comments, and responses, you will have an electronic conversation with a health information specialist.

Who are the people on the other end?

The people staffing AIDSinfo Live Help are trained health information specialists who are knowledgeable about HIV/AIDS, clinical trials for HIV treatment and prevention, hotlines, publications, websites, and other information about HIV/AIDS-related resources.

631

Do the people on the other end know who I am?

No. Before you start an AIDSinfo Live Help session, you must choose a nickname. The Live Help health information specialists will only know your nickname, the webpage you were on when you clicked the Live Help button, and whatever you choose to write them. They have no way of getting any other information about you. It is important to remember that the internet may not be secure, so you should not provide any information that identifies you.

What kind of information is available through AIDSinfo Live Help?

AIDSinfo Live Help health information specialists are prepared to answer your questions about HIV/AIDS and to help you navigate the AIDSinfo website. You can also get personalized information about HIV/AIDS clinical trials.

Can someone else on the internet listen in?

No. The session is strictly one-on-one only. AIDSinfo Live Help is not a "chat room". In addition, your AIDSinfo Live Help session is encrypted. Our encryption system is similar to the security techniques used to protect credit card numbers used for internet purchases.

Do I need special software or can I get a computer virus from AIDSinfo Live Help?

No. AIDSinfo Live Help works within the internet browser on your computer, and because AIDSinfo Live Help can only send text to your computer, it is impossible to send a virus.

Can I get the same information by telephone?

Yes. The AIDSinfo Information Service is available Monday through Friday between the hours of 12:00 p.m. and 5:00 p.m. Eastern Time. Call 800-448-0440 or 301-519-0459 (International) or 888-480-3739 (TTY/TDD). You can also send an e-mail to ContactUs@aidsinfo.nih.gov.

Live Help Disclaimer

Please note that although we can offer information, we are not health care providers and cannot provide medical advice. AIDSinfo is not a substitute for talking to your health care provider.

Chapter 75

Further Reading on HIV/AIDS

With a new HIV/AIDS treatment issue in the news each day, it is difficult for people living with HIV/AIDS and the health professionals who care for them to keep up with the latest breakthroughs. The purpose of this chapter is to identify websites that provide the most accurate and up-to-date information about HIV/AIDS treatment and research. Consulting quality HIV/AIDS websites is an efficient, inexpensive, and powerful way to find current information. Newspapers and television may break current developments, but often more in-depth information on the same topics—on the same day—can be found on a reputable HIV/AIDS website. It may take six to twelve months for new information to appear in a printed medical journal or newsletter, but some researchers, drug companies, HIV/AIDS organizations, and government agencies release important information on the internet within days. Additionally, many treatment newsletters are published on the internet.

Following is an annotated list of unique, high-quality websites that offer HIV/AIDS treatment information.

Acute HIV Infection and Early Diseases Research Program
http://aiedrp.org

The AIEDRP is a program funded by the National Institute of Allergy and Infectious Diseases (NIAID) that focuses on innovative ways to

Excerpted from "How to Find Reliable HIV/AIDS Treatment Information on the Internet," from the National Library of Medicine, prepared by the Medical Education and Outreach Group, Oak Ridge Institute for Science and Education (ORISE), November 2004. All contact information verified and updated May 2007.

study how HIV-1 causes disease in adults. Scientists will use interventions such as highly active antiretroviral therapy (HAART), given in the acute and early phases of infection, to increase their understanding of the mechanisms and course of HIV disease.

Adult AIDS Clinical Trials Group
http://aactg.s-3.com

The AACTG, the largest AIDS clinical trials organization in the world, assists in setting standards of care for HIV infection and related opportunistic diseases. The AACTG also provides data for the approval of therapeutic agents, and treatment and prevention strategies for opportunistic infections and malignancies. The management and core members of the AACTG consist of clinical scientists in the field of HIV/AIDS therapeutic research. The AACTG is funded by the Division of AIDS of the National Institute of Allergy and Infectious Diseases, part of the National Institutes of Health. This site would be of interest to clinicians conducting HIV/AIDS treatment research trials.

AIDS 2006: XVI International AIDS Conference
http://www.aids2006.org

The XVI International AIDS Conference was held in Toronto, Canada, August 13–18, 2006. The theme was "Time to Deliver" and focused on the promises and progress made to scale-up treatment, care, and prevention. Abstract presentations were built around five specialized tracks: "Biology and Pathogenesis of HIV," "Clinical Research, Treatment, and Care," "Epidemiology, Prevention, and Prevention Research," "Social, Behavioral, and Economic Science," and "Policy." Additional sessions included Cultural Program, Global Village, Youth Program, Outreach Program, and the Opening and Closing Plenaries.

AIDS Action Committee of Massachusetts, Inc.
http://www.aac.org

The AIDS Action Committee of Massachusetts, Inc. is a New England service organization. It provides services, educates, and is an advocate for people living with HIV/AIDS. Most of the committee's income is derived from non-government sources, including foundations, corporations, private donations, and special events. Individual donors are the largest source of financial support.

AIDS Nutrition Services Alliances
http://www.aidsnutrition.org

The AIDS Nutrition Service Alliance is a collaboration of nonprofit organizations that provide nutrition services for people living with HIV/AIDS. The mission of ANSA is to enhance the quality of life of people living with HIV/AIDS (PLWAs) by information sharing, technical assistance, education and advocacy, pooling resources, and collaboration. The home page contains links to over 30 fact sheets on topics related to nutrition and HIV treatment.

AIDS Research Institute
http://ari.ucsf.edu

ARI coordinates and integrates all AIDS research activities at the University of California, San Francisco. The institute brings together the resources of the university and affiliated labs and institutions, and works closely with affected communities to stimulate innovation and support interdisciplinary collaboration in all aspects of the epidemic domestically and around the world.

AIDS Treatment Data Network
http://www.atdn.org

The AIDS Treatment Data Network (commonly called the Network) is a national, not-for-profit, community-based organization sponsored by the Kaiser Family Foundation and several pharmaceutical companies. Treatment education and counseling services for men, women, and children with AIDS and HIV are supported by extensive, comprehensive, and up-to-date informational databases about AIDS treatments, research studies, services, and accessing care. Each link from the home page shows the date it was updated. Includes information in Spanish.

AIDSinfo
http://aidsinfo.nih.gov

This U.S. Department of Health and Human Services (DHHS) website provides information on HIV/AIDS clinical trials and treatment. It combines two previous DHHS projects: The AIDS Clinical Trials Information Service (ACTIS) and the HIV/AIDS Treatment Information Service (ATIS). AIDSinfo is a central resource for current information on federally and privately funded clinical trials for AIDS patients and others infected with HIV and a primary dissemination point for federally approved HIV treatment and prevention guidelines. The site also includes an HIV glossary.

aidsinfonyc.org
http://aidsinfonyc.org

"aidsinfonyc.org" is a series of information pages for people living with HIV/AIDS. The information is provided by community-based organizations. The website is supported by grants from nonprofit organizations and by donations from private organizations. Most of the information on this site seems current, but check the dates on each item.

AIDSMAP
http://www.aidsmap.com

The National AIDS Manual (NAM Publications), in collaboration with the British HIV Association and the International HIV/AIDS Alliance, produces this site. NAM is a community-based organization located in the United Kingdom supported by commercial and nonprofit organizations. Its mission is to develop and disseminate independent, accurate, accessible, and up-to-date HIV treatment information. NAM publishes a monthly newsletter entitled *AIDS Treatment Update*. Information is produced in both book form and as searchable databases. The websites can be searched in four languages (English, Spanish, French, and Portuguese). A medical advisory panel reviews the materials on the site.

AIDSmeds.com
http://www.aidsmeds.com

The mission of AIDSmeds is to provide people living with HIV the necessary information they need to make informed treatment decisions. A physician experienced in the treatment of HIV/AIDS reviews the content of this site. The organization is HIV-positive owned and operated. Sponsored by pharmaceutical and retail companies.

AIDS.ORG
http://aids.org

AIDS.org is a nonprofit organization dedicated to distributing HIV/AIDS information over the internet. AIDS.org includes the *AIDS Treatment News* archive, the AIDS BookStore with over 3,000 titles, independent AIDS book reviews, medical conference listings and abstracts, a resource directory, hotline phone numbers, and links to information on other websites. You can register to receive updates about the site via e-mail. Supported by various computer companies and HIV/AIDS organizations. Some resources are available in Spanish.

Alternative Medicine HomePage
http://www.pitt.edu/~cbw/altm.html

The Alternative Medicine home page is a jump station for sources of information on unconventional, unorthodox, unproven, alternative, complementary, innovative, and integrative therapies.

amfAR (American Foundation for AIDS Research)
http://www.amfar.org

The American Foundation for AIDS Research (amfAR) is a nonprofit organization dedicated to the support of HIV/AIDS research, AIDS prevention, treatment education, and the advocacy of sound AIDS-related public policy. The organization's mission is to prevent HIV infection and the disease and death associated with it, along with protecting the human rights of people with HIV/AIDS. Funding sources include contributions from individuals, foundations, and corporations.

Bastyr University AIDS Research Center
http://www.bastyr.edu/research/buarc

This research center was formed in 1994 with a grant from the National Institutes of Health's National Institute of Allergy and Infectious Diseases and the National Center on Complementary and Alternative Medicine (NCCAM). The center was established to document the use of alternative medicine in HIV/AIDS treatment, to screen and evaluate alternative medicine therapies, and to offer support to the medical field in evaluation of alternative therapies.

The Body
http://www.thebody.com

The Body's mission is to use the internet to lower barriers between patients and clinicians, demystify HIV/AIDS and its treatment, improve patients' quality of life, and foster community through human connection. The Body is a service of Body Health Resources Corporation and is sponsored in part by several drug companies. The Board of Advisers reviews links. Most of the information on this site is updated frequently. Links are organized in a logical, coherent manner. This is one of the larger HIV/AIDS websites, containing information on many topics. The emphasis is on inclusion of all HIV/AIDS resources, including older items, rather than selectively reviewing a smaller number of current items. Users may want to click on "Comprehensive Site Map" to see the 550 topic areas.

Canadian HIV Trials Network
http://www.hivnet.ubc.ca/e/home

The Canadian HIV Trials Network is a nonprofit clinical trials research organization committed to developing treatments, vaccines, and a cure for HIV/AIDS. The CTN is federally funded by Health Canada and jointly sponsored by the University of British Columbia and St. Paul's Hospital in Vancouver. Information is available in English and French.

Center for Mental Health Research on AIDS
http://www.nimh.nih.gov/dahbr/9a-as.cfm

Since 1983, the National Institute of Mental Health (NIMH) CMHRA has supported research activities related to the primary and secondary prevention of AIDS and the neurobehavioral sequelae that develop as a result of HIV infection.

Centers for Disease Control and Prevention (CDC), Divisions of HIV/AIDS Prevention
http://www.cdc.gov/hiv/dhap.htm

This is the website for CDC's National Center for HIV, STD and TB Prevention, Divisions of HIV/AIDS Prevention. It contains links to statistical, prevention, and treatment information on HIV/AIDS. You can subscribe to receive e-mail notification when the site is updated. Many items are also available in Spanish.

CenterWatch Clinical Trials Listing Service
http://www.centerwatch.com

CenterWatch is a commercial publishing company focusing on the clinical trials industry. The CenterWatch site provides information to patients and their advocates about ongoing clinical trials seeking study volunteers. Over 41,000 clinical trials are listed on the site. Clinical trial resources are available for patients as well as research professionals. The site offers a notification service for new clinical trials and drugs approved by the FDA, and a trial matching service in collaboration with thehealthexchange.org. Detailed profiles of more than 600 clinical research centers are listed. CenterWatch is a division of the Medical Economics Company.

ClinicalTrials.gov
http://clinicaltrials.gov

ClinicalTrials.gov is designed to provide patients, family members, health care professionals, and members of the public easy access to information on clinical trials for a wide range of diseases and conditions. The National Library of Medicine (NLM), an office of the U.S. National Institutes of Health (NIH), has developed this site in close and ongoing collaboration with all NIH Institutes and the Food and Drug Administration (FDA). This site currently [as of 2005] contains approximately 11,100 by the National Institutes of Health, other federal agencies, and private industry. Clinical trials can be searched by disease, location, treatment, and sponsor.

Community AIDS Treatment Information Exchange
http://www.catie.ca

The Community AIDS Treatment Information Exchange (CATIE) is a Canadian, community-based, nonprofit organization committed to improving the health and quality of life of all people living with HIV/AIDS. It is sometimes referred to as the Canadian AIDS Treatment Information Exchange. Some of the information on this site is provided in French.

Community Programs for Clinical Research on AIDS
http://www.cpcra.org

The CPCRA, founded in 1989 and called the Terry Beirn Community Programs for Clinical Research on AIDS since 1992, is a network of research units composed of community-based health care providers who offer their patients the opportunity to participate in research where they get their health care. The 15 CPCRA units comprise a variety of clinical settings, including private physicians' practices, university, and veterans' hospital clinics; drug treatment centers; and freestanding community clinics. Patients at these clinics are eligible for participation in CPCRA studies. The CPCRA, funded by the National Institute of Allergy and Infectious Diseases (NIAID), is targeted to serve populations underrepresented in previous clinical trials efforts. The research focus and scientific agenda of the CPCRA is identifying and improving treatment options in the day-to-day clinical care of people with HIV.

DIRLINE®
http://dirline.nlm.nih.gov

DIRLINE (Directory of Information Resources Online) is the National Library of Medicine's online database containing location and descriptive information about a wide variety of information resources including organizations, research resources, projects, and databases concerned with health and biomedicine. This information may not be readily available in bibliographic databases. Each record may contain information on the publications, holdings, and services provided. DIRLINE contains over 17,000 records and focuses primarily on health and biomedicine, although it also provides limited coverage of some other special interests. These information resources fall into many categories including federal, state, and local government agencies; information and referral centers; professional societies; self-help groups and voluntary associations; academic and research institutions and their programs; information systems and research facilities. Topics include HIV/AIDS, maternal and child health, most diseases and conditions including genetic and other rare diseases, health services research, and technology assessment.

Food and Drug Administration HIV and AIDS Activities
http://www.fda.gov/oashi/aids/hiv.html

The FDA's HIV/AIDS Program in the Office of Special Health Issues works with outside individuals and advocacy groups on issues related to HIV/AIDS, informs the HIV-affected community of activities and policies at FDA related to HIV/AIDS, represents patient and community views and concerns to the agency, serves as a resource for HIV/AIDS-related information, explains the regulatory processes affecting development and approval of new therapies, represents FDA at a range of public and government meetings related to serious and life-threatening illnesses, and assists in development of federal government policies and regulations related to HIV/AIDS.

Food and Nutrition Information Center—AIDS/HIV
http://www.nal.usda.gov/fnic/etext/000062.html#aids

Contains links to information about nutrition and HIV. Compiled by the Food and Nutrition Information Center at the National Agricultural Library of the U.S. Department of Agriculture.

Gay Men's Health Crisis (GMHC)
http://www.gmhc.org

GMHC is the oldest and largest not-for-profit AIDS organization in the U.S. GMHC offers hands-on support services to men, women, and children with AIDS and their families in New York City annually, as well as education and advocacy nationwide. Some information is available in Spanish.

Elizabeth Glaser Pediatric AIDS Foundation
http://www.pedaids.org

The Elizabeth Glaser Pediatric AIDS Foundation is a nonprofit organization. Its goals are to find therapies to prevent transmission from an infected mother to her newborn, to prolong and improve the lives of children with HIV, and to eliminate HIV in infected children.

Health Resources and Services Administration (HRSA), HIV/AIDS Bureau (HAB)
http://hab.hrsa.gov

This is the website of HRSA's HIV/AIDS Bureau. One of five bureaus of HRSA, it is the largest single source (except for the Medicaid program) of federal funding for HIV/AIDS care for low-income, uninsured, and underinsured individuals.

Healthology
http://www.healthology.com

Healthology produces and distributes physician-generated health and medical information on the internet including original, streaming health programs and physician-authored articles on a variety of health topics. From the home page, click "Health Topics," then "HIV and AIDS" for educational programs on AIDS and HIV symptoms and treatments.

HIV InSite
http://hivinsite.ucsf.edu

HIV InSite is a project of the University of California, San Francisco (UCSF). Within UCSF, the project is a collaboration among the San Francisco Veterans Affairs Medical Center, the Positive Health Program at San Francisco General Hospital, and the Center for AIDS

Prevention Studies of UCSF's AIDS Research Institute. The home page of this site contains recent news items. The editorial process at this site is independent of financial sponsors, which include several pharmaceutical companies. This is an information-dense site created primarily for clinicians.

HIV/AIDS Dietetic Practice Group (DPG)
http://hivaidsdpg.org

The HIV/AIDS Dietetic Practice Group is part of the American Dietetic Association. The group was founded in response to the overwhelming evidence that nutrition was an important factor in the treatment of HIV disease. The mission of HIV/AIDS DPG is to share information regarding the nutritional management of HIV, provide an avenue for national research projects, and advocate for nutrition intervention for all persons living with HIV. *Positive Communication* is the group's peer-reviewed quarterly publication, but it is not posted to the website.

HIVandHepatitis.com™
http://www.hivandhepatitis.com

The objective of HIVandHepatitis.com is to develop an online publication that provides accurate and timely treatment information to people living with HIV/AIDS, hepatitis B, hepatitis C, and co-infection. The staff consists of individuals who have years of combined experience in publishing, community education, and HIV treatment advocacy. The medical editor has a medical degree and is experienced in HIV/AIDS treatment, research, and education. This site is financially supported by grants from pharmaceutical companies and the majority of information is current. This site is dense with information, much of it written, and all of it reviewed, by medical doctors.

HIVDENT
http://www.hivdent.org

HIVDENT is a not-for-profit coalition of health care professionals committed to assuring access to high quality oral health care services for adults, adolescents, and children living with HIV. HIVDENT disseminates treatment information and shares expertise in advocacy, development, training, integration, and evaluation of oral health services for the HIV-infected population. The website contains several sections on the oral manifestations of HIV (including a large picture gallery) and information on infection control, post-exposure protocols, pediatric/adolescent care, medications, funding, and other resources. Support is provided through non-restricted educational grants and support from several pharmaceutical companies and a network of health centers.

How to Find Reliable HIV/AIDS Treatment Information on the Internet
http://www.orau.gov/meo/Materials/treatment

This online manual, available as PDF files, is for people living with HIV/AIDS and the health professionals who care for them. It includes descriptions of websites for the most accurate and up-to-date information about treatment and research, including clinical trials, HIV/AIDS drugs, treatment regimens, and medical literature.

International Association of Physicians in AIDS Care
http://www.iapac.org

The IAPAC website serves as a member resource and a public service for physicians and other health care professionals, nongovernmental and governmental agencies, communities of faith, and others throughout the world who care for and about the people infected and affected by the intersecting pandemics of life-threatening infectious diseases, poverty, and dehumanization. Much of the information on this site is not current; therefore, it is not recommended as a resource unless it is updated. The "What's New" link is a good guide to current information on this website.

International Bibliographic Information on Dietary Supplements
http://ods.od.nih.gov/databases/ibids.html

The IBIDS database is a cooperative project of the Office of Dietary Supplements (ODS) at the National Institutes of Health (NIH), and the Food and Nutrition Information Center at the National Agricultural Library of the U.S. Department of Agriculture. IBIDS was launched specifically to assist health care providers, researchers, and the general public with locating scientific information on dietary supplements.

Johns Hopkins AIDS Service
http://www.hopkins-aids.edu

This is the website of the faculty of Johns Hopkins University, Division of Infectious Diseases. The home page contains current news articles and a question/answer of the week.

Medem Medical Library
http://www.medem.com/MedLB/medlib_entry.cfm

Medem is an organization of professional medical societies. The Medical Library includes peer-reviewed (by physicians, probably, but not spelled out as such) patient education information from its partner societies, including the American Medical Association, the American Academy of Pediatrics, the American College of Allergy, Asthma and Immunology, and other sources. Under "Diseases and Conditions" on the home page, there is an HIV/AIDS link. A complexity indicator indicates the complexity of each item.

MedlinePlus®
http://medlineplus.gov

MedlinePlus is the National Library of Medicine's (NLM's) website for consumer health information. NLM's experienced staff of information experts review hundreds of government and nongovernment publications, brochures, databases, and websites in order to link the public with the most reliable and authoritative information. MedlinePlus is available on the World Wide Web from the NLM home page (http://www.nlm.nih.gov/) or directly at MedlinePlus (http://medlineplus.gov). MedlinePlus is not meant to be an exhaustive list of every health web resource. It is a selective list of appropriate, authoritative health information sources. MedlinePlus includes mostly U.S. resources. International sites may be included at a later date.

MEDLINE/PubMed®
http://pubmed.gov

PubMed is the National Library of Medicine's web search interface that provides access to over 10 million journal article abstracts/citations in MEDLINE, PreMEDLINE, and other related databases with links to participating online journals. The online journal providers usually charge a fee to read the entire journal article, but viewing the abstracts is free through PubMed. PubMed is also the free web interface to search

AIDS journal article abstracts/citations. To limit your search to only items in the AIDS subset of MEDLINE, click on the word "Limits" under the search box. On the lower right of the screen, click on the arrow to the right of "Subsets" and select "AIDS." Click in the search box and type in your search terms. A Spanish language tutorial for using PubMed, developed by the University of Florida Health Science Center Libraries, is available at http://www.sap.org.ar/staticfiles/med line/tutorial.

Medscape® HIV/AIDS
http://www.medscape.com/hiv-aidshome

Medscape offers health care providers online medical information and education tools concerning HIV/AIDS. The home page contains current HIV/AIDS news, recent conference coverage (that is actually recent), the latest additions to the Medscape HIV/AIDS website, many CMEs [continuing medical education units] concerning HIV/AIDS, and news from Reuters Health and MedscapeWire. This is a commercial site, but it is included in this text because it contains information of interest to clinicians and the conference summary information is current. Users must register (it is free) to access all of the information. The site is operated by Medscape, Inc.

National AIDS Treatment Advocacy Project
http://www.natap.org

The National AIDS Treatment Advocacy Project is a nonprofit organization dedicated to educating the diverse communities affected by HIV on the latest HIV and hepatitis treatments and advocating on treatment and policy issues for people with HIV. NATAP posts summary reports of conferences and conducts free community forums, usually at the New York University (NYU) Medical Center, to bridge the gap between the very latest research and the community by bringing in speakers who are conducting cutting-edge research. Proceedings from these forums are also posted to the NATAP website.

National Center for Complementary and Alternative Medicine
http://nccam.nih.gov

The National Center for Complementary and Alternative Medicine at the National Institutes of Health (NIH) conducts and supports basic and applied research and training and disseminates information on complementary and alternative medicine to practitioners and the public. The NCCAM does not serve as a referral agency for various alternative medical treatments or individual practitioners. The NCCAM facilitates and conducts biomedical research.

National Center for HIV, STD and TB Prevention —Divisions of HIV/AIDS Prevention
http://www.cdc.gov/nchstp/od/nchstp.html

The National Center for HIV, STD and TB Prevention is a component of the Centers for Disease Control and Prevention (CDC) that provides national leadership in preventing and controlling human immunodeficiency virus infection, sexually transmitted diseases, and tuberculosis.

National HIV/AIDS Clinicians' Consultation Center
http://www.ucsf.edu/hivcntr

The NCCC is funded by the University of California, San Francisco (UCSF) and the Health Resources and Services Administration (HRSA). It is an AIDS Education and Training Centers clinical resource for health care providers from the UCSF at San Francisco General Hospital. NCCC includes the National HIV Telephone Consultation Service (Warmline) and the National Clinician's Post-Exposure Prophylaxis Hotline (PEPline). These national services continue as programs of the AIDS Education and Training Centers (AETC) of the HIV/AIDS Bureau of HRSA, with additional funding from CDC.

National Institute of Allergy and Infectious Diseases, Division of Acquired Immunodeficiency Syndrome
http://www.niaid.nih.gov/daids

The mission of DAIDS is to increase basic knowledge of the pathogenesis, natural history, and transmission of HIV disease and to support research that promotes progress in its detection, treatment, and prevention. DAIDS accomplishes this through planning, implementing, managing, and evaluating programs in fundamental basic research, discovery and development of therapies for HIV infection and its complications, and discovery and development of vaccines and other prevention strategies.

National Institutes of Health Clinical Center Pharmacy Department
http://www.cc.nih.gov/phar

The NIH Clinical Center Pharmacy Department provides pharmaceutical care and research support to patients, health care providers, and investigators. Pharmacy staff members conduct and participate in research programs that enhance knowledge regarding optimal dosing and appropriate use of investigational and commercially available agents. Pharmacists at the NIH Clinical Center manage commercially available and investigational drugs in approximately 1,000 drug protocols.

National Institutes of Health Office of AIDS Research
http://www.oar.nih.gov

OAR is located within the Office of the Director of NIH and is responsible for the scientific, budgetary, legislative, and policy elements of the NIH AIDS research program. Congress has provided broad authority to OAR to plan, coordinate, evaluate, and fund all NIH AIDS research. OAR is responsible for the development of an annual comprehensive plan and budget for all NIH AIDS research. OAR supports trans-NIH Coordinating Committees to assist in these efforts in the following areas of program emphasis that have to do with treatment: therapeutics, vaccines, and information dissemination.

National Library of Medicine, National Institutes of Health, U.S. Department of Human Services
http://www.nlm.nih.gov

The NLM is the world's largest medical library. NLM's online AIDS resources and other NLM databases are searchable at libraries, other institutions, and via personal computers.

National Minority AIDS Council
http://www.nmac.org

NMAC, established in 1987, is dedicated to developing leadership within communities of color to address the challenge of HIV/AIDS. NMAC sponsors the U.S. Conference on AIDS and the North American AIDS Treatment Action Forum each year, along with regional training for community-based organizations.

647

National Prevention Information Network

http://www.cdcnpin.org

The Centers for Disease Control and Prevention's (CDC's) National Prevention Information Network is a reference, referral, and distribution service for information on HIV/AIDS, sexually transmitted diseases, and tuberculosis. This website is supported by the CDC and replaced the CDC National AIDS Clearinghouse.

New Mexico AIDS InfoNet

http://www.aidsinfonet.org

The New Mexico AIDS InfoNet is a project of the New Mexico AIDS Education and Training Center in the Infectious Diseases Division of the University of New Mexico School of Medicine. The InfoNet was originally designed to make information on HIV/AIDS services and treatments easily accessible in both English and Spanish for residents of New Mexico. Some InfoNet fact sheets have information that is specific to New Mexico; national references are provided when relevant. Major project funding has been provided by the National Library of Medicine; the New Mexico Department of Health, Public Health Division; and the Levi Strauss Foundation. Additional support has been provided by several pharmaceutical companies.

Pediatric AIDS Clinical Trials Group

http://pactg.s-3.com

The Pediatric AIDS Clinical Trials Group is a collaborative effort of the National Institute of Allergy and Infectious Diseases (NIAID) and the National Institute for Child Health and Human Development (NICHD). The PACTG specializes in evaluating treatments for HIV-infected children, developing new approaches for the interruption of mother-to-infant transmission, and establishing standards of care for children infected with HIV. This site would be of interest to clinicians conducting HIV/AIDS treatment research trials.

Physicians' Research Network, Inc.

http://www.prn.org

The mission of this not-for-profit organization is to provide peer support to health care providers who treat people with HIV disease. The organization works to improve the diagnosis, management, and prevention of all aspects of HIV disease and to enhance the skills of providers.

Clinical reports and scientific meeting summaries are published in a monthly journal entitled *The PRN Report*. Physicians review the content of the site. Several pharmaceutical companies provide unrestricted educational grants to support the site.

Project Inform
http://www.projectinform.org

Project Inform is a national, nonprofit, community-based organization based in San Francisco working to end the AIDS epidemic. Its mission is to provide vital information on the diagnosis and treatment of HIV to HIV-infected individuals, their caregivers, and their health care and service providers; to advocate enlightened regulatory, research, and funding policies affecting the development of, access to, and delivery of effective treatments, as well as to fund innovative research opportunities; to inspire people to make informed choices amid uncertainty, and to choose hope over despair. Funded by individuals, corporate and private foundations, individual bequests, and government sources. Some items are in Spanish.

San Francisco AIDS Foundation
http://www.sfaf.org

The goal of the San Francisco AIDS Foundation is to provide treatment information, support services, and advocacy for people living with HIV disease. *The Bulletin of Experimental Treatment for AIDS (BETA)* and *Treatment Flash* are treatment newsletters published by the Foundation. Resources on the site are available in Spanish. The San Francisco AIDS Foundation receives most of its funding from government grants and private donations.

Social Security Administration
http://www.ssa.gov

"Social Security Online" is the official home page of the SSA. Information on disability benefits may be helpful to HIV/AIDS patients.

Index

Index

653

National Herpes Hotline, contact
information 630
National HIV/AIDS Clinicians'
Consultation Center (NCCC),
website address 646
National HIV Behavioral
Surveillance system 124–25
National Institute of Aging, HIV/
AIDS publication 95n
National Institute of Allergy and
Infectious Diseases (NIAID)
contact information 624
publications
adolescents, HIV infection
461n
clinical trials 586n
genetic factors 77n
minorities, HIV/AIDS research
567n
pediatric HIV infection 445n
women, HIV infection 415n
website address 646
National Institute of Dental and
Craniofacial Research (NIDCR)
contact information 624
mouth problems publication
386n
National Institute of Mental
Health (NIMH)
contact information 624
depression publication 516n
National Institute of Neurological
Disorders and Stroke (NINDS)
contact information 624
neurological complications
publication 369n
National Institute on Aging (NIA),
contact information 624
National Institute on Alcohol Abuse
and Alcoholism (NIAAA), alcohol,
HIV/AIDS publication 145n
National Institute on Drug Abuse
(NIDA), contact information 625
National Institutes of Health (NIH),
publications
African Americans, HIV infection
118n
AIDS history 57n
AIDS vaccine 575n

National Library of Medicine (NLM)
publications
acronyms 593n
DIRLINE 640
online information 593n
website address 647
National Minority AIDS Council
contact information 628
website address 647
National Native American AIDS
Prevention Center, contact
information 630
National NeuroAIDS Tissue
Consortium, contact information
628
National Prevention Information
Network (NPIN)
contact information 630
sexually transmitted diseases
publication 630
National Prevention Information
Network, website address 648
National Runaway Switchboard,
contact information 630
National Sexually Transmitted
Diseases (STD) Hotline, contact
information 630
National Women's Health
Information Center (NWHIC),
publications
breast milk banks 443n
treatment options 259n
nausea, management 409–10
NCCAM *see* National Center for
Complementary and Alternative
Medicine
NCCC *see* National HIV/AIDS
Clinicians' Consultation Center
needle exchange programs
described 51
overview 181–84
needle sharing
alcohol use 146
HIV infection 4, 17, 46, 161, 174
prison populations 135–36
needle sticks
caregivers 546
HIV exposure 195
nelfinavir 10, 23, *263*, *278*, *281*

Health Reference Series

COMPLETE CATALOG

List price $87 per volume. **School and library price $78 per volume.**

Adolescent Health Sourcebook, 2nd Edition

Basic Consumer Health Information about the Physical, Mental, and Emotional Growth and Development of Adolescents, Including Medical Care, Nutritional and Physical Activity Requirements, Puberty, Sexual Activity, Acne, Tanning, Body Piercing, Common Physical Illnesses and Disorders, Eating Disorders, Attention Deficit Hyperactivity Disorder, Depression, Bullying, Hazing, and Adolescent Injuries Related to Sports, Driving, and Work

Along with Substance Abuse Information about Nicotine, Alcohol, and Drug Use, a Glossary, and Directory of Additional Resources

Edited by Joyce Brennfleck Shannon. 683 pages. 2006. 978-0-7808-0943-7.

"It is written in clear, nontechnical language aimed at general readers. . . . Recommended for public libraries, community colleges, and other agencies serving health care consumers."
— *American Reference Books Annual, 2003*

"Recommended for school and public libraries. Parents and professionals dealing with teens will appreciate the easy-to-follow format and the clearly written text. This could become a 'must have' for every high school teacher." — *E-Streams, Jan '03*

"A good starting point for information related to common medical, mental, and emotional concerns of adolescents." — *School Library Journal, Nov '02*

"This book provides accurate information in an easy to access format. It addresses topics that parents and caregivers might not be aware of and provides practical, useable information."
— *Doody's Health Sciences Book Review Journal, Sep-Oct '02*

"Recommended reference source."
— *Booklist, American Library Association, Sep '02*

AIDS Sourcebook, 3rd Edition

Basic Consumer Health Information about Acquired Immune Deficiency Syndrome (AIDS) and Human Immunodeficiency Virus (HIV) Infection, Including Facts about Transmission, Prevention, Diagnosis, Treatment, Opportunistic Infections, and Other Complications, with a Section for Women and Children, Including Details about Associated Gynecological Concerns, Pregnancy, and Pediatric Care

Along with Updated Statistical Information, Reports on Current Research Initiatives, a Glossary, and Directories of Internet, Hotline, and Other Resources

Edited by Dawn D. Matthews. 664 pages. 2003. 978-0-7808-0631-3.

"The 3rd edition of the *AIDS Sourcebook*, part of Omnigraphics' *Health Reference Series*, is a welcome update. . . . This resource is highly recommended for academic and public libraries."
— *American Reference Books Annual, 2004*

"Excellent sourcebook. This continues to be a highly recommended book. There is no other book that provides as much information as this book provides."
— *AIDS Book Review Journal, Dec-Jan '00*

"Recommended reference source."
— *Booklist, American Library Association, Dec '99*

Alcoholism Sourcebook, 2nd Edition

Basic Consumer Health Information about Alcohol Use, Abuse, and Dependence, Featuring Facts about the Physical, Mental, and Social Health Effects of Alcohol Addiction, Including Alcoholic Liver Disease, Pancreatic Disease, Cardiovascular Disease, Neurological Disorders, and the Effects of Drinking during Pregnancy

Along with Information about Alcohol Treatment, Medications, and Recovery Programs, in Addition to Tips for Reducing the Prevalence of Underage Drinking, Statistics about Alcohol Use, a Glossary of Related Terms, and Directories of Resources for More Help and Information

Edited by Amy L. Sutton. 653 pages. 2006. 978-0-7808-0942-0.

"This title is one of the few reference works on alcoholism for general readers. For some readers this will be a welcome complement to the many self-help books on the market. Recommended for collections serving general readers and consumer health collections."
— *E-Streams, Mar '01*

"This book is an excellent choice for public and academic libraries."
— *American Reference Books Annual, 2001*

"Recommended reference source."
— *Booklist, American Library Association, Dec '00*

"Presents a wealth of information on alcohol use and abuse and its effects on the body and mind, treatment, and prevention." — *SciTech Book News, Dec '00*

"Important new health guide which packs in the latest consumer information about the problems of alcoholism." — *Reviewer's Bookwatch, Nov '00*

SEE ALSO Drug Abuse Sourcebook

Allergies Sourcebook, 3rd Edition

Basic Consumer Health Information about Allergic Disorders, Such as Anaphylaxis, Hives, Eczema, Rhinitis, Sinusitis, and Conjunctivitis, and Their Triggers, Including Pollen, Mold, Dust Mites, Animal Dander, Insects, Chemicals, Food, Food Additives, and Medications;

Along with Advice about the Diagnosis and Treatment of Allergy Symptoms, a Glossary of Related Terms, a Directory of Resources for Help and Information, and Suggestions for Additional Reading

Edited by Amy L. Sutton. 598 pages. 2007. 978-0-7808-0950-5.

"This book brings a great deal of useful material together. . . . This is an excellent addition to public and consumer health library collections."
— *American Reference Books Annual, 2003*

"This second edition would be useful to laypersons with little or advanced knowledge of the subject matter. This book would also serve as a resource for nursing and other health care professions students. It would be useful in public, academic, and hospital libraries with consumer health collections." — *E-Streams, Jul '02*

■

Alternative Medicine Sourcebook

SEE Complementary & Alternative Medicine Sourcebook

■

Alzheimer's Disease Sourcebook, 3rd Edition

Basic Consumer Health Information about Alzheimer's Disease, Other Dementias, and Related Disorders, Including Multi-Infarct Dementia, AIDS Dementia Complex, Dementia with Lewy Bodies, Huntington's Disease, Wernicke-Korsakoff Syndrome (Alcohol-Related Dementia), Delirium, and Confusional States

Along with Information for People Newly Diagnosed with Alzheimer's Disease and Caregivers, Reports Detailing Current Research Efforts in Prevention, Diagnosis, and Treatment, Facts about Long-Term Care Issues, and Listings of Sources for Additional Information

Edited by Karen Bellenir. 645 pages. 2003. 978-0-7808-0666-5.

"This very informative and valuable tool will be a great addition to any library serving consumers, students and health care workers."
— *American Reference Books Annual, 2004*

"This is a valuable resource for people affected by dementias such as Alzheimer's. It is easy to navigate and includes important information and resources."
— *Doody's Review Service, Feb '04*

"Recommended reference source."
— *Booklist, American Library Association, Oct '99*

SEE ALSO *Brain Disorders Sourcebook*

Arthritis Sourcebook, 2nd Edition

Basic Consumer Health Information about Osteoarthritis, Rheumatoid Arthritis, Other Rheumatic Disorders, Infectious Forms of Arthritis, and Diseases with Symptoms Linked to Arthritis, Featuring Facts about Diagnosis, Pain Management, and Surgical Therapies

Along with Coping Strategies, Research Updates, a Glossary, and Resources for Additional Help and Information

Edited by Amy L. Sutton. 593 pages. 2004. 978-0-7808-0667-2.

"This easy-to-read volume is recommended for consumer health collections within public or academic libraries." — *E-Streams, May '05*

"As expected, this updated edition continues the excellent reputation of this series in providing sound, usable health information. . . . Highly recommended."
— *American Reference Books Annual, 2005*

"Excellent reference." — *The Bookwatch, Jan '05*

■

Asthma Sourcebook, 2nd Edition

Basic Consumer Health Information about the Causes, Symptoms, Diagnosis, and Treatment of Asthma in Infants, Children, Teenagers, and Adults, Including Facts about Different Types of Asthma, Common Co-Occurring Conditions, Asthma Management Plans, Triggers, Medications, and Medication Delivery Devices

Along with Asthma Statistics, Research Updates, a Glossary, a Directory of Asthma-Related Resources, and More

Edited by Karen Bellenir. 609 pages. 2006. 978-0-7808-0866-9.

"A worthwhile reference acquisition for public libraries and academic medical libraries whose readers desire a quick introduction to the wide range of asthma information." — *Choice, Association of College & Research Libraries, Jun '01*

"Recommended reference source."
— *Booklist, American Library Association, Feb '01*

"Highly recommended." — *The Bookwatch, Jan '01*

"There is much good information for patients and their families who deal with asthma daily."
— *American Medical Writers Association Journal, Winter '01*

"This informative text is recommended for consumer health collections in public, secondary school, and community college libraries and the libraries of universities with a large undergraduate population."
— *American Reference Books Annual, 2001*

■

Attention Deficit Disorder Sourcebook

Basic Consumer Health Information about Attention Deficit/Hyperactivity Disorder in Children and Adults,

Including Facts about Causes, Symptoms, Diagnostic Criteria, and Treatment Options Such as Medications, Behavior Therapy, Coaching, and Homeopathy

Along with Reports on Current Research Initiatives, Legal Issues, and Government Regulations, and Featuring a Glossary of Related Terms, Internet Resources, and a List of Additional Reading Material

Edited by Dawn D. Matthews. 470 pages. 2002. 978-0-7808-0624-5.

"Recommended reference source."
  — *Booklist, American Library Association, Jan '03*

"This book is recommended for all school libraries and the reference or consumer health sections of public libraries." — *American Reference Books Annual, 2003*

■

Back & Neck Sourcebook, 2nd Edition

Basic Consumer Health Information about Spinal Pain, Spinal Cord Injuries, and Related Disorders, Such as Degenerative Disk Disease, Osteoarthritis, Scoliosis, Sciatica, Spina Bifida, and Spinal Stenosis, and Featuring Facts about Maintaining Spinal Health, Self-Care, Pain Management, Rehabilitative Care, Chiropractic Care, Spinal Surgeries, and Complementary Therapies

Along with Suggestions for Preventing Back and Neck Pain, a Glossary of Related Terms, and a Directory of Resources

Edited by Amy L. Sutton. 633 pages. 2004. 978-0-7808-0738-9.

"Recommended . . . an easy to use, comprehensive medical reference book." — *E-Streams, Sep '05*

"The strength of this work is its basic, easy-to-read format. Recommended." — *Reference and User Services Quarterly, American Library Association, Winter '97*

■

Blood & Circulatory Disorders Sourcebook, 2nd Edition

Basic Consumer Health Information about the Blood and Circulatory System and Related Disorders, Such as Anemia and Other Hemoglobin Diseases, Cancer of the Blood and Associated Bone Marrow Disorders, Clotting and Bleeding Problems, and Conditions That Affect the Veins, Blood Vessels, and Arteries, Including Facts about the Donation and Transplantation of Bone Marrow, Stem Cells, and Blood and Tips for Keeping the Blood and Circulatory System Healthy

Along with a Glossary of Related Terms and Resources for Additional Help and Information

Edited by Amy L. Sutton. 659 pages. 2005. 978-0-7808-0746-4.

"Highly recommended pick for basic consumer health reference holdings at all levels."
  — *The Bookwatch, Aug '05*

"Recommended reference source."
  — *Booklist, American Library Association, Feb '99*

"An important reference sourcebook written in simple language for everyday, non-technical users. "
  — *Reviewer's Bookwatch, Jan '99*

■

Brain Disorders Sourcebook, 2nd Edition

Basic Consumer Health Information about Acquired and Traumatic Brain Injuries, Infections of the Brain, Epilepsy and Seizure Disorders, Cerebral Palsy, and Degenerative Neurological Disorders, Including Amyotrophic Lateral Sclerosis (ALS), Dementias, Multiple Sclerosis, and More

Along with Information on the Brain's Structure and Function, Treatment and Rehabilitation Options, Reports on Current Research Initiatives, a Glossary of Terms Related to Brain Disorders and Injuries, and a Directory of Sources for Further Help and Information

Edited by Sandra J. Judd. 625 pages. 2005. 978-0-7808-0744-0.

"Highly recommended pick for basic consumer health reference holdings at all levels."
  — *The Bookwatch, Aug '05*

"Belongs on the shelves of any library with a consumer health collection." — *E-Streams, Mar '00*

"Recommended reference source."
  — *Booklist, American Library Association, Oct '99*

SEE ALSO Alzheimer's Disease Sourcebook

■

Breast Cancer Sourcebook, 2nd Edition

Basic Consumer Health Information about Breast Cancer, Including Facts about Risk Factors, Prevention, Screening and Diagnostic Methods, Treatment Options, Complementary and Alternative Therapies, Post-Treatment Concerns, Clinical Trials, Special Risk Populations, and New Developments in Breast Cancer Research

Along with Breast Cancer Statistics, a Glossary of Related Terms, and a Directory of Resources for Additional Help and Information

Edited by Sandra J. Judd. 595 pages. 2004. 978-0-7808-0668-9.

"This book will be an excellent addition to public, community college, medical, and academic libraries."
  — *American Reference Books Annual, 2006*

"It would be a useful reference book in a library or on loan to women in a support group."
  — *Cancer Forum, Mar '03*

"Recommended reference source."
  — *Booklist, American Library Association, Jan '02*

"This reference source is highly recommended. It is quite informative, comprehensive and detailed in nature, and yet it offers practical advice in easy-to-read language. It could be thought of as the 'bible' of breast cancer for the consumer." — *E-Streams, Jan '02*

"From the pros and cons of different screening methods and results to treatment options, *Breast Cancer Sourcebook* provides the latest information on the subject."
— *Library Bookwatch, Dec '01*

"This thoroughgoing, very readable reference covers all aspects of breast health and cancer. . . . Readers will find much to consider here. Recommended for all public and patient health collections."
— *Library Journal, Sep '01*

SEE ALSO *Cancer Sourcebook for Women, Women's Health Concerns Sourcebook*

■

Breastfeeding Sourcebook

Basic Consumer Health Information about the Benefits of Breastmilk, Preparing to Breastfeed, Breastfeeding as a Baby Grows, Nutrition, and More, Including Information on Special Situations and Concerns Such as Mastitis, Illness, Medications, Allergies, Multiple Births, Prematurity, Special Needs, and Adoption

Along with a Glossary and Resources for Additional Help and Information

Edited by Jenni Lynn Colson. 388 pages. 2002. 978-0-7808-0332-9.

"Particularly useful is the information about professional lactation services and chapters on breastfeeding when returning to work. . . . *Breastfeeding Sourcebook* will be useful for public libraries, consumer health libraries, and technical schools offering nurse assistant training, especially in areas where Internet access is problematic."
— *American Reference Books Annual, 2003*

SEE ALSO *Pregnancy & Birth Sourcebook*

■

Burns Sourcebook

Basic Consumer Health Information about Various Types of Burns and Scalds, Including Flame, Heat, Cold, Electrical, Chemical, and Sun Burns

Along with Information on Short-Term and Long-Term Treatments, Tissue Reconstruction, Plastic Surgery, Prevention Suggestions, and First Aid

Edited by Allan R. Cook. 604 pages. 1999. 978-0-7808-0204-9.

"This is an exceptional addition to the series and is highly recommended for all consumer health collections, hospital libraries, and academic medical centers."
— *E-Streams, Mar '00*

"This key reference guide is an invaluable addition to all health care and public libraries in confronting this ongoing health issue."
— *American Reference Books Annual, 2000*

"Recommended reference source."
— *Booklist, American Library Association, Dec '99*

SEE ALSO *Dermatological Disorders Sourcebook*

Cancer Sourcebook, 5th Edition

Basic Consumer Health Information about Major Forms and Stages of Cancer, Featuring Facts about Head and Neck Cancers, Lung Cancers, Gastrointestinal Cancers, Genitourinary Cancers, Lymphomas, Blood Cell Cancers, Endocrine Cancers, Skin Cancers, Bone Cancers, Metastatic Cancers, and More

Along with Facts about Cancer Treatments, Cancer Risks and Prevention, a Glossary of Related Terms, Statistical Data, and a Directory of Resources for Additional Information

Edited by Karen Bellenir. 1,133 pages. 2007. 978-0-7808-0947-5.

"With cancer being the second leading cause of death for Americans, a prodigious work such as this one, which locates centrally so much cancer-related information, is clearly an asset to this nation's citizens and others."
— *Journal of the National Medical Association, 2004*

"This title is recommended for health sciences and public libraries with consumer health collections."
— *E-Streams, Feb '01*

". . . can be effectively used by cancer patients and their families who are looking for answers in a language they can understand. Public and hospital libraries should have it on their shelves."
— *American Reference Books Annual, 2001*

"Recommended reference source."
— *Booklist, American Library Association, Dec '00*

SEE ALSO *Breast Cancer Sourcebook, Cancer Sourcebook for Women, Pediatric Cancer Sourcebook, Prostate Cancer Sourcebook*

■

Cancer Sourcebook for Women, 3rd Edition

Basic Consumer Health Information about Leading Causes of Cancer in Women, Featuring Facts about Gynecologic Cancers and Related Concerns, Such as Breast Cancer, Cervical Cancer, Endometrial Cancer, Uterine Sarcoma, Vaginal Cancer, Vulvar Cancer, and Common Non-Cancerous Gynecologic Conditions, in Addition to Facts about Lung Cancer, Colorectal Cancer, and Thyroid Cancer in Women.

Along with Information about Cancer Risk Factors, Screening and Prevention, Treatment Options, and Tips on Coping with Life after Cancer Treatment, a Glossary of Cancer Terms, and a Directory of Resources for Additional Help and Information

Edited by Amy L. Sutton. 715 pages. 2006. 978-0-7808-0867-6.

"An excellent addition to collections in public, consumer health, and women's health libraries."
— *American Reference Books Annual, 2003*

"Overall, the information is excellent, and complex topics are clearly explained. As a reference book for the consumer it is a valuable resource to assist them to make informed decisions about cancer and its treatments."
— *Cancer Forum, Nov '02*

"Highly recommended for academic and medical reference collections."　　—Library Bookwatch, Sep '02

"This is a highly recommended book for any public or consumer library, being reader friendly and containing accurate and helpful information."
　　—E-Streams, Aug '02

"Recommended reference source."
　　—Booklist, American Library Association, Jul '02

SEE ALSO Breast Cancer Sourcebook, Women's Health Concerns Sourcebook

Cancer Survivorship Sourcebook

Basic Consumer Health Information about the Physical, Educational, Emotional, Social, and Financial Needs of Cancer Patients from Diagnosis, through Cancer Treatment, and Beyond, Including Facts about Researching Specific Types of Cancer and Learning about Clinical Trials and Treatment Options, and Featuring Tips for Coping with the Side Effects of Cancer Treatments and Adjusting to Life after Cancer Treatment Concludes

Along with Suggestions for Caregivers, Friends, and Family Members of Cancer Patients, a Glossary of Cancer Care Terms, and Directories of Related Resources

Edited by Karen Bellenir. 6561 pages. 2007. 978-0-7808-0985-7.

Cardiovascular Diseases & Disorders Sourcebook, 3rd Edition

Basic Consumer Health Information about Heart and Vascular Diseases and Disorders, Such as Angina, Heart Attacks, Arrhythmias, Cardiomyopathy, Valve Disease, Atherosclerosis, and Aneurysms, with Information about Managing Cardiovascular Risk Factors and Maintaining Heart Health, Medications and Procedures Used to Treat Cardiovascular Disorders, and Concerns of Special Significance to Women

Along with Reports on Current Research Initiatives, a Glossary of Related Medical Terms, and a Directory of Sources for Further Help and Information

Edited by Sandra J. Judd. 713 pages. 2005. 978-0-7808-0739-6.

"This updated sourcebook is still the best first stop for comprehensive introductory information on cardiovascular diseases."
　　—American Reference Books Annual, 2006

"Recommended for public libraries and libraries supporting health care professionals."
　　—E-Streams, Sep '05

"This should be a standard health library reference."
　　—The Bookwatch, Jun '05

"Recommended reference source."
　　—Booklist, American Library Association, Dec '00

"... comprehensive format provides an extensive overview on this subject."
　　—Choice, Association of College & Research Libraries

Caregiving Sourcebook

Basic Consumer Health Information for Caregivers, Including a Profile of Caregivers, Caregiving Responsibilities and Concerns, Tips for Specific Conditions, Care Environments, and the Effects of Caregiving

Along with Facts about Legal Issues, Financial Information, and Future Planning, a Glossary, and a Listing of Additional Resources

Edited by Joyce Brennfleck Shannon. 600 pages. 2001. 978-0-7808-0331-2.

"Essential for most collections."
　　—Library Journal, Apr 1, 2002

"An ideal addition to the reference collection of any public library. Health sciences information professionals may also want to acquire the Caregiving Sourcebook for their hospital or academic library for use as a ready reference tool by health care workers interested in aging and caregiving."　　—E-Streams, Jan '02

"Recommended reference source."
　　—Booklist, American Library Association, Oct '01

Child Abuse Sourcebook

Basic Consumer Health Information about the Physical, Sexual, and Emotional Abuse of Children, with Additional Facts about Neglect, Munchausen Syndrome by Proxy (MSBP), Shaken Baby Syndrome, and Controversial Issues Related to Child Abuse, Such as Withholding Medical Care, Corporal Punishment, and Child Maltreatment in Youth Sports, and Featuring Facts about Child Protective Services, Foster Care, Adoption, Parenting Challenges, and Other Abuse Prevention Efforts

Along with a Glossary of Related Terms and Resources for Additional Help and Information

Edited by Dawn D. Matthews. 620 pages. 2004. 978-0-7808-0705-1.

"A valuable and highly recommended resource for school, academic and public libraries whether used on its own or as a starting point for more in-depth research."　　—E-Streams, Apr '05

"Every week the news brings cases of child abuse or neglect, so it is useful to have a source that supplies so much helpful information. . . . Recommended. Public and academic libraries, and child welfare offices."
　　—Choice, Association of College & Research Libraries, Mar '05

"Packed with insights on all kinds of issues, from foster care and adoption to parenting and abuse prevention."
　　—The Bookwatch, Nov '04

SEE ALSO: Domestic Violence Sourcebook

Childhood Diseases & Disorders Sourcebook

Basic Consumer Health Information about Medical Problems Often Encountered in Pre-Adolescent Children, Including Respiratory Tract Ailments, Ear Infections, Sore Throats, Disorders of the Skin and Scalp, Digestive and Genitourinary Diseases, Infectious Diseases, Inflammatory Disorders, Chronic Physical and Developmental Disorders, Allergies, and More

Along with Information about Diagnostic Tests, Common Childhood Surgeries, and Frequently Used Medications, with a Glossary of Important Terms and Resource Directory

Edited by Chad T. Kimball. 662 pages. 2003. 978-0-7808-0458-6.

"This is an excellent book for new parents and should be included in all health care and public libraries."
—*American Reference Books Annual, 2004*

SEE ALSO: Healthy Children Sourcebook

∎

Colds, Flu & Other Common Ailments Sourcebook

Basic Consumer Health Information about Common Ailments and Injuries, Including Colds, Coughs, the Flu, Sinus Problems, Headaches, Fever, Nausea and Vomiting, Menstrual Cramps, Diarrhea, Constipation, Hemorrhoids, Back Pain, Dandruff, Dry and Itchy Skin, Cuts, Scrapes, Sprains, Bruises, and More

Along with Information about Prevention, Self-Care, Choosing a Doctor, Over-the-Counter Medications, Folk Remedies, and Alternative Therapies, and Including a Glossary of Important Terms and a Directory of Resources for Further Help and Information

Edited by Chad T. Kimball. 638 pages. 2001. 978-0-7808-0435-7.

"A good starting point for research on common illnesses. It will be a useful addition to public and consumer health library collections."
—*American Reference Books Annual, 2002*

"Will prove valuable to any library seeking to maintain a current, comprehensive reference collection of health resources. . . . Excellent reference."
—*The Bookwatch, Aug '01*

"Recommended reference source."
—*Booklist, American Library Association, Jul '01*

∎

Communication Disorders Sourcebook

Basic Information about Deafness and Hearing Loss, Speech and Language Disorders, Voice Disorders, Balance and Vestibular Disorders, and Disorders of Smell, Taste, and Touch

Edited by Linda M. Ross. 533 pages. 1996. 978-0-7808-0077-9.

"This is skillfully edited and is a welcome resource for the layperson. It should be found in every public and medical library." —*Booklist Health Sciences Supplement, American Library Association, Oct '97*

∎

Complementary & Alternative Medicine Sourcebook, 3rd Edition

Basic Consumer Health Information about Complementary and Alternative Medical Therapies, Including Acupuncture, Ayurveda, Traditional Chinese Medicine, Herbal Medicine, Homeopathy, Naturopathy, Biofeedback, Hypnotherapy, Yoga, Art Therapy, Aromatherapy, Clinical Nutrition, Vitamin and Mineral Supplements, Chiropractic, Massage, Reflexology, Crystal Therapy, Therapeutic Touch, and More

Along with Facts about Alternative and Complementary Treatments for Specific Conditions Such as Cancer, Diabetes, Osteoarthritis, Chronic Pain, Menopause, Gastrointestinal Disorders, Headaches, and Mental Illness, a Glossary, and a Resource List for Additional Help and Information

Edited by Sandra J. Judd. 657 pages. 2006. 978-0-7808-0864-5.

"Recommended for public, high school, and academic libraries that have consumer health collections. Hospital libraries that also serve the public will find this to be a useful resource." —*E-Streams, Feb '03*

"Recommended reference source."
—*Booklist, American Library Association, Jan '03*

"An important alternate health reference."
—*MBR Bookwatch, Oct '02*

"A great addition to the reference collection of every type of library." —*American Reference Books Annual, 2000*

∎

Congenital Disorders Sourcebook, 2nd Edition

Basic Consumer Health Information about Non-hereditary Birth Defects and Disorders Related to Prematurity, Gestational Injuries, Congenital Infections, and Birth Complications, Including Heart Defects, Hydrocephalus, Spina Bifida, Cleft Lip and Palate, Cerebral Palsy, and More

Along with Facts about the Prevention of Birth Defects, Fetal Surgery and Other Treatment Options, Research Initiatives, a Glossary of Related Terms, and Resources for Additional Information and Support

Edited by Sandra J. Judd. 647 pages. 2006. 978-0-7808-0945-1.

"Recommended reference source."
—*Booklist, American Library Association, Oct '97*

SEE ALSO Pregnancy & Birth Sourcebook

∎

Contagious Diseases Sourcebook

Basic Consumer Health Information about Infectious Diseases Spread by Person-to-Person Contact through

Direct Touch, Airborne Transmission, Sexual Contact, or Contact with Blood or Other Body Fluids, Including Hepatitis, Herpes, Influenza, Lice, Measles, Mumps, Pinworm, Ringworm, Severe Acute Respiratory Syndrome (SARS), Streptococcal Infections, Tuberculosis, and Others

Along with Facts about Disease Transmission, Antimicrobial Resistance, and Vaccines, with a Glossary and Directories of Resources for More Information

Edited by Karen Bellenir. 643 pages. 2004. 978-0-7808-0736-5.

"This easy-to-read volume is recommended for consumer health collections within public or academic libraries." *— E-Streams, May '05*

"This informative book is highly recommended for public libraries, consumer health collections, and secondary schools and undergraduate libraries." *— American Reference Books Annual, 2005*

"Excellent reference." *— The Bookwatch, Jan '05*

■

Death & Dying Sourcebook, 2nd Edition

Basic Consumer Health Information about End-of-Life Care and Related Perspectives and Ethical Issues, Including End-of-Life Symptoms and Treatments, Pain Management, Quality-of-Life Concerns, the Use of Life Support, Patients' Rights and Privacy Issues, Advance Directives, Physician-Assisted Suicide, Caregiving, Organ and Tissue Donation, Autopsies, Funeral Arrangements, and Grief

Along with Statistical Data, Information about the Leading Causes of Death, a Glossary, and Directories of Support Groups and Other Resources

Edited by Joyce Brennfleck Shannon. 653 pages. 2006. 978-0-7808-0871-3.

"Public libraries, medical libraries, and academic libraries will all find this sourcebook a useful addition to their collections." *— American Reference Books Annual, 2001*

"An extremely useful resource for those concerned with death and dying in the United States." *— Respiratory Care, Nov '00*

"Recommended reference source." *—Booklist, American Library Association, Aug '00*

"This book is a definite must for all those involved in end-of-life care." *— Doody's Review Service, 2000*

■

Dental Care & Oral Health Sourcebook, 2nd Edition

Basic Consumer Health Information about Dental Care, Including Oral Hygiene, Dental Visits, Pain Management, Cavities, Crowns, Bridges, Dental Implants, and Fillings, and Other Oral Health Concerns, Such as Gum Disease, Bad Breath, Dry Mouth, Genetic and Developmental Abnormalities, Oral Cancers, Orthodontics, and Temporomandibular Disorders

Along with Updates on Current Research in Oral Health, a Glossary, a Directory of Dental and Oral Health Organizations, and Resources for People with Dental and Oral Health Disorders

Edited by Amy L. Sutton. 609 pages. 2003. 978-0-7808-0634-4.

"This book could serve as a turning point in the battle to educate consumers in issues concerning oral health." *— American Reference Books Annual, 2004*

"Unique source which will fill a gap in dental sources for patients and the lay public. A valuable reference tool even in a library with thousands of books on dentistry. Comprehensive, clear, inexpensive, and easy to read and use. It fills an enormous gap in the health care literature." *— Reference & User Services Quarterly, American Library Association, Summer '98*

"Recommended reference source." *—Booklist, American Library Association, Dec '97*

■

Depression Sourcebook

Basic Consumer Health Information about Unipolar Depression, Bipolar Disorder, Postpartum Depression, Seasonal Affective Disorder, and Other Types of Depression in Children, Adolescents, Women, Men, the Elderly, and Other Selected Populations

Along with Facts about Causes, Risk Factors, Diagnostic Criteria, Treatment Options, Coping Strategies, Suicide Prevention, a Glossary, and a Directory of Sources for Additional Help and Information

Edited by Karen Bellenir. 602 pages. 2002. 978-0-7808-0611-5.

"*Depression Sourcebook* is of a very high standard. Its purpose, which is to serve as a reference source to the lay reader, is very well served." *— Journal of the National Medical Association, 2004*

"Invaluable reference for public and school library collections alike." *— Library Bookwatch, Apr '03*

"Recommended for purchase." *— American Reference Books Annual, 2003*

■

Dermatological Disorders Sourcebook, 2nd Edition

Basic Consumer Health Information about Conditions and Disorders Affecting the Skin, Hair, and Nails, Such as Acne, Rosacea, Rashes, Dermatitis, Pigmentation Disorders, Birthmarks, Skin Cancer, Skin Injuries, Psoriasis, Scleroderma, and Hair Loss, Including Facts about Medications and Treatments for Dermatological Disorders and Tips for Maintaining Healthy Skin, Hair, and Nails

Along with Information about How Aging Affects the Skin, a Glossary of Related Terms, and a Directory of Resources for Additional Help and Information

Edited by Amy L. Sutton. 645 pages. 2005. 978-0-7808-0795-2.

■

Diabetes Sourcebook, 3rd Edition

Basic Consumer Health Information about Type 1 Diabetes (Insulin-Dependent or Juvenile-Onset Diabetes), Type 2 Diabetes (Noninsulin-Dependent or Adult-Onset Diabetes), Gestational Diabetes, Impaired Glucose Tolerance (IGT), and Related Complications, Such as Amputation, Eye Disease, Gum Disease, Nerve Damage, and End-Stage Renal Disease, Including Facts about Insulin, Oral Diabetes Medications, Blood Sugar Testing, and the Role of Exercise and Nutrition in the Control of Diabetes

Along with a Glossary and Resources for Further Help and Information

Edited by Dawn D. Matthews. 622 pages. 2003. 978-0-7808-0629-0.

■

Diet & Nutrition Sourcebook, 3rd Edition

Basic Consumer Health Information about Dietary Guidelines and the Food Guidance System, Recommended Daily Nutrient Intakes, Serving Proportions, Weight Control, Vitamins and Supplements, Nutrition Issues for Different Life Stages and Lifestyles, and the Needs of People with Specific Medical Concerns, Including Cancer, Celiac Disease, Diabetes, Eating Disorders, Food Allergies, and Cardiovascular Disease

Along with Facts about Federal Nutrition Support Programs, a Glossary of Nutrition and Dietary Terms, and Directories of Additional Resources for More Information about Nutrition

Edited by Joyce Brennfleck Shannon. 633 pages. 2006. 978-0-7808-0800-3.

■

Digestive Diseases & Disorders Sourcebook

Basic Consumer Health Information about Diseases and Disorders that Impact the Upper and Lower Digestive System, Including Celiac Disease, Constipation, Crohn's Disease, Cyclic Vomiting Syndrome, Diarrhea, Diverticulosis and Diverticulitis, Gallstones, Heartburn, Hemorrhoids, Hernias, Indigestion (Dyspepsia), Irritable Bowel Syndrome, Lactose Intolerance, Ulcers, and More

Along with Information about Medications and Other Treatments, Tips for Maintaining a Healthy Digestive Tract, a Glossary, and Directory of Digestive Diseases Organizations

Edited by Karen Bellenir. 335 pages. 2000. 978-0-7808-0327-5.

■

Disabilities Sourcebook

Basic Consumer Health Information about Physical and Psychiatric Disabilities, Including Descriptions of Major Causes of Disability, Assistive and Adaptive Aids, Workplace Issues, and Accessibility Concerns

Along with Information about the Americans with Disabilities Act, a Glossary, and Resources for Additional Help and Information

Edited by Dawn D. Matthews. 616 pages. 2000. 978-0-7808-0389-3.

"A much needed addition to the Omnigraphics *Health Reference Series*. A current reference work to provide people with disabilities, their families, caregivers or those who work with them, a broad range of information in one volume, has not been available until now. . . . It is recommended for all public and academic library reference collections." —*E-Streams, May '01*

"An excellent source book in easy-to-read format covering many current topics; highly recommended for all libraries." —*Choice, Association of College & Research Libraries, Jan '01*

"Recommended reference source." —*Booklist, American Library Association, Jul '00*

■

Domestic Violence Sourcebook, 2nd Edition

Basic Consumer Health Information about the Causes and Consequences of Abusive Relationships, Including Physical Violence, Sexual Assault, Battery, Stalking, and Emotional Abuse, and Facts about the Effects of Violence on Women, Men, Young Adults, and the Elderly, with Reports about Domestic Violence in Selected Populations, and Featuring Facts about Medical Care, Victim Assistance and Protection, Prevention Strategies, Mental Health Services, and Legal Issues

Along with a Glossary of Related Terms and Resources for Additional Help and Information

Edited by Dawn D. Matthews. 628 pages. 2004. 978-0-7808-0669-6.

"Educators, clergy, medical professionals, police, and victims and their families will benefit from this realistic and easy-to-understand resource." —*American Reference Books Annual, 2005*

"Recommended for all collections supporting consumer health information. It should also be considered for any collection needing general, readable information on domestic violence." —*E-Streams, Jan '05*

"This sourcebook complements other books in its field, providing a one-stop resource . . . Recommended." —*Choice, Association of College & Research Libraries, Jan '05*

"Interested lay persons should find the book extremely beneficial. . . . A copy of *Domestic Violence and Child Abuse Sourcebook* should be in every public library in the United States." —*Social Science & Medicine, No. 56, 2003*

"This is important information. The Web has many resources but this sourcebook fills an important societal need. I am not aware of any other resources of this type." —*Doody's Review Service, Sep '01*

"Recommended reference source." —*Booklist, American Library Association, Apr '01*

"Important pick for college-level health reference libraries." —*The Bookwatch, Mar '01*

"Because this problem is so widespread and because this book includes a lot of issues within one volume, this work is recommended for all public libraries." —*American Reference Books Annual, 2001*

SEE ALSO Child Abuse Sourcebook

■

Drug Abuse Sourcebook, 2nd Edition

Basic Consumer Health Information about Illicit Substances of Abuse and the Misuse of Prescription and Over-the-Counter Medications, Including Depressants, Hallucinogens, Inhalants, Marijuana, Stimulants, and Anabolic Steroids

Along with Facts about Related Health Risks, Treatment Programs, Prevention Programs, a Glossary of Abuse and Addiction Terms, a Glossary of Drug-Related Street Terms, and a Directory of Resources for More Information

Edited by Catherine Ginther. 607 pages. 2004. 978-0-7808-0740-2.

"Commendable for organizing useful, normally scattered government and association-produced data into a logical sequence." —*American Reference Books Annual, 2006*

"This easy-to-read volume is recommended for consumer health collections within public or academic libraries." —*E-Streams, Sep '05*

"An excellent library reference." —*The Bookwatch, May '05*

"Containing a wealth of information, this book will be useful to the college student just beginning to explore the topic of substance abuse. This resource belongs in libraries that serve a lower-division undergraduate or community college clientele as well as the general public." —*Choice, Association of College & Research Libraries, Jun '01*

"Recommended reference source." —*Booklist, American Library Association, Feb '01*

SEE ALSO Alcoholism Sourcebook

■

Ear, Nose & Throat Disorders Sourcebook, 2nd Edition

Basic Consumer Health Information about Disorders of the Ears, Hearing Loss, Vestibular Disorders, Nasal and Sinus Problems, Throat and Vocal Cord Disorders, and Otolaryngologic Cancers, Including Facts about Ear Infections and Injuries, Genetic and Congenital Deafness, Sensorineural Hearing Disorders, Tinnitus, Vertigo, Ménière Disease, Rhinitis, Sinusitis, Snoring, Sore Throats, Hoarseness, and More

Along with Reports on Current Research Initiatives, a Glossary of Related Medical Terms, and a Directory of Sources for Further Help and Information

Edited by Sandra J. Judd. 659 pages. 2006. 978-0-7808-0872-0.

"Overall, this sourcebook is helpful for the consumer seeking information on ENT issues. It is recommended for public libraries."
— *American Reference Books Annual, 1999*

"Recommended reference source."
— *Booklist, American Library Association, Dec '98*

■

Eating Disorders Sourcebook, 2nd Edition

Basic Consumer Health Information about Anorexia Nervosa, Bulimia Nervosa, Binge Eating, Compulsive Exercise, Female Athlete Triad, and Other Eating Disorders, Including Facts about Body Image and Other Cultural and Age-Related Risk Factors, Prevention Efforts, Adverse Health Effects, Treatment Options, and the Recovery Process

Along with Guidelines for Healthy Weight Control, a Glossary, and Directories of Additional Resources

Edited by Joyce Brennfleck Shannon. 585 pages. 2007. 978-0-7808-0948-2.

"Recommended for health science libraries that are open to the public, as well as hospital libraries. This book is a good resource for the consumer who is concerned about eating disorders." — *E-Streams, Mar '02*

"This volume is another convenient collection of excerpted articles. Recommended for school and public library patrons; lower-division undergraduates; and two-year technical program students."
— *Choice, Association of College & Research Libraries, Jan '02*

"Recommended reference source."
— *Booklist, American Library Association, Oct '01*

SEE ALSO *Diet & Nutrition Sourcebook, Digestive Diseases & Disorders Sourcebook, Gastrointestinal Diseases & Disorders Sourcebook*

■

Emergency Medical Services Sourcebook

Basic Consumer Health Information about Preventing, Preparing for, and Managing Emergency Situations, When and Who to Call for Help, What to Expect in the Emergency Room, the Emergency Medical Team, Patient Issues, and Current Topics in Emergency Medicine

Along with Statistical Data, a Glossary, and Sources of Additional Help and Information

Edited by Jenni Lynn Colson. 494 pages. 2002. 978-0-7808-0420-3.

"Handy and convenient for home, public, school, and college libraries. Recommended."
— *Choice, Association of College & Research Libraries, Apr '03*

"This reference can provide the consumer with answers to most questions about emergency care in the United States, or it will direct them to a resource where the answer can be found."
— *American Reference Books Annual, 2003*

"Recommended reference source."
— *Booklist, American Library Association, Feb '03*

■

Endocrine & Metabolic Disorders Sourcebook

Basic Information for the Layperson about Pancreatic and Insulin-Related Disorders Such as Pancreatitis, Diabetes, and Hypoglycemia; Adrenal Gland Disorders Such as Cushing's Syndrome, Addison's Disease, and Congenital Adrenal Hyperplasia; Pituitary Gland Disorders Such as Growth Hormone Deficiency, Acromegaly, and Pituitary Tumors; Thyroid Disorders Such as Hypothyroidism, Graves' Disease, Hashimoto's Disease, and Goiter; Hyperparathyroidism; and Other Diseases and Syndromes of Hormone Imbalance or Metabolic Dysfunction

Along with Reports on Current Research Initiatives

Edited by Linda M. Shin. 574 pages. 1998. 978-0-7808-0207-0.

"Omnigraphics has produced another needed resource for health information consumers."
— *American Reference Books Annual, 2000*

"Recommended reference source."
— *Booklist, American Library Association, Dec '98*

■

Environmental Health Sourcebook, 2nd Edition

Basic Consumer Health Information about the Environment and Its Effect on Human Health, Including the Effects of Air Pollution, Water Pollution, Hazardous Chemicals, Food Hazards, Radiation Hazards, Biological Agents, Household Hazards, Such as Radon, Asbestos, Carbon Monoxide, and Mold, and Information about Associated Diseases and Disorders, Including Cancer, Allergies, Respiratory Problems, and Skin Disorders

Along with Information about Environmental Concerns for Specific Populations, a Glossary of Related Terms, and Resources for Further Help and Information

Edited by Dawn D. Matthews. 673 pages. 2003. 978-0-7808-0632-0.

"This recently updated edition continues the level of quality and the reputation of the numerous other volumes in Omnigraphics' *Health Reference Series*."
— *American Reference Books Annual, 2004*

"An excellent updated edition."
— *The Bookwatch, Oct '03*

"Recommended reference source."
— *Booklist, American Library Association, Sep '98*

"This book will be a useful addition to anyone's library." — *Choice Health Sciences Supplement, Association of College & Research Libraries, May '98*

". . . a good survey of numerous environmentally induced physical disorders . . . a useful addition to anyone's library."
— *Doody's Health Sciences Book Reviews, Jan '98*

Ethnic Diseases Sourcebook

Basic Consumer Health Information for Ethnic and Racial Minority Groups in the United States, Including General Health Indicators and Behaviors, Ethnic Diseases, Genetic Testing, the Impact of Chronic Diseases, Women's Health, Mental Health Issues, and Preventive Health Care Services

Along with a Glossary and a Listing of Additional Resources

Edited by Joyce Brennfleck Shannon. 664 pages. 2001. 978-0-7808-0336-7.

"Recommended for health sciences libraries where public health programs are a priority."
— *E-Streams, Jan '02*

"Not many books have been written on this topic to date, and the *Ethnic Diseases Sourcebook* is a strong addition to the list. It will be an important introductory resource for health consumers, students, health care personnel, and social scientists. It is recommended for public, academic, and large hospital libraries."
— *American Reference Books Annual, 2002*

"Recommended reference source."
— *Booklist, American Library Association, Oct '01*

"Will prove valuable to any library seeking to maintain a current, comprehensive reference collection of health resources.... An excellent source of health information about genetic disorders which affect particular ethnic and racial minorities in the U.S."
— *The Bookwatch, Aug '01*

Eye Care Sourcebook, 2nd Edition

Basic Consumer Health Information about Eye Care and Eye Disorders, Including Facts about the Diagnosis, Prevention, and Treatment of Common Refractive Problems Such as Myopia, Hyperopia, Astigmatism, and Presbyopia, and Eye Diseases, Including Glaucoma, Cataract, Age-Related Macular Degeneration, and Diabetic Retinopathy

Along with a Section on Vision Correction and Refractive Surgeries, Including LASIK and LASEK, a Glossary, and Directories of Resources for Additional Help and Information

Edited by Amy L. Sutton. 543 pages. 2003. 978-0-7808-0635-1.

". . . a solid reference tool for eye care and a valuable addition to a collection."
— *American Reference Books Annual, 2004*

Family Planning Sourcebook

Basic Consumer Health Information about Planning for Pregnancy and Contraception, Including Traditional Methods, Barrier Methods, Hormonal Methods, Permanent Methods, Future Methods, Emergency Contraception, and Birth Control Choices for Women at Each Stage of Life

Along with Statistics, a Glossary, and Sources of Additional Information

Edited by Amy Marcaccio Keyzer. 520 pages. 2001. 978-0-7808-0379-4.

"Recommended for public, health, and undergraduate libraries as part of the circulating collection."
— *E-Streams, Mar '02*

"Information is presented in an unbiased, readable manner, and the sourcebook will certainly be a necessary addition to those public and high school libraries where Internet access is restricted or otherwise problematic." — *American Reference Books Annual, 2002*

"Recommended reference source."
— *Booklist, American Library Association, Oct '01*

"Will prove valuable to any library seeking to maintain a current, comprehensive reference collection of health resources.... Excellent reference."
— *The Bookwatch, Aug '01*

SEE ALSO Pregnancy & Birth Sourcebook

Fitness & Exercise Sourcebook, 3rd Edition

Basic Consumer Health Information about the Physical and Mental Benefits of Fitness, Including Cardiorespiratory Endurance, Muscular Strength, Muscular Endurance, and Flexibility, with Facts about Sports Nutrition and Exercise-Related Injuries and Tips about Physical Activity and Exercises for People of All Ages and for People with Health Concerns

Along with Advice on Selecting and Using Exercise Equipment, Maintaining Exercise Motivation, a Glossary of Related Terms, and a Directory of Resources for More Help and Information

Edited by Amy L. Sutton. 663 pages. 2007. 978-0-7808-0946-8.

"This work is recommended for all general reference collections."
— *American Reference Books Annual, 2002*

"Highly recommended for public, consumer, and school grades fourth through college." — *E-Streams, Nov '01*

"Recommended reference source."
— *Booklist, American Library Association, Oct '01*

"The information appears quite comprehensive and is considered reliable. . . . This second edition is a welcomed addition to the series."
— *Doody's Review Service, Sep '01*

Food Safety Sourcebook

Basic Consumer Health Information about the Safe Handling of Meat, Poultry, Seafood, Eggs, Fruit Juices, and Other Food Items, and Facts about Pesticides, Drinking Water, Food Safety Overseas, and the Onset, Duration, and Symptoms of Foodborne Illnesses, Including Types of Pathogenic Bacteria, Parasitic Protozoa, Worms, Viruses, and Natural Toxins

Along with the Role of the Consumer, the Food Handler, and the Government in Food Safety; a Glossary, and Resources for Additional Help and Information

Edited by Dawn D. Matthews. 339 pages. 1999. 978-0-7808-0326-8.

"This book is recommended for public libraries and universities with home economic and food science programs." — E-Streams, Nov '00

"Recommended reference source."
— Booklist, American Library Association, May '00

"This book takes the complex issues of food safety and foodborne pathogens and presents them in an easily understood manner. [It does] an excellent job of covering a large and often confusing topic."
— American Reference Books Annual, 2000

■

Forensic Medicine Sourcebook

Basic Consumer Information for the Layperson about Forensic Medicine, Including Crime Scene Investigation, Evidence Collection and Analysis, Expert Testimony, Computer-Aided Criminal Identification, Digital Imaging in the Courtroom, DNA Profiling, Accident Reconstruction, Autopsies, Ballistics, Drugs and Explosives Detection, Latent Fingerprints, Product Tampering, and Questioned Document Examination

Along with Statistical Data, a Glossary of Forensics Terminology, and Listings of Sources for Further Help and Information

Edited by Annemarie S. Muth. 574 pages. 1999. 978-0-7808-0232-2.

"Given the expected widespread interest in its content and its easy to read style, this book is recommended for most public and all college and university libraries."
— E-Streams, Feb '01

"Recommended for public libraries."
— Reference & User Services Quarterly, American Library Association, Spring 2000

"Recommended reference source."
— Booklist, American Library Association, Feb '00

"A wealth of information, useful statistics, references are up-to-date and extremely complete. This wonderful collection of data will help students who are interested in a career in any type of forensic field. It is a great resource for attorneys who need information about types of expert witnesses needed in a particular case. It also offers useful information for fiction and nonfiction writers whose work involves a crime. A fascinating compilation. All levels."
— Choice, Association of College & Research Libraries, Jan '00

"There are several items that make this book attractive to consumers who are seeking certain forensic data. . . . This is a useful current source for those seeking general forensic medical answers."
— American Reference Books Annual, 2000

Gastrointestinal Diseases & Disorders Sourcebook, 2nd Edition

Basic Consumer Health Information about the Upper and Lower Gastrointestinal (GI) Tract, Including the Esophagus, Stomach, Intestines, Rectum, Liver, and Pancreas, with Facts about Gastroesophageal Reflux Disease, Gastritis, Hernias, Ulcers, Celiac Disease, Diverticulitis, Irritable Bowel Syndrome, Hemorrhoids, Gastrointestinal Cancers, and Other Diseases and Disorders Related to the Digestive Process

Along with Information about Commonly Used Diagnostic and Surgical Procedures, Statistics, Reports on Current Research Initiatives and Clinical Trials, a Glossary, and Resources for Additional Help and Information

Edited by Sandra J. Judd. 681 pages. 2006. 978-0-7808-0798-3.

". . . very readable form. The successful editorial work that brought this material together into a useful and understandable reference makes accessible to all readers information that can help them more effectively understand and obtain help for digestive tract problems."
— Choice, Association of College & Research Libraries, Feb '97

SEE ALSO Diet & Nutrition Sourcebook, Digestive Diseases & Disorders Sourcebook, Eating Disorders Sourcebook

■

Genetic Disorders Sourcebook, 3rd Edition

Basic Consumer Health Information about Hereditary Diseases and Disorders, Including Facts about the Human Genome, Genetic Inheritance Patterns, Disorders Associated with Specific Genes, Such as Sickle Cell Disease, Hemophilia, and Cystic Fibrosis, Chromosome Disorders, Such as Down Syndrome, Fragile X Syndrome, and Turner Syndrome, and Complex Diseases and Disorders Resulting from the Interaction of Environmental and Genetic Factors, Such as Allergies, Cancer, and Obesity

Along with Facts about Genetic Testing, Suggestions for Parents of Children with Special Needs, Reports on Current Research Initiatives, a Glossary of Genetic Terminology, and Resources for Additional Help and Information

Edited by Karen Bellenir. 777 pages. 2004. 978-0-7808-0742-6.

"This text is recommended for any library with an interest in providing consumer health resources."
— E-Streams, Aug '05

"This is a valuable resource for anyone wishing to have an understandable description of any of the topics or disorders included. The editor succeeds in making complex genetic issues understandable."
— Doody's Book Review Service, May '05

"A good acquisition for public libraries."
— American Reference Books Annual, 2005

■

Head Trauma Sourcebook

Basic Information for the Layperson about Open-Head and Closed-Head Injuries, Treatment Advances, Recovery, and Rehabilitation

Along with Reports on Current Research Initiatives

Edited by Karen Bellenir. 414 pages. 1997. 978-0-7808-0208-7.

Headache Sourcebook

Basic Consumer Health Information about Migraine, Tension, Cluster, Rebound and Other Types of Headaches, with Facts about the Cause and Prevention of Headaches, the Effects of Stress and the Environment, Headaches during Pregnancy and Menopause, and Childhood Headaches

Along with a Glossary and Other Resources for Additional Help and Information

Edited by Dawn D. Matthews. 362 pages. 2002. 978-0-7808-0337-4.

■

Healthy Aging Sourcebook

Basic Consumer Health Information about Maintaining Health through the Aging Process, Including Advice on Nutrition, Exercise, and Sleep, Help in Making Decisions about Midlife Issues and Retirement, and Guidance Concerning Practical and Informed Choices in Health Consumerism

Along with Data Concerning the Theories of Aging, Different Experiences in Aging by Minority Groups, and Facts about Aging Now and Aging in the Future; and Featuring a Glossary, a Guide to Consumer Help, Additional Suggested Reading, and Practical Resource Directory

Edited by Jenifer Swanson. 536 pages. 1999. 978-0-7808-0390-9.

SEE ALSO *Physical & Mental Issues in Aging Sourcebook*

■

Healthy Children Sourcebook

Basic Consumer Health Information about the Physical and Mental Development of Children between the Ages of 3 and 12, Including Routine Health Care, Preventative Health Services, Safety and First Aid,

Healthy Sleep, Dental Care, Nutrition, and Fitness, and Featuring Parenting Tips on Such Topics as Bedwetting, Choosing Day Care, Monitoring TV and Other Media, and Establishing a Foundation for Substance Abuse Prevention

Along with a Glossary of Commonly Used Pediatric Terms and Resources for Additional Help and Information.

Edited by Chad T. Kimball. 647 pages. 2003. 978-0-7808-0247-6.

SEE ALSO *Childhood Diseases & Disorders Sourcebook*

■

Healthy Heart Sourcebook for Women

Basic Consumer Health Information about Cardiac Issues Specific to Women, Including Facts about Major Risk Factors and Prevention, Treatment and Control Strategies, and Important Dietary Issues

Along with a Special Section Regarding the Pros and Cons of Hormone Replacement Therapy and Its Impact on Heart Health, and Additional Help, Including Recipes, a Glossary, and a Directory of Resources

Edited by Dawn D. Matthews. 336 pages. 2000. 978-0-7808-0329-9.

SEE ALSO *Cardiovascular Diseases & Disorders Sourcebook, Women's Health Concerns Sourcebook*

■

Hepatitis Sourcebook

Basic Consumer Health Information about Hepatitis A, Hepatitis B, Hepatitis C, and Other Forms of Hepatitis, Including Autoimmune Hepatitis, Alcoholic Hepatitis, Nonalcoholic Steatohepatitis, and Toxic Hepatitis, with

Facts about Risk Factors, Screening Methods, Diagnostic Tests, and Treatment Options

Along with Information on Liver Health, Tips for People Living with Chronic Hepatitis, Reports on Current Research Initiatives, a Glossary of Terms Related to Hepatitis, and a Directory of Sources for Further Help and Information

Edited by Sandra J. Judd. 597 pages. 2005. 978-0-7808-0749-5.

"Highly recommended."
— American Reference Books Annual, 2006

■

Household Safety Sourcebook

Basic Consumer Health Information about Household Safety, Including Information about Poisons, Chemicals, Fire, and Water Hazards in the Home

Along with Advice about the Safe Use of Home Maintenance Equipment, Choosing Toys and Nursery Furniture, Holiday and Recreation Safety, a Glossary, and Resources for Further Help and Information

Edited by Dawn D. Matthews. 606 pages. 2002. 978-0-7808-0338-1.

"This work will be useful in public libraries with large consumer health and wellness departments."
— American Reference Books Annual, 2003

"As a sourcebook on household safety this book meets its mark. It is encyclopedic in scope and covers a wide range of safety issues that are commonly seen in the home."
— E-Streams, Jul '02

■

Hypertension Sourcebook

Basic Consumer Health Information about the Causes, Diagnosis, and Treatment of High Blood Pressure, with Facts about Consequences, Complications, and Co-Occurring Disorders, Such as Coronary Heart Disease, Diabetes, Stroke, Kidney Disease, and Hypertensive Retinopathy, and Issues in Blood Pressure Control, Including Dietary Choices, Stress Management, and Medications

Along with Reports on Current Research Initiatives and Clinical Trials, a Glossary, and Resources for Additional Help and Information

Edited by Dawn D. Matthews and Karen Bellenir. 613 pages. 2004. 978-0-7808-0674-0.

"Academic, public, and medical libraries will want to add the Hypertension Sourcebook to their collections."
— E-Streams, Aug '05

"The strength of this source is the wide range of information given about hypertension."
— American Reference Books Annual, 2005

■

Immune System Disorders Sourcebook, 2nd Edition

Basic Consumer Health Information about Disorders of the Immune System, Including Immune System Function and Response, Diagnosis of Immune Disorders, Information about Inherited Immune Disease, Acquired Immune Disease, and Autoimmune Diseases, Including Primary Immune Deficiency, Acquired Immunodeficiency Syndrome (AIDS), Lupus, Multiple Sclerosis, Type 1 Diabetes, Rheumatoid Arthritis, and Graves' Disease

Along with Treatments, Tips for Coping with Immune Disorders, a Glossary, and a Directory of Additional Resources.

Edited by Joyce Brennfleck Shannon. 671 pages. 2005. 978-0-7808-0748-8.

"Highly recommended for academic and public libraries." — American Reference Books Annual, 2006

"The updated second edition is a 'must' for any consumer health library seeking a solid resource covering the treatments, symptoms, and options for immune disorder sufferers. . . . An excellent guide."
— MBR Bookwatch, Jan '06

■

Infant & Toddler Health Sourcebook

Basic Consumer Health Information about the Physical and Mental Development of Newborns, Infants, and Toddlers, Including Neonatal Concerns, Nutrition Recommendations, Immunization Schedules, Common Pediatric Disorders, Assessments and Milestones, Safety Tips, and Advice for Parents and Other Caregivers

Along with a Glossary of Terms and Resource Listings for Additional Help

Edited by Jenifer Swanson. 585 pages. 2000. 978-0-7808-0246-9.

"As a reference for the general public, this would be useful in any library." — E-Streams, May '01

"Recommended reference source."
— Booklist, American Library Association, Feb '01

"This is a good source for general use."
— American Reference Books Annual, 2001

■

Infectious Diseases Sourcebook

Basic Consumer Health Information about Non-Contagious Bacterial, Viral, Prion, Fungal, and Parasitic Diseases Spread by Food and Water, Insects and Animals, or Environmental Contact, Including Botulism, E. Coli, Encephalitis, Legionnaires' Disease, Lyme Disease, Malaria, Plague, Rabies, Salmonella, Tetanus, and Others, and Facts about Newly Emerging Diseases, Such as Hantavirus, Mad Cow Disease, Monkeypox, and West Nile Virus

Along with Information about Preventing Disease Transmission, the Threat of Bioterrorism, and Current Research Initiatives, with a Glossary and Directory of Resources for More Information

Edited by Karen Bellenir. 634 pages. 2004. 978-0-7808-0675-7.

"This reference continues the excellent tradition of the *Health Reference Series* in consolidating a wealth of information on a selected topic into a format that is easy to use and accessible to the general public."
— *American Reference Books Annual, 2005*

"Recommended for public and academic libraries."
— *E-Streams, Jan '05*

■

Injury & Trauma Sourcebook

Basic Consumer Health Information about the Impact of Injury, the Diagnosis and Treatment of Common and Traumatic Injuries, Emergency Care, and Specific Injuries Related to Home, Community, Workplace, Transportation, and Recreation

Along with Guidelines for Injury Prevention, a Glossary, and a Directory of Additional Resources

Edited by Joyce Brennfleck Shannon. 696 pages. 2002. 978-0-7808-0421-0.

"This publication is the most comprehensive work of its kind about injury and trauma."
— *American Reference Books Annual, 2003*

"This sourcebook provides concise, easily readable, basic health information about injuries. . . . This book is well organized and an easy to use reference resource suitable for hospital, health sciences and public libraries with consumer health collections."
— *E-Streams, Nov '02*

"Practitioners should be aware of guides such as this in order to facilitate their use by patients and their families."
— *Doody's Health Sciences Book Review Journal, Sep-Oct '02*

"Recommended reference source."
— *Booklist, American Library Association, Sep '02*

"Highly recommended for academic and medical reference collections."
— *Library Bookwatch, Sep '02*

■

Kidney & Urinary Tract Diseases & Disorders Sourcebook

SEE Urinary Tract & Kidney Diseases & Disorders Sourcebook

■

Learning Disabilities Sourcebook, 2nd Edition

Basic Consumer Health Information about Learning Disabilities, Including Dyslexia, Developmental Speech and Language Disabilities, Non-Verbal Learning Disorders, Developmental Arithmetic Disorder, Developmental Writing Disorder, and Other Conditions That Impede Learning Such as Attention Deficit/Hyperactivity Disorder, Brain Injury, Hearing Impairment, Klinefelter Syndrome, Dyspraxia, and Tourette's Syndrome

Along with Facts about Educational Issues and Assistive Technology, Coping Strategies, a Glossary of Related Terms, and Resources for Further Help and Information

Edited by Dawn D. Matthews. 621 pages. 2003. 978-0-7808-0626-9.

"The second edition of Learning Disabilities Sourcebook far surpasses the earlier edition in that it is more focused on information that will be useful as a consumer health resource."
— *American Reference Books Annual, 2004*

"Teachers as well as consumers will find this an essential guide to understanding various syndromes and their latest treatments. [An] invaluable reference for public and school library collections alike."
— *Library Bookwatch, Apr '03*

Named "Outstanding Reference Book of 1999."
— *New York Public Library, Feb '00*

"An excellent candidate for inclusion in a public library reference section. It's a great source of information. Teachers will also find the book useful. Definitely worth reading."
— *Journal of Adolescent & Adult Literacy, Feb 2000*

"Readable . . . provides a solid base of information regarding successful techniques used with individuals who have learning disabilities, as well as practical suggestions for educators and family members. Clear language, concise descriptions, and pertinent information for contacting multiple resources add to the strength of this book as a useful tool."
— *Choice, Association of College & Research Libraries, Feb '99*

"Recommended reference source."
— *Booklist, American Library Association, Sep '98*

"A useful resource for libraries and for those who don't have the time to identify and locate the individual publications."
— *Disability Resources Monthly, Sep '98*

■

Leukemia Sourcebook

Basic Consumer Health Information about Adult and Childhood Leukemias, Including Acute Lymphocytic Leukemia (ALL), Chronic Lymphocytic Leukemia (CLL), Acute Myelogenous Leukemia (AML), Chronic Myelogenous Leukemia (CML), and Hairy Cell Leukemia, and Treatments Such as Chemotherapy, Radiation Therapy, Peripheral Blood Stem Cell and Marrow Transplantation, and Immunotherapy

Along with Tips for Life During and After Treatment, a Glossary, and Directories of Additional Resources

Edited by Joyce Brennfleck Shannon. 587 pages. 2003. 978-0-7808-0627-6.

"Unlike other medical books for the layperson, . . . the language does not talk down to the reader. . . . This volume is highly recommended for all libraries."
— *American Reference Books Annual, 2004*

". . . a fine title which ranges from diagnosis to alternative treatments, staging, and tips for life during and after diagnosis."
— *The Bookwatch, Dec '03*

Liver Disorders Sourcebook

Basic Consumer Health Information about the Liver and How It Works; Liver Diseases, Including Cancer, Cirrhosis, Hepatitis, and Toxic and Drug Related Diseases; Tips for Maintaining a Healthy Liver; Laboratory Tests, Radiology Tests, and Facts about Liver Transplantation

Along with a Section on Support Groups, a Glossary, and Resource Listings

Edited by Joyce Brennfleck Shannon. 591 pages. 2000. 978-0-7808-0383-1.

"A valuable resource."
—American Reference Books Annual, 2001

"This title is recommended for health sciences and public libraries with consumer health collections."
—E-Streams, Oct '00

"Recommended reference source."
—Booklist, American Library Association, Jun '00

■

Lung Disorders Sourcebook

Basic Consumer Health Information about Emphysema, Pneumonia, Tuberculosis, Asthma, Cystic Fibrosis, and Other Lung Disorders, Including Facts about Diagnostic Procedures, Treatment Strategies, Disease Prevention Efforts, and Such Risk Factors as Smoking, Air Pollution, and Exposure to Asbestos, Radon, and Other Agents

Along with a Glossary and Resources for Additional Help and Information

Edited by Dawn D. Matthews. 678 pages. 2002. 978-0-7808-0339-8.

"This title is a great addition for public and school libraries because it provides concise health information on the lungs."
—American Reference Books Annual, 2003

"Highly recommended for academic and medical reference collections." *—Library Bookwatch, Sep '02*

SEE ALSO *Respiratory Diseases & Disorders Sourcebook*

■

Medical Tests Sourcebook, 2nd Edition

Basic Consumer Health Information about Medical Tests, Including Age-Specific Health Tests, Important Health Screenings and Exams, Home-Use Tests, Blood and Specimen Tests, Electrical Tests, Scope Tests, Genetic Testing, and Imaging Tests, Such as X-Rays, Ultrasound, Computed Tomography, Magnetic Resonance Imaging, Angiography, and Nuclear Medicine

Along with a Glossary and Directory of Additional Resources

Edited by Joyce Brennfleck Shannon. 654 pages. 2004. 978-0-7808-0670-2.

"Recommended for hospital and health sciences

libraries with consumer health collections."
—E-Streams, Mar '00

"This is an overall excellent reference with a wealth of general knowledge that may aid those who are reluctant to get vital tests performed."
—Today's Librarian, Jan '00

"A valuable reference guide."
—American Reference Books Annual, 2000

■

Men's Health Concerns Sourcebook, 2nd Edition

Basic Consumer Health Information about the Medical and Mental Concerns of Men, Including Theories about the Shorter Male Lifespan, the Leading Causes of Death and Disability, Physical Concerns of Special Significance to Men, Reproductive and Sexual Concerns, Sexually Transmitted Diseases, Men's Mental and Emotional Health, and Lifestyle Choices That Affect Wellness, Such as Nutrition, Fitness, and Substance Use

Along with a Glossary of Related Terms and a Directory of Organizational Resources in Men's Health

Edited by Robert Aquinas McNally. 644 pages. 2004. 978-0-7808-0671-9.

"A very accessible reference for non-specialist general readers and consumers." *—The Bookwatch, Jun '04*

"This comprehensive resource and the series are highly recommended."
—American Reference Books Annual, 2000

"Recommended reference source."
—Booklist, American Library Association, Dec '98

■

Mental Health Disorders Sourcebook, 3rd Edition

Basic Consumer Health Information about Mental and Emotional Health and Mental Illness, Including Facts about Depression, Bipolar Disorder, and Other Mood Disorders, Phobias, Post-Traumatic Stress Disorder (PTSD), Obsessive-Compulsive Disorder, and Other Anxiety Disorders, Impulse Control Disorders, Eating Disorders, Personality Disorders, and Psychotic Disorders, Including Schizophrenia and Dissociative Disorders

Along with Statistical Information, a Special Section Concerning Mental Health Issues in Children and Adolescents, a Glossary, and Directories of Resources for Additional Help and Information

Edited by Karen Bellenir. 661 pages. 2005. 978-0-7808-0747-1.

"Recommended for public libraries and academic libraries with an undergraduate program in psychology."
—American Reference Books Annual, 2006

"Recommended reference source."
—Booklist, American Library Association, Jun '00

Mental Retardation Sourcebook

Basic Consumer Health Information about Mental Retardation and Its Causes, Including Down Syndrome, Fetal Alcohol Syndrome, Fragile X Syndrome, Genetic Conditions, Injury, and Environmental Sources

Along with Preventive Strategies; Parenting Issues, Educational Implications, Health Care Needs, Employment and Economic Matters, Legal Issues, a Glossary, and a Resource Listing for Additional Help and Information

Edited by Joyce Brennfleck Shannon. 642 pages. 2000. 978-0-7808-0377-0.

"Public libraries will find the book useful for reference and as a beginning research point for students, parents, and caregivers."
— American Reference Books Annual, 2001

"The strength of this work is that it compiles many basic fact sheets and addresses for further information in one volume. It is intended and suitable for the general public. This sourcebook is relevant to any collection providing health information to the general public."
— E-Streams, Nov '00

"From preventing retardation to parenting and family challenges, this covers health, social and legal issues and will prove an invaluable overview."
— Reviewer's Bookwatch, Jul '00

Movement Disorders Sourcebook

Basic Consumer Health Information about Neurological Movement Disorders, Including Essential Tremor, Parkinson's Disease, Dystonia, Cerebral Palsy, Huntington's Disease, Myasthenia Gravis, Multiple Sclerosis, and Other Early-Onset and Adult-Onset Movement Disorders, Their Symptoms and Causes, Diagnostic Tests, and Treatments

Along with Mobility and Assistive Technology Information, a Glossary, and a Directory of Additional Resources

Edited by Joyce Brennfleck Shannon. 655 pages. 2003. 978-0-7808-0628-3.

". . . a good resource for consumers and recommended for public, community college and undergraduate libraries." *— American Reference Books Annual, 2004*

Muscular Dystrophy Sourcebook

Basic Consumer Health Information about Congenital, Childhood-Onset, and Adult-Onset Forms of Muscular Dystrophy, Such as Duchenne, Becker, Emery-Dreifuss, Distal, Limb-Girdle, Facioscapulohumeral (FSHD), Myotonic, and Ophthalmoplegic Muscular Dystrophies, Including Facts about Diagnostic Tests, Medical and Physical Therapies, Management of Co-Occurring Conditions, and Parenting Guidelines

Along with Practical Tips for Home Care, a Glossary, and Directories of Additional Resources

Edited by Joyce Brennfleck Shannon. 577 pages. 2004. 978-0-7808-0676-4.

"This book is highly recommended for public and academic libraries as well as health care offices that support the information needs of patients and their families."
— E-Streams, Apr '05

"Excellent reference." *— The Bookwatch, Jan '05*

Obesity Sourcebook

Basic Consumer Health Information about Diseases and Other Problems Associated with Obesity, and Including Facts about Risk Factors, Prevention Issues, and Management Approaches

Along with Statistical and Demographic Data, Information about Special Populations, Research Updates, a Glossary, and Source Listings for Further Help and Information

Edited by Wilma Caldwell and Chad T. Kimball. 376 pages. 2001. 978-0-7808-0333-6.

"The book synthesizes the reliable medical literature on obesity into one easy-to-read and useful resource for the general public."
— American Reference Books Annual, 2002

"This is a very useful resource book for the lay public."
— Doody's Review Service, Nov '01

"Well suited for the health reference collection of a public library or an academic health science library that serves the general population." *— E-Streams, Sep '01*

"Recommended reference source."
— Booklist, American Library Association, Apr '01

"Recommended pick both for specialty health library collections and any general consumer health reference collection." *— The Bookwatch, Apr '01*

Oral Health Sourcebook

SEE *Dental Care & Oral Health Sourcebook*

Osteoporosis Sourcebook

Basic Consumer Health Information about Primary and Secondary Osteoporosis and Juvenile Osteoporosis and Related Conditions, Including Fibrous Dysplasia, Gaucher Disease, Hyperthyroidism, Hypophosphatasia, Myeloma, Osteopetrosis, Osteogenesis Imperfecta, and Paget's Disease

Along with Information about Risk Factors, Treatments, Traditional and Non-Traditional Pain Management, a Glossary of Related Terms, and a Directory of Resources

Edited by Allan R. Cook. 584 pages. 2001. 978-0-7808-0239-1.

"This would be a book to be kept in a staff or patient library. The targeted audience is the layperson, but the therapist who needs a quick bit of information on a particular topic will also find the book useful."
— Physical Therapy, Jan '02

"This resource is recommended as a great reference source for public, health, and academic libraries, and is another triumph for the editors of Omnigraphics."
— *American Reference Books Annual, 2002*

"Recommended for all public libraries and general health collections, especially those supporting patient education or consumer health programs."
— *E-Streams, Nov '01*

"Will prove valuable to any library seeking to maintain a current, comprehensive reference collection of health resources. . . . From prevention to treatment and associated conditions, this provides an excellent survey."
— *The Bookwatch, Aug '01*

"Recommended reference source."
— *Booklist, American Library Association, Jul '01*

SEE ALSO *Healthy Aging Sourcebook, Physical & Mental Issues in Aging Sourcebook, Women's Health Concerns Sourcebook*

Pain Sourcebook, 2nd Edition

Basic Consumer Health Information about Specific Forms of Acute and Chronic Pain, Including Muscle and Skeletal Pain, Nerve Pain, Cancer Pain, and Disorders Characterized by Pain, Such as Fibromyalgia, Shingles, Angina, Arthritis, and Headaches

Along with Information about Pain Medications and Management Techniques, Complementary and Alternative Pain Relief Options, Tips for People Living with Chronic Pain, a Glossary, and a Directory of Sources for Further Information

Edited by Karen Bellenir. 670 pages. 2002. 978-0-7808-0612-2.

"A source of valuable information. . . . This book offers help to nonmedical people who need information about pain and pain management. It is also an excellent reference for those who participate in patient education."
— *Doody's Review Service, Sep '02*

"Highly recommended for academic and medical reference collections." — *Library Bookwatch, Sep '02*

"The text is readable, easily understood, and well indexed. This excellent volume belongs in all patient education libraries, consumer health sections of public libraries, and many personal collections."
— *American Reference Books Annual, 1999*

"The information is basic in terms of scholarship and is appropriate for general readers. Written in journalistic style . . . intended for non-professionals. Quite thorough in its coverage of different pain conditions and summarizes the latest clinical information regarding pain treatment." — *Choice, Association of College and Research Libraries, Jun '98*

"Recommended reference source."
— *Booklist, American Library Association, Mar '98*

Pediatric Cancer Sourcebook

Basic Consumer Health Information about Leukemias, Brain Tumors, Sarcomas, Lymphomas, and Other Cancers in Infants, Children, and Adolescents, Including Descriptions of Cancers, Treatments, and Coping Strategies

Along with Suggestions for Parents, Caregivers, and Concerned Relatives, a Glossary of Cancer Terms, and Resource Listings

Edited by Edward J. Prucha. 587 pages. 1999. 978-0-7808-0245-2.

"An excellent source of information. Recommended for public, hospital, and health science libraries with consumer health collections." — *E-Streams, Jun '00*

"Recommended reference source."
— *Booklist, American Library Association, Feb '00*

"A valuable addition to all libraries specializing in health services and many public libraries."
— *American Reference Books Annual, 2000*

SEE ALSO *Childhood Diseases & Disorders Sourcebook, Healthy Children Sourcebook*

Physical & Mental Issues in Aging Sourcebook

Basic Consumer Health Information on Physical and Mental Disorders Associated with the Aging Process, Including Concerns about Cardiovascular Disease, Pulmonary Disease, Oral Health, Digestive Disorders, Musculoskeletal and Skin Disorders, Metabolic Changes, Sexual and Reproductive Issues, and Changes in Vision, Hearing, and Other Senses

Along with Data about Longevity and Causes of Death, Information on Acute and Chronic Pain, Descriptions of Mental Concerns, a Glossary of Terms, and Resource Listings for Additional Help

Edited by Jenifer Swanson. 660 pages. 1999. 978-0-7808-0233-9.

"This is a treasure of health information for the layperson." — *Choice Health Sciences Supplement, Association of College & Research Libraries, May '00*

"Recommended for public libraries."
— *American Reference Books Annual, 2000*

"Recommended reference source."
— *Booklist, American Library Association, Oct '99*

SEE ALSO *Healthy Aging Sourcebook*

Podiatry Sourcebook, 2nd Edition

Basic Consumer Health Information about Disorders, Diseases, Deformities, and Injuries that Affect the Foot and Ankle, Including Sprains, Corns, Calluses, Bunions, Plantar Warts, Plantar Fasciitis, Neuromas, Clubfoot, Flat Feet, Achilles Tendonitis, and Much More

Along with Information about Selecting a Foot Care Specialist, Foot Fitness, Shoes and Socks, Diagnostic Tests and Corrective Procedures, Financial Assistance for Corrective Devices, a Glossary of Related Terms, and a Directory of Resources for Additional Help and Information

Edited by Ivy L. Alexander. 543 pages. 2007. 978-0-7808-0944-4.

"Recommended reference source."
— *Booklist, American Library Association, Feb '02*

"There is a lot of information presented here on a topic that is usually only covered sparingly in most larger comprehensive medical encyclopedias."
— *American Reference Books Annual, 2002*

■

Pregnancy & Birth Sourcebook, 2nd Edition

Basic Consumer Health Information about Conception and Pregnancy, Including Facts about Fertility, Infertility, Pregnancy Symptoms and Complications, Fetal Growth and Development, Labor, Delivery, and the Postpartum Period, as Well as Information about Maintaining Health and Wellness during Pregnancy and Caring for a Newborn

Along with Information about Public Health Assistance for Low-Income Pregnant Women, a Glossary, and Directories of Agencies and Organizations Providing Help and Support

Edited by Amy L. Sutton. 626 pages. 2004. 978-0-7808-0672-6.

"Will appeal to public and school reference collections strong in medicine and women's health. . . . Deserves a spot on any medical reference shelf."
— *The Bookwatch, Jul '04*

"A well-organized handbook. Recommended."
— *Choice, Association of College & Research Libraries, Apr '98*

"Recommended reference source."
— *Booklist, American Library Association, Mar '98*

"Recommended for public libraries."
— *American Reference Books Annual, 1998*

SEE ALSO *Breastfeeding Sourcebook, Congenital Disorders Sourcebook, Family Planning Sourcebook*

■

Prostate & Urological Disorders Sourcebook

Basic Consumer Health Information about Urogenital and Sexual Disorders in Men, Including Prostate and Other Andrological Cancers, Prostatitis, Benign Prostatic Hyperplasia, Testicular and Penile Trauma, Cryptorchidism, Peyronie Disease, Erectile Dysfunction, and Male Factor Infertility, and Facts about Commonly Used Tests and Procedures, Such as Prostatectomy, Vasectomy, Vasectomy Reversal, Penile Implants, and Semen Analysis

Along with a Glossary of Andrological Terms and a Directory of Resources for Additional Information

Edited by Karen Bellenir. 631 pages. 2005. 978-0-7808-0797-6.

Prostate Cancer Sourcebook

Basic Consumer Health Information about Prostate Cancer, Including Information about the Associated Risk Factors, Detection, Diagnosis, and Treatment of Prostate Cancer

Along with Information on Non-Malignant Prostate Conditions, and Featuring a Section Listing Support and Treatment Centers and a Glossary of Related Terms

Edited by Dawn D. Matthews. 358 pages. 2001. 978-0-7808-0324-4.

"Recommended reference source."
— *Booklist, American Library Association, Jan '02*

"A valuable resource for health care consumers seeking information on the subject. . . . All text is written in a clear, easy-to-understand language that avoids technical jargon. Any library that collects consumer health resources would strengthen their collection with the addition of the *Prostate Cancer Sourcebook*."
— *American Reference Books Annual, 2002*

SEE ALSO *Men's Health Concerns Sourcebook*

■

Reconstructive & Cosmetic Surgery Sourcebook

Basic Consumer Health Information on Cosmetic and Reconstructive Plastic Surgery, Including Statistical Information about Different Surgical Procedures, Things to Consider Prior to Surgery, Plastic Surgery Techniques and Tools, Emotional and Psychological Considerations, and Procedure-Specific Information

Along with a Glossary of Terms and a Listing of Resources for Additional Help and Information

Edited by M. Lisa Weatherford. 374 pages. 2001. 978-0-7808-0214-8.

"An excellent reference that addresses cosmetic and medically necessary reconstructive surgeries. . . . The style of the prose is calm and reassuring, discussing the many positive outcomes now available due to advances in surgical techniques."
— *American Reference Books Annual, 2002*

"Recommended for health science libraries that are open to the public, as well as hospital libraries that are open to the patients. This book is a good resource for the consumer interested in plastic surgery."
— *E-Streams, Dec '01*

"Recommended reference source."
— *Booklist, American Library Association, Jul '01*

■

Rehabilitation Sourcebook

Basic Consumer Health Information about Rehabilitation for People Recovering from Heart Surgery, Spinal Cord Injury, Stroke, Orthopedic Impairments, Amputation, Pulmonary Impairments, Traumatic Injury, and More, Including Physical Therapy, Occupational Therapy, Speech/Language Therapy, Massage Therapy, Dance Therapy, Art Therapy, and Recreational Therapy

Along with Information on Assistive and Adaptive Devices, a Glossary, and Resources for Additional Help and Information

Edited by Dawn D. Matthews. 531 pages. 1999. 978-0-7808-0236-0.

"This is an excellent resource for public library reference and health collections."
— American Reference Books Annual, 2001

"Recommended reference source."
— Booklist, American Library Association, May '00

■

Respiratory Diseases & Disorders Sourcebook

Basic Information about Respiratory Diseases and Disorders, Including Asthma, Cystic Fibrosis, Pneumonia, the Common Cold, Influenza, and Others, Featuring Facts about the Respiratory System, Statistical and Demographic Data, Treatments, Self-Help Management Suggestions, and Current Research Initiatives

Edited by Allan R. Cook and Peter D. Dresser. 771 pages. 1995. 978-0-7808-0037-3.

"Designed for the layperson and for patients and their families coping with respiratory illness. . . . an extensive array of information on diagnosis, treatment, management, and prevention of respiratory illnesses for the general reader." — Choice, Association of College & Research Libraries, Jun '96

"A highly recommended text for all collections. It is a comforting reminder of the power of knowledge that good books carry between their covers."
— Academic Library Book Review, Spring '96

"A comprehensive collection of authoritative information presented in a nontechnical, humanitarian style for patients, families, and caregivers."
— Association of Operating Room Nurses, Sep/Oct '95

SEE ALSO Lung Disorders Sourcebook

■

Sexually Transmitted Diseases Sourcebook, 3rd Edition

Basic Consumer Health Information about Chlamydial Infections, Gonorrhea, Hepatitis, Herpes, HIV/AIDS, Human Papillomavirus, Pubic Lice, Scabies, Syphilis, Trichomoniasis, Vaginal Infections, and Other Sexually Transmitted Diseases, Including Facts about Risk Factors, Symptoms, Diagnosis, Treatment, and the Prevention of Sexually Transmitted Infections

Along with Updates on Current Research Initiatives, a Glossary of Related Terms, and Resources for Additional Help and Information

Edited by Amy L. Sutton. 629 pages. 2006. 978-0-7808-0824-9.

"Recommended for consumer health collections in public libraries, and secondary school and community college libraries."
— American Reference Books Annual, 2002

"Every school and public library should have a copy of this comprehensive and user-friendly reference book."
— Choice, Association of College & Research Libraries, Sep '01

"This is a highly recommended book. This is an especially important book for all school and public libraries."
— AIDS Book Review Journal, Jul-Aug '01

"Recommended reference source."
— Booklist, American Library Association, Apr '01

■

Sleep Disorders Sourcebook, 2nd Edition

Basic Consumer Health Information about Sleep and Sleep Disorders, Including Insomnia, Sleep Apnea, Restless Legs Syndrome, Narcolepsy, Parasomnias, and Other Health Problems That Affect Sleep, Plus Facts about Diagnostic Procedures, Treatment Strategies, Sleep Medications, and Tips for Improving Sleep Quality

Along with a Glossary of Related Terms and Resources for Additional Help and Information

Edited by Amy L. Sutton. 567 pages. 2005. 978-0-7808-0743-3.

"This book will be useful for just about everybody, especially the 40 million Americans with sleep disorders."
— American Reference Books Annual, 2006

"Recommended for public libraries and libraries supporting health care professionals." — E-Streams, Sep '05

". . . key medical library acquisition."
— The Bookwatch, Jun '05

■

Smoking Concerns Sourcebook

Basic Consumer Health Information about Nicotine Addiction and Smoking Cessation, Featuring Facts about the Health Effects of Tobacco Use, Including Lung and Other Cancers, Heart Disease, Stroke, and Respiratory Disorders, Such as Emphysema and Chronic Bronchitis

Along with Information about Smoking Prevention Programs, Suggestions for Achieving and Maintaining a Smoke-Free Lifestyle, Statistics about Tobacco Use, Reports on Current Research Initiatives, a Glossary of Related Terms, and Directories of Resources for Additional Help and Information

Edited by Karen Bellenir. 621 pages. 2004. 978-0-7808-0323-7.

"Provides everything needed for the student or general reader seeking practical details on the effects of tobacco use." — The Bookwatch, Mar '05

"Public libraries and consumer health care libraries will find this work useful."
— American Reference Books Annual, 2005

Sports Injuries Sourcebook, 3rd Edition

Basic Consumer Health Information about Sprains and Strains, Fractures, Growth Plate Injuries, Overtraining Injuries, and Injuries to the Head, Face, Shoulders, Elbows, Hands, Spinal Column, Knees, Ankles, and Feet, and with Facts about Heat-Related Illness, Steroids and Sport Supplements, Protective Equipment, Diagnostic Procedures, Treatment Options, and Rehabilitation

Along with a Glossary of Related Terms and a Directory of Resources for Additional Help and Information

Edited by Sandra J. Judd. 651 pages. 2007. 978-0-7808-0949-9.

"This is an excellent reference for consumers and it is recommended for public, community college, and undergraduate libraries."
— *American Reference Books Annual, 2003*

"Recommended reference source."
— *Booklist, American Library Association, Feb '03*

■

Stress-Related Disorders Sourcebook

Basic Consumer Health Information about Stress and Stress-Related Disorders, Including Stress Origins and Signals, Environmental Stress at Work and Home, Mental and Emotional Stress Associated with Depression, Post-Traumatic Stress Disorder, Panic Disorder, Suicide, and the Physical Effects of Stress on the Cardiovascular, Immune, and Nervous Systems

Along with Stress Management Techniques, a Glossary, and a Listing of Additional Resources

Edited by Joyce Brennfleck Shannon. 610 pages. 2002. 978-0-7808-0560-6.

"Well written for a general readership, the *Stress-Related Disorders Sourcebook* is a useful addition to the health reference literature."
— *American Reference Books Annual, 2003*

"I am impressed by the amount of information. It offers a thorough overview of the causes and consequences of stress for the layperson. . . . A well-done and thorough reference guide for professionals and nonprofessionals alike." — *Doody's Review Service, Dec '02*

■

Stroke Sourcebook

Basic Consumer Health Information about Stroke, Including Ischemic, Hemorrhagic, Transient Ischemic Attack (TIA), and Pediatric Stroke, Stroke Triggers and Risks, Diagnostic Tests, Treatments, and Rehabilitation Information

Along with Stroke Prevention Guidelines, Legal and Financial Information, a Glossary, and a Directory of Additional Resources

Edited by Joyce Brennfleck Shannon. 606 pages. 2003. 978-0-7808-0630-6.

"This volume is highly recommended and should be in every medical, hospital, and public library."
— *American Reference Books Annual, 2004*

"Highly recommended for the amount and variety of topics and information covered." — *Choice, Nov '03*

■

Surgery Sourcebook

Basic Consumer Health Information about Inpatient and Outpatient Surgeries, Including Cardiac, Vascular, Orthopedic, Ocular, Reconstructive, Cosmetic, Gynecologic, and Ear, Nose, and Throat Procedures and More

Along with Information about Operating Room Policies and Instruments, Laser Surgery Techniques, Hospital Errors, Statistical Data, a Glossary, and Listings of Sources for Further Help and Information

Edited by Annemarie S. Muth and Karen Bellenir. 596 pages. 2002. 978-0-7808-0380-0.

"Large public libraries and medical libraries would benefit from this material in their reference collections."
— *American Reference Books Annual, 2004*

"Invaluable reference for public and school library collections alike." — *Library Bookwatch, Apr '03*

■

Thyroid Disorders Sourcebook

Basic Consumer Health Information about Disorders of the Thyroid and Parathyroid Glands, Including Hypothyroidism, Hyperthyroidism, Graves Disease, Hashimoto Thyroiditis, Thyroid Cancer, and Parathyroid Disorders, Featuring Facts about Symptoms, Risk Factors, Tests, and Treatments

Along with Information about the Effects of Thyroid Imbalance on Other Body Systems, Environmental Factors That Affect the Thyroid Gland, a Glossary, and a Directory of Additional Resources

Edited by Joyce Brennfleck Shannon. 599 pages. 2005. 978-0-7808-0745-7.

"Recommended for consumer health collections."
— *American Reference Books Annual, 2006*

"Highly recommended pick for basic consumer health reference holdings at all levels."
— *The Bookwatch, Aug '05*

■

Transplantation Sourcebook

Basic Consumer Health Information about Organ and Tissue Transplantation, Including Physical and Financial Preparations, Procedures and Issues Relating to Specific Solid Organ and Tissue Transplants, Rehabilitation, Pediatric Transplant Information, the Future of Transplantation, and Organ and Tissue Donation

Along with a Glossary and Listings of Additional Resources

Edited by Joyce Brennfleck Shannon. 628 pages. 2002. 978-0-7808-0322-0.

"Along with these advances [in transplantation technology] have come a number of daunting questions for potential transplant patients, their families, and their health care providers. This reference text is the best single tool to address many of these questions. . . . It will be a much-needed addition to the reference collections in health care, academic, and large public libraries."
— *American Reference Books Annual, 2003*

"Recommended for libraries with an interest in offering consumer health information." — *E-Streams, Jul '02*

"This is a unique and valuable resource for patients facing transplantation and their families."
— *Doody's Review Service, Jun '02*

■

Traveler's Health Sourcebook

Basic Consumer Health Information for Travelers, Including Physical and Medical Preparations, Transportation Health and Safety, Essential Information about Food and Water, Sun Exposure, Insect and Snake Bites, Camping and Wilderness Medicine, and Travel with Physical or Medical Disabilities

Along with International Travel Tips, Vaccination Recommendations, Geographical Health Issues, Disease Risks, a Glossary, and a Listing of Additional Resources

Edited by Joyce Brennfleck Shannon. 613 pages. 2000. 978-0-7808-0384-8.

"Recommended reference source."
— *Booklist, American Library Association, Feb '01*

"This book is recommended for any public library, any travel collection, and especially any collection for the physically disabled."
— *American Reference Books Annual, 2001*

SEE ALSO Worldwide Health Sourcebook

■

Urinary Tract & Kidney Diseases & Disorders Sourcebook, 2nd Edition

Basic Consumer Health Information about the Urinary System, Including the Bladder, Urethra, Ureters, and Kidneys, with Facts about Urinary Tract Infections, Incontinence, Congenital Disorders, Kidney Stones, Cancers of the Urinary Tract and Kidneys, Kidney Failure, Dialysis, and Kidney Transplantation

Along with Statistical and Demographic Information, Reports on Current Research in Kidney and Urologic Health, a Summary of Commonly Used Diagnostic Tests, a Glossary of Related Terms, and a Directory of Resources for Additional Help and Information

Edited by Ivy L. Alexander. 649 pages. 2005. 978-0-7808-0750-1.

"A good choice for a consumer health information library or for a medical library needing information to refer to their patients."
— *American Reference Books Annual, 2006*

Vegetarian Sourcebook

Basic Consumer Health Information about Vegetarian Diets, Lifestyle, and Philosophy, Including Definitions of Vegetarianism and Veganism, Tips about Adopting Vegetarianism, Creating a Vegetarian Pantry, and Meeting Nutritional Needs of Vegetarians, with Facts Regarding Vegetarianism's Effect on Pregnant and Lactating Women, Children, Athletes, and Senior Citizens

Along with a Glossary of Commonly Used Vegetarian Terms and Resources for Additional Help and Information

Edited by Chad T. Kimball. 360 pages. 2002. 978-0-7808-0439-5.

"Organizes into one concise volume the answers to the most common questions concerning vegetarian diets and lifestyles. This title is recommended for public and secondary school libraries." — *E-Streams, Apr '03*

"Invaluable reference for public and school library collections alike." — *Library Bookwatch, Apr '03*

"The articles in this volume are easy to read and come from authoritative sources. The book does not necessarily support the vegetarian diet but instead provides the pros and cons of this important decision. The Vegetarian Sourcebook is recommended for public libraries and consumer health libraries."
— *American Reference Books Annual, 2003*

SEE ALSO Diet & Nutrition Sourcebook

■

Women's Health Concerns Sourcebook, 2nd Edition

Basic Consumer Health Information about the Medical and Mental Concerns of Women, Including Maintaining Health and Wellness, Gynecological Concerns, Breast Health, Sexuality and Reproductive Issues, Menopause, Cancer in Women, Leading Causes of Death and Disability among Women, Physical Concerns of Special Significance to Women, and Women's Mental and Emotional Health

Along with a Glossary of Related Terms and Directories of Resources for Additional Help and Information

Edited by Amy L. Sutton. 746 pages. 2004. 978-0-7808-0673-3.

"This is a useful reference book, which makes the reader knowledgeable about several issues that concern women's health. It is recommended for public libraries and home library collections." — *E-Streams, May '05*

"A useful addition to public and consumer health library collections."
— *American Reference Books Annual, 2005*

"A highly recommended title."
— *The Bookwatch, May '04*

"Handy compilation. There is an impressive range of diseases, devices, disorders, procedures, and other physical and emotional issues covered . . . well organized, illustrated, and indexed." — *Choice, Association of College & Research Libraries, Jan '98*

SEE ALSO *Breast Cancer Sourcebook, Cancer Sourcebook for Women, Healthy Heart Sourcebook for Women, Osteoporosis Sourcebook*

■

Workplace Health & Safety Sourcebook

Basic Consumer Health Information about Workplace Health and Safety, Including the Effect of Workplace Hazards on the Lungs, Skin, Heart, Ears, Eyes, Brain, Reproductive Organs, Musculoskeletal System, and Other Organs and Body Parts

Along with Information about Occupational Cancer, Personal Protective Equipment, Toxic and Hazardous Chemicals, Child Labor, Stress, and Workplace Violence

Edited by Chad T. Kimball. 626 pages. 2000. 978-0-7808-0231-5.

"As a reference for the general public, this would be useful in any library." — *E-Streams, Jun '01*

"Provides helpful information for primary care physicians and other caregivers interested in occupational medicine. . . . General readers; professionals."
— *Choice, Association of College & Research Libraries, May '01*

"Recommended reference source."
— *Booklist, American Library Association, Feb '01*

"Highly recommended." — *The Bookwatch, Jan '01*

■

Worldwide Health Sourcebook

Basic Information about Global Health Issues, Including Malnutrition, Reproductive Health, Disease Dispersion and Prevention, Emerging Diseases, Risky Health Behaviors, and the Leading Causes of Death

Along with Global Health Concerns for Children, Women, and the Elderly, Mental Health Issues, Research and Technology Advancements, and Economic, Environmental, and Political Health Implications, a Glossary, and a Resource Listing for Additional Help and Information

Edited by Joyce Brennfleck Shannon. 614 pages. 2001. 978-0-7808-0330-5.

"Named an Outstanding Academic Title."
— *Choice, Association of College & Research Libraries, Jan '02*

"Yet another handy but also unique compilation in the extensive *Health Reference Series*, this is a useful work because many of the international publications reprinted or excerpted are not readily available. Highly recommended." — *Choice, Association of College & Research Libraries, Nov '01*

"Recommended reference source."
— *Booklist, American Library Association, Oct '01*

SEE ALSO *Traveler's Health Sourcebook*

Teen Health Series

Helping Young Adults Understand, Manage, and Avoid Serious Illness

List price $65 per volume. **School and library price $58 per volume.**

Alcohol Information for Teens
Health Tips about Alcohol and Alcoholism
Including Facts about Underage Drinking, Preventing Teen Alcohol Use, Alcohol's Effects on the Brain and the Body, Alcohol Abuse Treatment, Help for Children of Alcoholics, and More

Edited by Joyce Brennfleck Shannon. 370 pages. 2005. 978-0-7808-0741-9.

"Boxed facts and tips add visual interest to the well-researched and clearly written text."
— *Curriculum Connection, Apr '06*

Allergy Information for Teens
Health Tips about Allergic Reactions Such as Anaphylaxis, Respiratory Problems, and Rashes
Including Facts about Identifying and Managing Allergies to Food, Pollen, Mold, Animals, Chemicals, Drugs, and Other Substances

Edited by Karen Bellenir. 410 pages. 2006. 978-0-7808-0799-0.

Asthma Information for Teens
Health Tips about Managing Asthma and Related Concerns
Including Facts about Asthma Causes, Triggers, Symptoms, Diagnosis, and Treatment

Edited by Karen Bellenir. 386 pages. 2005. 978-0-7808-0770-9.

"Highly recommended for medical libraries, public school libraries, and public libraries."
— *American Reference Books Annual, 2006*

"It is so clearly written and well organized that even hesitant readers will be able to find the facts they need, whether for reports or personal information. . . . A succinct but complete resource."
— *School Library Journal, Sep '05*

Body Information for Teens
Health Tips about Maintaining Well-Being for a Lifetime
Including Facts about the Development and Functioning of the Body's Systems, Organs, and Structures and the Health Impact of Lifestyle Choices

Edited by Sandra Augustyn Lawton. 458 pages. 2007. 978-0-7808-0443-2.

Cancer Information for Teens
Health Tips about Cancer Awareness, Prevention, Diagnosis, and Treatment
Including Facts about Frequently Occurring Cancers, Cancer Risk Factors, and Coping Strategies for Teens Fighting Cancer or Dealing with Cancer in Friends or Family Members

Edited by Wilma R. Caldwell. 428 pages. 2004. 978-0-7808-0678-8.

"Recommended for school libraries, or consumer libraries that see a lot of use by teens."
— *E-Streams, May '05*

"A valuable educational tool."
— *American Reference Books Annual, 2005*

"Young adults and their parents alike will find this new addition to the *Teen Health Series* an important reference to cancer in teens."
— *Children's Bookwatch, Feb '05*

Complementary and Alternative Medicine Information for Teens
Health Tips about Non-Traditional and Non-Western Medical Practices
Including Information about Acupuncture, Chiropractic Medicine, Dietary and Herbal Supplements, Hypnosis, Massage Therapy, Prayer and Spirituality, Reflexology, Yoga, and More

Edited by Sandra Augustyn Lawton. 405 pages. 2006. 978-0-7808-0966-6.

Diabetes Information for Teens
Health Tips about Managing Diabetes and Preventing Related Complications
Including Information about Insulin, Glucose Control, Healthy Eating, Physical Activity, and Learning to Live with Diabetes

Edited by Sandra Augustyn Lawton. 410 pages. 2006. 978-0-7808-0811-9.

Diet Information for Teens, 2nd Edition

Health Tips about Diet and Nutrition

Including Facts about Dietary Guidelines, Food Groups, Nutrients, Healthy Meals, Snacks, Weight Control, Medical Concerns Related to Diet, and More

Edited by Karen Bellenir. 432 pages. 2006. 978-0-7808-0820-1.

"Full of helpful insights and facts throughout the book. . . . An excellent resource to be placed in public libraries or even in personal collections."
— *American Reference Books Annual, 2002*

"Recommended for middle and high school libraries and media centers as well as academic libraries that educate future teachers of teenagers. It is also a suitable addition to health science libraries that serve patrons who are interested in teen health promotion and education." — *E-Streams, Oct '01*

"This comprehensive book would be beneficial to collections that need information about nutrition, dietary guidelines, meal planning, and weight control. . . . This reference is so easy to use that its purchase is recommended." — *The Book Report, Sep-Oct '01*

"This book is written in an easy to understand format describing issues that many teens face every day, and then provides thoughtful explanations so that teens can make informed decisions. This is an interesting book that provides important facts and information for today's teens." — *Doody's Health Sciences Book Review Journal, Jul-Aug '01*

"A comprehensive compendium of diet and nutrition. The information is presented in a straightforward, plain-spoken manner. This title will be useful to those working on reports on a variety of topics, as well as to general readers concerned about their dietary health."
— *School Library Journal, Jun '01*

Drug Information for Teens, 2nd Edition

Health Tips about the Physical and Mental Effects of Substance Abuse

Including Information about Marijuana, Inhalants, Club Drugs, Stimulants, Hallucinogens, Opiates, Prescription and Over-the-Counter Drugs, Herbal Products, Tobacco, Alcohol, and More

Edited by Sandra Augustyn Lawton. 468 pages. 2006. 978-0-7808-0862-1.

"A clearly written resource for general readers and researchers alike." — *School Library Journal*

"This book is well-balanced. . . . a must for public and school libraries."
— *VOYA: Voice of Youth Advocates, Dec '03*

"The chapters are quick to make a connection to their teenage reading audience. The prose is straightforward and the book lends itself to spot reading. It should be useful both for practical information and for research, and it is suitable for public and school libraries."
— *American Reference Books Annual, 2003*

"Recommended reference source."
— *Booklist, American Library Association, Feb '03*

"This is an excellent resource for teens and their parents. Education about drugs and substances is key to discouraging teen drug abuse and this book provides this much needed information in a way that is interesting and factual." — *Doody's Review Service, Dec '02*

Eating Disorders Information for Teens

Health Tips about Anorexia, Bulimia, Binge Eating, and Other Eating Disorders

Including Information on the Causes, Prevention, and Treatment of Eating Disorders, and Such Other Issues as Maintaining Healthy Eating and Exercise Habits

Edited by Sandra Augustyn Lawton. 337 pages. 2005. 978-0-7808-0783-9.

"An excellent resource for teens and those who work with them."
— *VOYA: Voice of Youth Advocates, Apr '06*

"A welcome addition to high school and undergraduate libraries." — *American Reference Books Annual, 2006*

"This book covers the topic in a lucid manner but delves deeper into every aspect of an eating disorder. A solid addition for any nonfiction or reference collection." — *School Library Journal, Dec '05*

Fitness Information for Teens

Health Tips about Exercise, Physical Well-Being, and Health Maintenance

Including Facts about Aerobic and Anaerobic Conditioning, Stretching, Body Shape and Body Image, Sports Training, Nutrition, and Activities for Non-Athletes

Edited by Karen Bellenir. 425 pages. 2004. 978-0-7808-0679-5.

"Another excellent offering from Omnigraphics in their *Teen Health Series*. . . . This book will be a great addition to any public, junior high, senior high, or secondary school library."
— *American Reference Books Annual, 2005*

Learning Disabilities Information for Teens

Health Tips about Academic Skills Disorders and Other Disabilities That Affect Learning

Including Information about Common Signs of Learning Disabilities, School Issues, Learning to Live with a Learning Disability, and Other Related Issues

Edited by Sandra Augustyn Lawton. 337 pages. 2005. 978-0-7808-0796-9.

"This book provides a wealth of information for any reader interested in the signs, causes, and consequences

of learning disabilities, as well as related legal rights and educational interventions. . . . Public and academic libraries should want this title for both students and general readers."
— *American Reference Books Annual, 2006*

Mental Health Information for Teens, 2nd Edition
Health Tips about Mental Wellness and Mental Illness

Including Facts about Mental and Emotional Health, Depression and Other Mood Disorders, Anxiety Disorders, Behavior Disorders, Self-Injury, Psychosis, Schizophrenia, and More

Edited by Karen Bellenir. 400 pages. 2006. 978-0-7808-0863-8.

"In both language and approach, this user-friendly entry in the *Teen Health Series* is on target for teens needing information on mental health concerns."
— *Booklist, American Library Association, Jan '02*

"Readers will find the material accessible and informative, with the shaded notes, facts, and embedded glossary insets adding appropriately to the already interesting and succinct presentation."
— *School Library Journal, Jan '02*

"This title is highly recommended for any library that serves adolescents and parents/caregivers of adolescents."
— *E-Streams, Jan '02*

"Recommended for high school libraries and young adult collections in public libraries. Both health professionals and teenagers will find this book useful."
— *American Reference Books Annual, 2002*

"This is a nice book written to enlighten the society, primarily teenagers, about common teen mental health issues. It is highly recommended to teachers and parents as well as adolescents."
— *Doody's Review Service, Dec '01*

Sexual Health Information for Teens
Health Tips about Sexual Development, Human Reproduction, and Sexually Transmitted Diseases

Including Facts about Puberty, Reproductive Health, Chlamydia, Human Papillomavirus, Pelvic Inflammatory Disease, Herpes, AIDS, Contraception, Pregnancy, and More

Edited by Deborah A. Stanley. 391 pages. 2003. 978-0-7808-0445-6.

"This work should be included in all high school libraries and many larger public libraries. . . . highly recommended."
— *American Reference Books Annual, 2004*

"*Sexual Health* approaches its subject with appropriate seriousness and offers easily accessible advice and information."
— *School Library Journal, Feb '04*

Skin Health Information for Teens
Health Tips about Dermatological Concerns and Skin Cancer Risks

Including Facts about Acne, Warts, Hives, and Other Conditions and Lifestyle Choices, Such as Tanning, Tattooing, and Piercing, That Affect the Skin, Nails, Scalp, and Hair

Edited by Robert Aquinas McNally. 429 pages. 2003. 978-0-7808-0446-3.

"This volume, as with others in the series, will be a useful addition to school and public library collections."
— *American Reference Books Annual, 2004*

"There is no doubt that this reference tool is valuable."
— *VOYA: Voice of Youth Advocates, Feb '04*

"This volume serves as a one-stop source and should be a necessity for any health collection."
— *Library Media Connection*

Sports Injuries Information for Teens
Health Tips about Sports Injuries and Injury Protection

Including Facts about Specific Injuries, Emergency Treatment, Rehabilitation, Sports Safety, Competition Stress, Fitness, Sports Nutrition, Steroid Risks, and More

Edited by Joyce Brennfleck Shannon. 405 pages. 2003. 978-0-7808-0447-0.

"This work will be useful in the young adult collections of public libraries as well as high school libraries."
— *American Reference Books Annual, 2004*

Suicide Information for Teens
Health Tips about Suicide Causes and Prevention

Including Facts about Depression, Risk Factors, Getting Help, Survivor Support, and More

Edited by Joyce Brennfleck Shannon. 368 pages. 2005. 978-0-7808-0737-2.

Tobacco Information for Teens
Health Tips about the Hazards of Using Cigarettes, Smokeless Tobacco, and Other Nicotine Products

Including Facts about Nicotine Addiction, Immediate and Long-Term Health Effects of Tobacco Use, Related Cancers, Smoking Cessation, Tobacco Use Prevention, and Tobacco Use Statistics

Edited by Karen Bellenir. 440 pages. 2007. 978-0-7808-0976-5.

Health Reference Series